MINDFULNESS AND PSYCHOTHERAPY

Mindfulness
and Psychotherapy

Edited by

CHRISTOPHER K. GERMER
RONALD D. SIEGEL
PAUL R. FULTON

THE GUILFORD PRESS
New York   London

© 2005 The Guilford Press
A Division of Guilford Publications, Inc.
72 Spring Street, New York, NY 10012
www.guilford.com

Printed in the United States of America

This book is printed on acid-free paper.

Last digit is print number: 9 8 7 6 5 4

Library of Congress Cataloging-in-Publication Data

Mindfulness and psychotherapy / Christopher K. Germer, Ronald D.
Siegel, Paul R. Fulton, editors.— 1st ed.
    p. cm.
  Includes bibliographical references and index.
  ISBN-10: 1-59385-139-1   ISBN-13: 978-1-59385-139-2
  1. Meditation—Therapeutic use. 2. Meditation—Buddhism. 3.
Psychotherapy. I. Germer, Christopher K. II. Siegel, Ronald D. III.
Fulton, Paul R.
  RC489.M43M56 2005
  615.8′52—dc22
                                                    2004028821

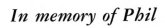

In memory of Phil

About the Editors

Christopher K. Germer, PhD, is a clinical psychologist in private practice, specializing in mindfulness-based treatment of anxiety and panic. He has been integrating meditation and mindfulness principles into psychotherapy since 1978. Dr. Germer has taken over a dozen trips to India to explore the varieties of meditation and yoga. He is currently the Director of Continuing Education for the Institute for Meditation and Psychotherapy and is a clinical instructor in psychology at Harvard Medical School.

Ronald D. Siegel, PsyD, is a clinical psychologist, a member of the clinical faculty of Harvard Medical School for over 20 years, and a long-term student of mindfulness meditation. His personal recovery from disabling back pain led him to develop the *Back Sense* program, a step-by-step mind–body approach to treating chronic back pain, which integrates Western psychological and medical interventions with mindfulness practice. He teaches nationally about mind–body treatment and maintains a private clinical practice in Lincoln, Massachusetts. Dr. Siegel is coauthor, with Michael H. Urdang and Douglas R. Johnson, of *Back Sense: A Revolutionary Approach to Halting the Cycle of Chronic Back Pain* (Broadway Books).

Paul R. Fulton, EdD, is the Director of Mental Health for Tufts Health Plan in Massachusetts, a clinical psychologist in private psychotherapy practice, and a forensic psychologist. He received lay ordination as a Zen Buddhist in 1972, and has been a student of psychology and meditation for 35 years. He was the clinical director of a large state psychiatric facility, and later the program director for a private psychiatric hospital. Dr. Fulton has been teaching about psychology and meditation for many years, is on the board of directors of the Barre Center for Buddhist Studies, and is President of the Institute for Meditation and Psychotherapy.

Contributors

Paul R. Fulton, EdD (see "About the Editors").

Christopher K. Germer, PhD (see "About the Editors").

Trudy A. Goodman, EdM, LMFT, studied child development with Jean Piaget in Geneva. She was a dharma teacher with Zen Master Seung Sahn, and studied with Maurine Stuart Roshi until her death. Ms. Goodman was an early mindfulness meditation student of Joseph Goldstein and Sharon Salzberg, and she received additional training as a teacher with Jack Kornfield. She began teaching about the integration of psychotherapy and meditation in 1976, and is the Guiding Teacher of the Institute for Meditation and Psychotherapy. After years at the Cambridge Buddhist Association teaching Zen, Ms. Goodman now teaches mindfulness meditation at the Spirit Rock Meditation Center, the Barre Center for Buddhist Studies, and the Insight Meditation Society. She founded Insight LA in Los Angeles.

Sara W. Lazar, PhD, is a scientist in the Psychiatry Department at Massachusetts General Hospital and an instructor in psychology at Harvard Medical School. The focus of her research is the neurobiology of meditation. Dr. Lazar uses functional magnetic resonance imaging to investigate the neural correlates of changes in autonomic function during the practice of meditation. She has been practicing yoga and mindfulness meditation since 1994, and serves as Science Advisor to the Institute for Meditation and Psychotherapy.

Stephanie P. Morgan, PsyD, MSW, is a clinical psychologist and social worker. She has been a student of meditation in the mindfulness and Zen traditions for the past 25 years. She was an instructor in psychology at Harvard Medical School from 1990 to 1994, training psychology interns in mindfulness and self-care skills. Dr. Morgan is currently in private practice in Manchester, Massachusetts, specializing in depression treatment and consultation to meditation communities on mental health issues.

Susan T. Morgan, MSN, RN, CS, is a clinical nurse specialist in private practice in Cambridge, Massachusetts. She was Coordinator of the Yale Adult Pervasive Developmental Disorders Research Clinic for 5 years. Following this, she became a clinician at the Harvard University Health Services and introduced mindfulness meditation to college students in the context of psychotherapy. Ms. Morgan participates in a 6-week silent mindfulness retreat each year. When not practicing psychotherapy, she is mindfully throwing clay pots.

William D. Morgan, PsyD, is a clinical psychologist in private practice in Cambridge and Braintree, Massachusetts. He has participated in intensive retreats in the Theravadin, Zen, and Tibetan schools of Buddhism during his 30 years of meditation practice. Dr. Morgan's graduate research focused on the meaning of making progress in meditation. Since 1987, he has led retreats and taught mindfulness meditation, most recently to psychotherapists.

Andrew Olendzki, PhD, a scholar of the early Buddhist tradition, trained at Lancaster University (England), Harvard University, and at the University of Sri Lanka (Perediniya). In addition to teaching at various New England colleges, he was the Executive Director of the Insight Meditation Society for 6 years, and is currently the Executive Director and core faculty member of the Barre Center for Buddhist Studies, Barre, Massachusetts. Dr. Olendzki is also the editor of the *Insight Journal*.

Ronald D. Siegel, PsyD (see "About the Editors").

Charles W. Styron, PsyD, is a clinical psychologist in private practice in Watertown, Massachusetts, as well as a consulting psychologist for Caritas Norwood Hospital in Norwood, Massachusetts. He is the founder of Everest Coaching, for which he does professional and executive coaching, and he is also a former architect. Dr. Styron has been a practitioner and teacher in the Shambhala and Tibetan Vajrayana Buddhist traditions for 25 years. He is married, has a 9-year-old daughter, and is a collagist and an amateur mountain climber.

Janet L. Surrey, PhD, is a clinical psychologist and a Founding Scholar of the Jean Baker Miller Training Institute at the Stone Center, Wellesley College. She is on the faculty of the Institute for Meditation and Psychotherapy and the Andover–Newton Theological School. Dr. Surrey has been consulting and teaching relational–cultural theory nationally and internationally for over 20 years, and has been working to synthesize Buddhist and relational psychology. Her publications include *Women's Growth in Connection* (coauthored with Judith V. Jordan, Alexandra G. Kaplan, Jean Baker Miller, and Irene P. Stiver; Guilford Press), *Mothering Against the Odds: Diverse Voices of Contemporary Mothers* (coedited with Cynthia García Coll and Kathy Weingarten; Guilford Press), *We Have to Talk: Healing Dialogues between Women and Men* (coauthored with Samuel Shem; Basic Books), and *Bill W. and Dr. Bob: The Story of the Founding of Alcoholics Anonymous* (coauthored with Samuel Shem; Samuel French).

Preface

This book is not about anything special. It is about a simple form of awareness—mindfulness—that is available to everyone at any moment. As you start to read this preface, for example, your attention may be absorbed in the words or you may be wondering whether this book will be worth your trouble. Do you know where your attention is? Has it already wandered from this page? It is natural for the mind to wander, but are you aware when it does so, and what you are thinking about? Mindfulness is simply about being aware of where your mind is from one moment to the next, with gentle acceptance. This kind of simple attention can have a deeply transformative effect on our daily lives. We can learn to enjoy very ordinary things, such as the flavor of an apple, or tolerate great hardship, such as the death of a loved one, just by learning to be aware.

This is also a book by clinicians for clinicians. It is the fruit of over 20 years of monthly meetings by a small group of psychotherapists who found themselves drawn to the twin practices of mindfulness meditation and psychotherapy. Most of our meditation practices have evolved over somewhat longer periods of time than our therapy practices. Some of the authors managed to write dissertations in graduate school on subjects related to Buddhist psychology or meditation. Over the years, a robust conversation on a wide range of professional topics developed. Many of the fruits of this exchange are shared in this volume.

Although the authors of this book have grown older over the past two decades, the experience of mindfulness has not grown old. Mindfulness is a renewable source of energy and delight. It can easily be experienced by anyone but cannot adequately be described. Mindful awareness is mostly experiential and nonverbal (i.e., sensory, somatic, intuitive, emotional), and it requires some practice to develop. Like any acquired skill, the experience of mindfulness becomes steadier with increased practice.

Our little group of therapists originally drew together to discuss members' research and personal experience at the interface between meditation and psychotherapy. As curiosity about mindfulness grew in the psychotherapy community and other clinicians asked to participate in our discussions, we decided to expand the discourse into the public arena. Our first conference was held in 1994, and 2 years later, spurred on by the energy and leadership of Phillip Aranow, we formed the Institute for Meditation and Psychotherapy (IMP). IMP now sponsors retreats and other training opportunities under its own auspices and with the Barre Center for Buddhist Studies, Barre, Massachusetts.

In February 2000, Phil was tragically killed in a car accident after an IMP conference in Florida. This book was his idea and it is written in his honor. Phil was and is an enormous inspiration to us. The institute that Phil started remains committed to his practice-based vision. Phil believed that clinical theory, the therapy relationship, and strategic interventions are guided most meaningfully by a therapist's own daily mindfulness practice.

The question that seems to arise most often in the minds of clinicians is how to *integrate* mindfulness into our daily practice of psychotherapy. This question soon leads to many others at the interface of mindfulness and psychotherapy:

- What is mindfulness, really?
- Is mindfulness a new therapy, or a common factor in all therapy?
- What does sitting on a cushion in meditation have to do with relating in psychotherapy?
- What can a mindfulness approach offer to patients suffering from particular conditions, such as anxiety or depression?
- How and when should mindfulness be introduced into psychotherapy?
- Can mindfulness help with severe conditions, such as trauma, personality disorders, or psychosis?
- What can mindfulness meditation accomplish that therapy cannot, and vice versa?
- What is the role of ethics in mindfulness practice and healing in general?
- Can modern brain science contribute to our understanding of mindfulness?
- Is mindfulness in therapy incompatible with its ancient roots?

This book surely will raise many more questions than it answers. We hope it will contribute to a rich dialogue in which we can all share over the coming years.

Some readers may be wondering about the link between mindfulness and Buddhist psychology or philosophy. Mindfulness is the heart of Buddhist psychology. Most of the authors of this volume consider themselves students of Buddhist psychology and meditation rather than Buddhists. None of us were raised in countries with a Buddhist culture. Similarly, when mindfulness skills are taught in therapy, patients do not need to take up a new religion or exotic lifestyle to benefit from them. As mindfulness theory and practice are increasingly adopted by Western psychology, concern about this issue will probably diminish.

A challenge of this book has been to maintain a consistent voice as we present a broad range of perspectives from 11 different authors on the subtle matter of mindfulness. Our most optimistic goal was to stitch together an attractive patchwork quilt. This was a labor of love, not without struggle, but we hope that in the process something essential about the subject has revealed itself.

Part of stitching this book together was to arrive at a consistent use of the word "client" or "patient." Our profession has not settled that discussion yet, and we will not either. However, after some exploration, we decided upon "patient." Etymologically, patient means "one who bears suffering," while client means "one who puts himself under the protection of a patron." Since doctor means "teacher," it can be said that we are doctoring patients, or "teaching people who bear suffering." This meaning is parallel to the original use of mindfulness 2,500 years ago: It is a teaching that alleviates suffering.

Mindfulness practice inspired and transformed countless lives before Western psychotherapists discovered it. Our science community is currently investigating the subject with great enthusiasm. The intelligent, critical, relatively dogma-free exploration of mindfulness by clinical researchers is in keeping with the ancient spirit of Buddhist inquiry. However, we are just beginning; our scientific understanding is preliminary and promising. Therefore, many ideas in this book are provisional and, we hope, will serve as an invitation for further study.

Finally, mindfulness is an opportunity to be fully alive and awake to our own lives. Most therapists do not forget what a privilege it is to participate so deeply in the lives of our fellow human beings. We love, laugh, and cry together; yearn and fear together; succeed and fail together; and, on good days, heal together. As the years go by, the fleeting nature of each precious encounter becomes more apparent. We want to make the most of each moment of therapy. It is in this spirit that we offer this book to our colleagues.

CHRISTOPHER K. GERMER
RONALD D. SIEGEL
PAUL R. FULTON

Acknowledgments

Many people have contributed to the creation of this book. Each of the authors has had the privilege of learning over many years from teachers and colleagues in the clinical world as well as the world of meditation practice. While the efforts found in these pages are our own, they are based on the insights of others. We would like to thank, in particular, a few of the many individuals who have been influential to one or more of us in our development as psychotherapists and meditation students: Dan Brown, Richard Chasin, Jay Efran, Jack Engler, Robert Fox, Joseph Goldstein, Narayan Liebenson-Grady, Rob Guerette, Thich Nhat Hanh, Les Havens, Judith Jordan, Jon Kabat-Zinn, Anna Klegon, Jack Kornfield, Joanna Macy, Florence Meyers, Jean Baker Miller, Norby Mintz, Sakyong Mipham, Paul Russell, Seung Sahn, Sharon Salzberg, Irene Stiver, Larry Strasburger, Maurine Stuart, Vimala Thaker, Chogyam Trungpa, and Rama Jyoti Vernon.

We are particularly grateful to our editor, Jim Nageotte, at The Guilford Press, who has worked patiently to shepherd this book through its development, and whose insights and innumerable suggestions have contributed greatly to the final manuscript.

We are also very indebted to our patients, who have trusted us with their minds and hearts, and have taught us most of what we know about clinical work.

Finally, we cannot say enough to thank our families and friends for their love, support, and sacrifice during the process of bringing this book to fruition.

Contents

PART IV. PAST AND PROMISE

APPENDICES

PART I

The Meaning of Mindfulness

CHAPTER 1

Mindfulness

What Is It? What Does It Matter?

CHRISTOPHER K. GERMER

To live is so startling, it leaves but little room for other
occupations. . . .
                              —EMILY DICKINSON (1872/2004)

Psychotherapists are in the business of alleviating emotional
suffering. Suffering arrives in innumerable guises: stress, anxiety, depression, behavior problems, interpersonal conflict, confusion,
despair. It is the common denominator of all clinical diagnoses and is en-
demic to the human condition. Some of our suffering is existential, such
as sickness, old age, and dying. Some suffering has a more personal flavor. The cause of our individual difficulties may include past conditioning, present circumstances, genetic predisposition, or any number of in-
teracting factors. *Mindfulness*, a deceptively simple way of relating to
experience, has long been used to lessen the sting of life's difficulties, especially those that are seemingly self-imposed. In this volume, we illustrate the potential of mindfulness for enhancing psychotherapy.

People are clear about one thing when they enter therapy: *They
want to feel better.* They often have a number of ideas about how to ac-

complish this goal, although therapy does not necessarily proceed as expected.

For example, a young woman with panic disorder—let's call her Lynn—might call a therapist, hoping to escape the emotional turmoil of her condition. Lynn may be seeking freedom *from* her anxiety, but as therapy progresses, Lynn actually discovers freedom *in* her anxiety. How does this occur? A strong therapeutic alliance may provide Lynn with courage and safety to begin to explore her panic more closely. Through self-monitoring, Lynn becomes aware of the sensations of anxiety in her body and the thoughts associated with them. She learns how to cope with panic by talking herself through it. When Lynn feels ready, she directly experiences the sensations of anxiety that trigger a panic attack and tests herself in a mall or on an airplane. This whole process requires that Lynn first turn *toward* the anxiety. A compassionate bait and switch has occurred.

Therapists who work in a more relational or psychodynamic model may observe a similar process. As connection deepens between the patient and the therapist, the conversation becomes more spontaneous and authentic, and the patient acquires the freedom to explore what is really troubling him or her in a more open, curious way. With the support of the relationship, the patient is gently exposed to what is going on inside. The patient discovers that he or she need not avoid experience to feel better.

We know that many seemingly dissimilar forms of psychotherapy work (Seligman, 1995). Is there an essential ingredient active across various modalities that can be isolated and refined? Mindfulness may prove to be that ingredient.

MINDFULNESS:
A SPECIAL RELATIONSHIP TO SUFFERING

Successful therapy changes the patient's *relationship* to his or her particular form of suffering. Obviously, if we are less upset by events in our lives, then our suffering will decrease. But how can we become less disturbed by *unpleasant* experiences? Life includes pain. Do the body and mind not instinctively react to painful experiences? Mindfulness is a skill that allows us to be less reactive to what is happening in the moment. It is a way of relating to *all* experience—positive, negative, and neutral—such that our overall level of suffering is reduced and our sense of well-being increases.

To be mindful is to wake up, to recognize what is happening in the present moment. We are rarely mindful. We are usually caught up in distracting thoughts or in opinions about what is happening in the moment. This is mind*less*ness. Examples of mindlessness (adapted from Brown & Ryan, 2003) include:

- Rushing through activities without being attentive to them.
- Breaking or spilling things because of carelessness, inattention, or thinking of something else.
- Failing to notice subtle feelings of physical tension or discomfort.
- Forgetting a person's name almost as soon as we have heard it.
- Finding ourselves preoccupied with the future or the past.
- Snacking without being aware of eating.

Mind*ful*ness, in contrast, focuses our attention on the task at hand. When we are mindful, our attention is not entangled in the past or future, and we are not judging or rejecting what is occurring at the moment. We are present. This kind of attention generates energy, clearheadedness, and joy. Fortunately, it is a skill that can be cultivated by anyone.

When Gertrude Stein (1922/1993, p. 187) wrote, "A rose is a rose is a rose is a rose," she was bringing the reader back again and again to the simple rose. She was suggesting, perhaps, what a rose is *not*. It is not a romantic relationship that ended tragically 4 years ago; it is not an imperative to trim the hedges over the weekend—it is just a rose. Perceiving with this kind of "bare attention" is an example of mindfulness.

Most people in psychotherapy are preoccupied with past or future events. For example, people who are depressed often feel regret, sadness, or guilt about the past, and people who are anxious fear the future. Suffering seems to increase as we stray from the present moment. As our attention gets absorbed in mental activity and we begin to daydream, unaware that we are indeed daydreaming, our daily lives can become a nightmare. Some of our patients feel as if they are stuck in a movie theater, watching the same upsetting movie their whole lives, unable to leave. Mindfulness can help us to step out of our conditioning and see things freshly—to see the rose as it is.

DEFINITIONS OF MINDFULNESS

The term *mindfulness* is an English translation of the Pali word *sati*. Pali was the language of Buddhist psychology 2,500 years ago, and mindfulness is the core teaching of this tradition. *Sati* connotes *awareness, attention*, and *remembering*.

What is awareness? Brown and Ryan (2003) define *awareness* and *attention* under the umbrella of consciousness:

Consciousness encompasses both awareness and attention. *Awareness* is the background "radar" of consciousness, continually monitoring the inner and outer environment. One may be aware of stimuli without them being at the center of attention. *Attention* is a process of focusing conscious awareness, providing heightened sensitivity to a limited range of experience (Westen, 1999). In actuality, awareness and attention are intertwined, such that attention continually pulls "figures" out of the "ground" of awareness, holding them focally for varying lengths of time. (p. 822)

You are using both awareness and attention to read these words. A tea-kettle whistling in the background may eventually command your attention when it gets loud enough, particularly if you would like a cup of tea. Similarly, we may drive a familiar route "on autopilot," vaguely aware of the road, but respond immediately if a child runs in front of us. Mindfulness is the opposite of being on autopilot; the opposite of daydreaming, it is paying attention to what is salient in the present moment.

Mindfulness also involves *remembering*, but not dwelling in memories. It involves remembering to reorient our attention and awareness to current experience in a wholehearted, receptive manner. This requires the *intention* to disentangle from our reverie and fully experience the moment.

Therapeutic Mindfulness

The word *mindfulness* can be used to describe a theoretical construct (mindfulness), a practice of cultivating mindfulness (such as meditation), or a psychological process (being mindful). A basic definition of *mindfulness* is "moment-by-moment awareness." Other definitions include "keeping one's consciousness alive to the present reality" (Hanh, 1976, p. 11); "the clear and single-minded awareness of what actually happens to us and in us at the successive moments of perception" (Nyanaponika Thera, 1972, p. 5); attentional control (Teasdale, Segal, & Williams, 1995); "keeping one's complete attention to the experience on a moment-to-moment basis" (Marlatt & Kristeller, 1999, p. 68); and, from a more Western psychological perspective, a cognitive process that employs creation of new categories, openness to new information, and awareness of more than one perspective (Langer, 1989). Ultimately, mindfulness cannot be fully captured with words, because it is a subtle, nonverbal experience (Gunaratana, 2002).

When mindfulness is transported to the therapeutic arena, its definition often expands to include *nonjudgment*: "the awareness that emerges through paying attention on purpose, in the present moment, and nonjudgmentally to the unfolding of experience moment to moment" (Kabat-Zinn, 2003, p. 145). In her summary of the mindfulness and psychotherapy literature, Baer (2003, p. 125) defines *mindfulness* as "the non-judgmental observation of the ongoing stream of internal and external stimuli as they arise." Nonjudgment fosters mindfulness when we are dealing with difficult physical or emotional states. By not judging our experience, we are more likely to see it as it is.

Mindfulness and Acceptance

"Acceptance" is an extension of nonjudgment. It adds a measure of kindness or friendliness. When therapists are working with intense emotions, such as shame, anger, fear, or grief, it is essential that we maintain an open, compassionate, and accepting attitude. Empathy and positive regard are important relational aspects of successful therapy (Norcross, 2001, 2002) that overlap with acceptance. If either the therapist or the patient turns away from unpleasant experience with anxiety or revulsion, the ability to understand the problem is likely to be compromised.

From the mindfulness perspective, *acceptance* refers to a willingness to let things be just as they are the moment we become aware of them—accepting pleasurable and painful experiences as they arise. Acceptance is not about endorsing maladaptive behavior. Rather, acceptance precedes behavior change. "Change is the brother of acceptance, but it is the younger brother" (Christensen & Jacobson, 2000, p. 11). Mindfulness-oriented clinicians see "radical acceptance" as part of therapy practice (Brach, 2003; Linehan, 1993b).

Mindfulness in Psychotherapy

The short definition of *mindfulness* we use in this volume is (1) *awareness*, (2) *of present experience*, (3) *with acceptance*. These three elements can be found in most discussions of mindfulness in both the psychotherapy and the Buddhist literature. (For detailed consideration of the contruct of mindfulness within psychology, see Bishop et al., 2004; Brown & Ryan, 2004; and Hayes & Feldman, 2004.) Although our definition has these three distinct components, they are irreducibly intertwined in the experience of mindfulness.

The presence of one aspect of mindfulness does not automatically imply the presence of others. For example, awareness may be absorbed in the past, such as in blind rage about a perceived injustice. Awareness may also be present without acceptance, such as in disowned shame. Likewise, acceptance can exist without awareness, as in premature forgiveness; while present-centeredness without awareness may exist in a moment of intoxication. All components of mindfulness—awareness, present-centeredness, and acceptance—are required for a moment of full mindfulness. Therapists can use these three elements as a touchstone for identifying mindfulness in therapy.

The value of a stripped-down, operational definition of *therapeutic mindfulness* is twofold. First, if mindfulness indeed reveals itself to be a key ingredient of effective psychotherapy (Martin, 1997), then clinicians will want a conceptual tool to guide their movements in the consultation room. Second, if outcome research continues to show mindfulness to be a promising treatment strategy (Baer, 2003), then researchers will need a definition with clearly defined component parts to design new interventions.

Mindfulness and Levels of Practice

Mindfulness has to be experienced to be known. People may practice mindfulness with varying degrees of intensity. At one end of a continuum of practice is everyday mindfulness. Even in our often pressured and distracted daily lives, it is possible to have mindful moments. We can momentarily disengage from our activities by taking a long, conscious breath. After gathering our attention, we can ask ourselves: "What am I feeling right now? What am I doing right now? What is most compelling to my awareness right now?" This is mindfulness in daily life, and it is how mindfulness commonly occurs in psychotherapy.

At the other end of the continuum we find monks, nuns, and laypeople who spend a considerable amount of time in meditation. When we have the opportunity to sit over sustained periods of time with closed eyes, in a silent place, and sharpen concentration on one thing (such as the breath), the mind becomes like a microscope and can detect minute mental activity. This is illustrated by the following meditation instruction:

> Should an itching sensation be felt in any part of the body, keep the mind on that part and make a mental note *itching*. . . . Should the itching continue and become too strong and you intend to rub the itching part, be sure to make a mental note *intending*. Slowly lift the hand, simultaneously noting the action of *lifting*, and *touching* when the hand touches the part that itches. Rub slowly in complete awareness of *rubbing*. When the itching sensation has disappeared and you intend to discontinue the rubbing, be mindful of making the usual mental note of *intending*. Slowly withdraw the hand, concurrently making a mental note of the action, *withdrawing*. When the hand rests in its usual place touching the leg, *touching*. (Sayadaw, 1971, pp. 5–6)

This level of precise and subtle awareness, in which we can even detect "intending," clearly requires an unusual level of dedication on the part of the practitioner. Remarkably, the instruction above is considered a "basic" instruction. Sayadaw writes that, at more advanced stages, "some meditators perceive distinctly three phases: noticing an object, its ceasing, and the passing away of the consciousness that cognizes that ceasing—all in quick succession" (1971, p. 15).

Moments of mindfulness have certain common aspects regardless of where they lie on the practice continuum. The actual moment of awakening, of mindfulness, is the same for the experienced meditator as for the beginner practicing mindfulness in everyday life. The experience is simply more continuous for experienced meditators. Mindful moments are:

- *Nonconceptual*. Mindfulness is awareness without absorption in our thought processes.
- *Present-centered*. Mindfulness is always in the present moment. Thoughts *about* our experience are one step removed from the present moment.
- *Nonjudgmental*. Awareness cannot occur freely if we would like our experience to be other than it is.
- *Intentional*. Mindfulness always includes an intention to direct attention somewhere. Returning attention to the present moment gives mindfulness continuity over time.
- *Participant observation*. Mindfulness is not detached witnessing. It is experiencing the mind and body *more* intimately.
- *Nonverbal*. The experience of mindfulness cannot be captured in words, because awareness occurs before words arise in the mind.
- *Exploratory*. Mindful awareness is always investigating subtler levels of perception.
- *Liberating*. Every moment of mindful awareness provides freedom from conditioned suffering.

These qualities occur simultaneously in each moment of mindfulness. Mindfulness practice is a conscious attempt to return awareness more frequently to the present, with all the qualities of awareness listed. Mindfulness per se is not unusual; *continuity* of mindfulness is rare indeed.

Everyday mindfulness allows us to develop insight into psychological functioning and to respond skillfully to new situations. Mindfulness in deep meditation provides insights into the nature of mind and the causes of suffering. These insights, such as awareness of how impermanent things really are, help us become less entangled in our ruminations and thereby foster more mindfulness.

PSYCHOTHERAPISTS AND MINDFULNESS

Clinicians are drawn to the subject of mindfulness and psychotherapy from a variety of directions: clinical, scientific, theoretical, and personal. In addition, psychotherapy patients are increasingly seeking therapists who might understand their meditation practice. These developments are not surprising given that Buddhist psychology and its core practice, mindfulness, have been growing in popular appeal in the West.

A Brief History of Mindfulness in Psychotherapy

The field of psychoanalysis has flirted with Buddhist psychology for some time. Freud exchanged letters with a friend in 1930, in which he admitted that Eastern philosophy was alien to him and perhaps "beyond the limits of [his] nature" (cited in Epstein, 1995, p. 2). That did not stop Freud from writing in *Civilization and Its Discontents* (1930/ 1961b) that the "oceanic feeling" in meditation was an essentially regressive experience. Franz Alexander (1931) wrote a paper entitled "Buddhist Training as an Artificial Catatonia." Other psychodynamic theorists were more complimentary, notably Carl Jung (1939/1992), who wrote a commentary on the *Tibetan Book of the Dead* in 1939 and had a lifelong curiosity about Eastern psychology. Later, Erich Fromm and Karen Horney dialogued with Zen scholar, D. T. Suzuki (Fromm, Suzuki, & DeMartino, 1960; Horney, 1945). In 1995, Mark Epstein wrote *Thoughts without a Thinker*, which triggered new interest in Buddhist psychology among psychodynamic clinicians.

Many practicing therapists took to Eastern philosophy or meditation as a way of improving their lives before beginning their professional careers. Some started to meditate in the late 1960s, at a time when ideas of enlightenment followed the Beatles and other famous pilgrims back to the West from India. Former Harvard psychologist Ram Dass's book, *Be Here Now* (1971), a mixture of Hindu and Buddhist ideas, sold over 1 million copies. Yoga, which is essentially mindfulness in movement (Boccio, 2004; Hartranft, 2003), also traveled West at the time. Some therapists began trying to connect their personal practice of meditation with their clinical work.

Studies on meditation flourished, including cardiologist Herbert Benson's (1975) use of meditation to treat heart disease. Clinical psychology kept pace with numerous articles on meditation as an adjunct to psychotherapy or as psychotherapy itself (Smith, 1975). In 1977, the American Psychiatric Association called for an examination of the clinical effectiveness of meditation. The majority of the journal articles at the time studied concentration meditation, such as transcendental meditation and Benson's program. In the last 10 years, the preponderance of studies has switched to mindfulness meditation (Smith, 2004). Jon Kabat-Zinn established the Center for Mindfulness in 1979, at the University of Massachusetts Medical School, to treat chronic conditions for which physicians could offer no further help. Over 15,000 patients have completed this mindfulness-based stress reduction (MBSR) program, not counting participants in over 250 MBSR programs around the world (Davidson & Kabat-Zinn, 2004).

An exciting, more recent area of integration for mindfulness and psychotherapy is in scientifically validated, mindfulness-based interventions. The original impetus seems to stem from the pioneering work of Kabat-Zinn's (1990) MBSR program and Marsha Linehan's Zen-inspired dialectical behavior therapy (1993a). The publication by Teasdale et al. in 2000 of an effective mindfulness-based treatment for chronic depression kindled interest in mindfulness among cognitive-behavioral researchers. The potential of these mindfulness and acceptance-based approaches is ushering in a new wave of empirically based treatments for familiar problems (Hayes, Follette, & Linehan, 2004; Hayes, Masuda, Bissett, Luoma, & Guerrero, 2004).

Where is the current interest in mindfulness heading? We may be witnessing the emergence of a more unified model of psychotherapy. We are likely to see more research that identifies mindfulness as a key element in treatment protocols, as a crucial ingredient in the therapy relationship, and as a technology for psychotherapists to cultivate personal therapeutic qualities and general well-being. Mindfulness might become a construct that draws clinical theory, research, and practice closer together, and helps integrate the private and professional lives of therapists.

THERAPIST WELL-BEING

Although mindfulness appears to enhance general well-being (Brown & Ryan, 2003; Reibel, Greeson, Brainard, & Rosenzweig, 2001; Rosenzweig, Reibel, Greeson, Brainard, & Hojat, 2003), therapists may be drawn to mindfulness for the simple reason that they would like to enjoy their work more fully. Psychotherapists choose to witness and share human conflict and despair many of their waking hours. Sometimes we are asked by a sympathetic patient, "How do you do it?" What *do* we do when a clinical situation appears impossible to handle? How do we stay calm and think clearly?

Doing psychotherapy is an opportunity to practice mindfulness in everyday life. The therapy office can be like a meditation room in which we invite our moment-to-moment experience to become known to us, openly and wholeheartedly. As the therapist learns to identify and disentangle from his or her own conditioned patterns of thought and feeling that arise in the therapy relationship, the patient may discover the same emotional freedom. The reverse is also true; we can be moved and inspired by our patients' capacity for mindfulness under especially trying circumstances.

Practicing clinicians are reminded regularly about the importance of the therapy relationship in treatment outcome (Crits-Christoph et al., 1991; Luborsky et al., 1986, 2002; Wampold, 2001). Clinicians also struggle with "transfer of technology"—making a bridge between treatment protocols developed in our universities and their application in the field. When focused primarily on implementing an empirically derived protocol, to the exclusion of a vital, interesting, and supportive therapy relationship, therapists and their patients can both lose interest in the work. In the coming years, mindfulness practice may prove to be a tangible means for building empirically supported relationship skills. This may help return our focus to the therapeutic connection, since there is something we can *do* to improve it. How we plan interventions may even be guided by a common therapeutic principle—the simple mechanism of mindfulness.

A Word about Buddhism

Mindfulness lies at the heart of Buddhist psychology. Psychotherapists are likely to find Buddhist psychology familiar, because it shares with psychotherapy the goal of alleviating suffering and the value of empirical inquiry. Whereas Western science explores phenomena through objective, third-person observation, Buddhist psychology is a highly-disciplined, systematic, first-person approach.

It cannot be overemphasized that Buddhist psychology is not a religion in the familiar, theistic sense, although some Eastern cultures continue to worship the Buddha's teachings and image. The historical Buddha is understood to have been a human being, not a God, and his life's work was dedicated to alleviating psychological suffering. According to Buddhist tradition, when he discovered this path to freedom, he decided (reluctantly at first) to teach others what he had learned.

According to legend, when people met the Buddha after his realization, he did not seem quite like other men. When they asked him who he was, he replied that he was "Buddha," which simply meant a person who is awake. He reportedly taught for a total of 45 years and had many students, rich and poor. He spoke in simple language, using stories and ideas from the popular Indian culture. In his first sermon on the Four Noble Truths, he put forth four basic ideas: (1) The human condition involves suffering; (2) the conflict between how things are and how we desire them to be causes this suffering; (3) suffering can be reduced or even eliminated by changing our attitude toward unpleasant experience; and, (4) there are eight general strategies (the Eightfold Path) to bring suffering to an end (see Chapter 2 and Appendix B). The Buddha died at age 80, probably from contaminated food at the home of a poor follower.

The Buddha is said to have discovered how to end suffering, without any props or religious rituals. Cultures have venerated his image, but the Buddha enjoined his students not to do so. He asked students to discover the truth of his teachings in their own experience—inviting them to "come and see." Belief in notions such as karma or rebirth are unnecessary to derive full benefit from Buddhist psychology (Batchelor, 1997). Buddhist psychology is primarily a practical way to know the mind, shape the mind, and free the mind (Nyanaponika Thera, 1965). Mindfulness is the core practice of Buddhist psychology, and the body of Buddhist psychology, including the Buddha's original teachings and later writings of the *Abhidharma*, may be considered the theoretical basis for mindfulness (Bhikkhu Bodhi, 2000; Nyanaponika Thera, 1949/1998).

Reading early Buddhist texts will convince the clinician that the Buddha was essentially a psychologist. William James, an American introspectionist psychologist, appreciated the Buddhist tradition. Epstein (1995) writes:

> While lecturing at Harvard in the early 1900's, James suddenly stopped when he recognized a visiting Buddhist monk from Sri Lanka in his audience. "Take my chair," he is reported to have said. "You are better equipped to lecture on psychology than I. This is the psychology everybody will be studying twenty-five years from now." (pp. 1–2)

William James's prediction may be coming true, although it is off by a number of years.

Chapter 12 of this book provides a more comprehensive historical and conceptual background to mindfulness practice, and resources for learning more about mindfulness in the context of Buddhist psychology can be found in the appendixes.

MINDFULNESS PRACTICE

Mindfulness is a naturally occurring event of everyday life but requires practice to be maintained. We all periodically wake up to our present experience, only to slip quickly back into ordinary discursive thinking. Even when we feel particularly attentive while doing therapy, we are only *intermittently* mindful. Our minds may become absorbed in associations to what our patients are saying or doing. We may then have a moment of awakening from our reverie, reorient our attention to the patient, and resume our exploration of what the patient is trying to communicate. Soon, however, we again slip away in distracted thinking. Sometimes the content of our distraction is a meaningful clue to what is occurring in the therapy room. Other times it is not. Continuity of mindfulness requires commitment and hard work.

Formal and Informal Practice

Mindfulness can be learned. Mindfulness practice can be organized in two general categories: formal and informal. *Formal* mindfulness training refers to mindfulness meditation and is an opportunity to experience mindfulness at its deepest levels. Sustained, disciplined introspection allows the practitioner to learn how the mind works and to systematically observe its contents. More will be said about meditation in the next section.

Informal mindfulness training refers to the application of mindfulness skills in everyday life. Any exercise that alerts us to the present moment, with acceptance, cultivates mindfulness. Examples are directing attention to one's breathing, listening to ambient sounds in the environment, paying attention to our posture at a given moment, labeling feelings, and so forth. The list is endless. This sort of mindfulness practice is being developed by therapists to help particular patients disentangle from disruptive patterns of thinking, feeling, and behaving, and to feel the relief of moment-to-moment awareness. Each patient may get hooked in a particular way by particular thoughts or feelings, for which a special mindfulness exercise can be developed (see Chapter 6).

Two common exercises for cultivating mindfulness in daily life, which are also used in intensive practice, involve slow walking and slow eating. In walking meditation, we attend to the sequential, moment-to-moment, kinesthetic sense of walking. From the outside, it looks like a slow-motion movie. From the inside, we are silently noting "lifting . . . stepping forward . . . heel touching . . . toe touching . . . lifting. . . . " In eating meditation, we eat silently, more slowly than usual, and notice the sight of the food on the plate, the use of utensils to bring the food to the mouth, the feel of the food in the mouth, the muscle movements of chewing, the flavors of the food, and the process of swallowing. This can make an ordinary meal exceptionally interesting and is used in mindfulness-based strategies to manage compulsive eating (Kristeller & Hallett, 1999).

Any mental event may be an object of mindful awareness. Traditionally, in Buddhist psychology, the mindfulness practitioner may focus on different parts of the body; the pleasant, unpleasant, or neutral quality of sensations; states of mind, such as distraction or the arising of pride; and various qualities that foster well-being, such as energy and tranquility, or qualities that inhibit wellness, such as anger and sloth. While the distinction between thoughts and emotions apparently did not exist in the East at the time of the Buddha, mindfulness of emotions is very important in psychotherapy.

Mindfulness and Concentration Meditation

Most therapists are familiar with meditation as a relaxation technique (Benson, 1975). Some meditation may be relaxing, but the style and the purpose of meditation partly determine its effect. Buddhist psychology distinguishes between two distinct methods of meditation: insight (*vipassana*) and concentration (*samatha*). Research suggests that the two forms of meditation are neurologically different practices (see Chapter 11). *Vipassana* meditation is usually called "mindfulness meditation" in the psychological literature, rather than "insight meditation," and we continue this usage here.

Concentration Meditation

Concentration meditation can be compared to a *laser* light beam, which illuminates whatever object to which it is directed. The benefit of concentration meditation is a calm, unruffled mind, detached from emotional and interpersonal involvement. (The Pali word, *samatha*, connotes both tranquility and concentration.) Any object of awareness, internal or external, may be an object of concentration. Examples of internal objects of meditation include words (mantra), an image (often religious), a spot on the body (such as the tip of the nose), or a kinesthetic feeling (such as the breath). Concentration is generally easier when the object is pleasant. Objects for external concentration might be a candle flame, a beloved image, a mandala, or even a dot on the wall. In concentration meditation, the mind is gently returned to the object of meditation when we notice that it has wandered.

Mindfulness Meditation

Mindfulness meditation can be compared to a *searchlight* that illumines a wider range of objects as they arise in awareness, one at a time. The benefits are greater awareness of the personal conditioning of our minds and an understanding of the nature of mind itself. The meditation instruction is to "notice whatever predominates in awareness from moment to moment." Mindfulness meditation helps us to develop the capacity for relaxed, choiceless awareness in which conscious attention moves instantly and naturally among the changing elements of experience. (Even choiceless awareness includes intention; in this case, the intention not to choose, but to stay aware of where our attention resides.) Mindfulness meditation can also be somewhat more directed. For example, an early exercise in mindfulness is to "sit with closed eyes and listen to sounds, allowing them to come to you." (People who like to walk in the woods do this naturally.) Meditation can be practiced sitting, standing, lying down, or moving. Mindfulness meditation is not hard to learn; and anyone can practice it.

Beginning meditators often misunderstand what mindfulness meditation is and does. Mindfulness meditation is not a relaxation exercise; sometimes its effect is quite the opposite when the object of awareness is disturbing. It is not a way to avoid difficulties in life, because it brings us closer to our difficulties before we disentangle from them. It does not bypass our personality problems; it is a slow, gentle process of coming to grips with who we are. Finally, mindfulness meditation is not about achieving a different state of mind; it is about settling into our current experience in a relaxed, alert, and openhearted way.

Mindfulness practice may include any sense—sight, sound, touch, smell, taste, and hearing—as well as mindfulness of thoughts and feelings. However, due to the seductive and evanescent nature of thoughts and feelings, it is often easier to start mindfulness practice by exploring the five senses.

In typical practice, mindfulness meditation begins with concentration on the breath. When sufficient stability of mind has been achieved, after minutes or days, we direct awareness—ply the searchlight—to include other experiences. If the mind loses its stability by becoming entangled in the objects of perception, we can take refuge in the breath anytime, strengthening concentration. An unstable mind is like an unstable camera; we get a fuzzy picture.

The basic mindfulness meditation instructions are deceptively simple (see p. 17, Exercise 1). When we focus on the breath, we are focusing on a perceptual event in the present. It is sometimes difficult to *find* the breath through the continuous buzz of compelling thoughts and feelings. Counting breaths sometimes helps. The instruction given in Exercise 1, "Notice what it was that took you away," is the heart of mindfulness practice and is what distinguishes it from concentration meditation. The searchlight goes out to notice the distraction. The distraction is no more or less an opportunity for mindfulness than the breath, but in the begin-

Exercise 1

1. Assume a comfortable posture lying on your back or sitting; keep the spine straight and let your shoulders drop.

2. Close your eyes, if it feels comfortable.

3. Bring your attention to your belly, feeling it rise or expand gently on the inbreath and fall or recede on the outbreath.

4. Keep the focus on your breathing, "being with" each inbreath for its full duration and with each outbreath for its full duration, as if you were riding the waves of your own breathing.

5. Every time you notice that your mind has wandered off the breath, notice what it was that took you away and then gently bring your attention back to your belly and the feeling of the breath coming in and out.

6. If your mind wanders away from your breath a thousand times, then your "job" is simply to bring it back to the breath every time, no matter what preoccupies it.

7. Practice this exercise for 15 minutes at a convenient time every day, whether you feel like it or not, for 1 week, and see how it feels to incorporate a disciplined meditation practice into your life. Be aware of how it feels to spend some time each day just being with your breath, without having to *do* anything.

Exercise 2

1. Tune in to your breathing at different times during the day, feeling the belly go through one or two risings and fallings.

2. Become aware of your thoughts and feelings at these moments, just observing them without judging them or yourself.

3. At the same time, be aware of any changes in the way you are seeing things and feeling about yourself.

ning, we first want to stabilize the mind by returning gently and quickly to the breath. Exercise 2 supports mindfulness throughout the day.

Concentration and mindfulness actually complement one another. Concentration requires more effort and may create tension if it is not blended with a mindful attitude of inviting and accepting whatever appears on our perceptual screen. Mindfulness may uncover difficult memories that can hijack the mind if we do not return to the refuge of concentration. Most of us can only practice concentration in quiet places, whereas moments of mindfulness may take place anywhere. Mindfulness meditation is a dance between mindfulness and concentration.

Mindfulness and concentration meditation practitioners both are actually learning mindfulness; they are learning to awaken from unconscious absorption in thoughts and feelings, and to intentionally redirect attention. The difference is that in mindfulness meditation, we are intentionally exploring a broader array of mental contents and, over time, may find it easier to recognize and disentangle from them in daily life.

Mindfulness-Oriented Psychotherapy

There many ways to integrate mindfulness into therapeutic work, and they are not mutually exclusive. A therapist may (1) personally practice mindfulness meditation or everyday mindfulness to cultivate a more *mindful presence* in psychotherapy; (2) use a theoretical frame of reference informed by insights derived from mindfulness practice, recent psychological literature on mindfulness, or Buddhist psychology (mindfulness-*informed* psychotherapy); or (3) may explicitly teach patients how to practice mindfulness (mindfulness-*based* psychotherapy). Collectively, we refer to this range of approaches as *mindfulness-oriented* psychotherapy.

Practicing Therapist

Mindfulness appears to be a cognitive style; part state and part trait (Sternberg, 2000). While different life experiences and genetic predispositions probably account for natural variance among individuals, mindfulness can be cultivated through daily meditation (ideally 20–45 minutes per day) and/or practicing informal mindfulness exercises.

Meditating therapists often report feeling more "present," relaxed and receptive with their patients if they meditate earlier in the day. While this effect has not yet been studied experimentally, indirect evidence for the benefits of meditation includes a study by Ryan and Brown (2003), who found that Zen meditators had higher levels of mindfulness than a matched sample of adults; and the work of Davidson et al. (2003), who discovered that mindfulness meditation practice increases activation in an area of the brain associated with compassion.

The meditating therapist can relate mindfully to his or her patients within *any* theoretical frame of reference, including psychodynamic, cognitive-behavioral, family systems, or narrative psychotherapy. Chapter 3 of this book explores this topic further.

Mindfulness-Informed Psychotherapy

Mindfulness-informed psychotherapy borrows ideas from both Buddhist and Western psychology, as well as from the practical experience of practitioners. As mentioned earlier, direct experience is necessary to truly understand mindfulness because it is nonconceptual in nature. Therapists who practice mindfulness-informed psychotherapy may identify with a theoretical frame of reference based on mindfulness, but they do not explicitly teach patients how to practice mindfulness. There are a number of works that conceptually integrate Buddhist psychology and psychotherapy in this way, including those of Brazier (1995), Epstein (1995, 1998), Goleman, 2003), Kawai (1996), Ladner (2004), Magid (2002), Molino (1998), Rosenbaum (1999), Rubin (1996), Safran (2003), Segall (2003), Suler (1993), Watts (1963), Welwood (2000), and Young-Eisendrath and Muramoto (2002).

Mindfulness-Based Psychotherapy

The integration of mindfulness into cognitive-behavioral therapy has led to new mindfulness exercises and multicomponent treatment protocols. These mindfulness-based psychotherapies involve teaching patients specific mindfulness skills, such as breath awareness, mindful eating, and other ways of regulating attention (see Chapter 6). The proliferation of treatment protocols is encouraging clinicians to experiment with mindfulness techniques, even if therapists do not implement the entire protocol. Work in this category includes that by Bennett-Goleman (2001); Bien and Bien (2002); Brach (2003); Brantley (2003); Fishman (2002); Goleman (1997); Hayes et al. (2004); Hayes, Strosahl, and Wilson (1999); Kabat-Zinn (1990, 1994); Linehan (1993a, 1993b); Martin (1999); McQuaid and Carmona (2004); Schwartz (1996); Schwartz and Begley (2002); Segal, Williams, and Teasdale (2002); and Siegel, Urdang, and Johnson (2001).

AN EMERGING, NEW MODEL OF PSYCHOTHERAPY?

We may be on the threshold of a new, mindfulness-oriented model of psychotherapy. There is a clear philosophical paradigm that supports such a model (discussed later in this chapter). Treatment strategies can be derived from the basic elements of mindfulness—awareness, of present experience, with acceptance. The strategies are distinguishable from those of other models and are beginning to be tested for effectiveness. A review of the empirical literature by Baer (2003) suggests that mindfulness-based treatments are "probably efficacious" and en route to becoming "well established."

We will have a developed new model of psychotherapy, if the outcome literature further confirms its usefulness, when we elaborate and refine relevant aspects of mindfulness for different settings and diagnostic categories, when we specify the limitations of the approach, and when the different areas of scholarly investigation are brought under a consistent theoretical umbrella.

The emerging mindfulness model offers intriguing possibilities to diverse areas of psychology and psychotherapy. Its scope is wide, because mindfulness is a very simple and universal human capacity, and because it can find its way into psychology both as a theoretical construct and as a practice. Mindfulness is already making strange bedfellows of far-ranging fields such as behaviorism, psychoanalysis, humanistic psychotherapy, brain science, ethics, spirituality, health psychology, and positive psychology.

Cognitive-Behavioral Therapy

There has been a surge of literature on mindfulness and acceptance-based cognitive-behavioral treatment (Baer, 2003; Campos, 2002; Hayes et al., 2004; Roemer & Orsillo, 2002). Unlike change-based therapies, mindfulness- and acceptance-based treatments cultivate a relaxed, nonadversarial relationship to symptoms, in which disturbing sensations, feelings, or thoughts are allowed to come and go. Acceptance-based therapies address the familiar paradox of symptoms intensifying when we try to remove them, such as when trying to go to sleep or struggling to relax.

The four leading approaches are (1) dialectical behavior therapy (DBT; Linehan, 1993a, 1993b), which has become the preferred treatment for borderline personality disorder and is being used for affect regulation in general; (2) mindfulness-based stress reduction (MBSR; Kabat-Zinn, 1990), an 8- to 10-week mindfulness training course with multiple applications to physical and mental health; (3) mindfulness-based cognitive therapy (MBCT; Segal, Williams, & Teasdale, 2002), an application of MBSR to cognitive therapy and depression, which teaches patients to observe their thoughts; and (4) acceptance and commitment therapy (ACT; Hayes, Strosahl, et al., 1999; Hayes, Strosahl, & Houts, 2005), which encourages patients to accept, rather than control, unpleasant sensations. For a review of the promising outcome literature, see Baer (2003), Hayes, Masuda, et al. (2004), and Chapter 11 of this book.

Other mindfulness- and acceptance-based treatment programs include integrative behavioral couple therapy (Jacobson, Christensen, Prince, Cordove, & Eldridge, 2000), Roemer and Orsillo's (2002) treatment of generalized anxiety disorder, Schwartz's (1996) treatment of obsessive–compulsive disorder, Marlatt's (2002) work with substance abuse, Kohlenberg's functional analytic psychotherapy (Kohlenberg & Tsai, 1991), Kristeller and Hallett's (1999) approach to eating disorders, and Martell, Addis, & Jacobson's (2001) guided strategies for treating depression.

Cognitive psychology is undergoing a "second cognitive revolution": a new understanding that much of what we think, feel and do is the consequence of unconscious, "implicit" processes (Westen, 2000a). The task of therapy, then, is to *access* implicit, automatic, dysfunctional thought patterns (Friedman & Whisman, 2004; Palfai & Wagner, 2004). Mindfulness practice will probably grow in importance over the coming years as a "technology of access."

Psychodynamic Psychotherapy

As mentioned earlier, psychodynamic theorists saw the value of Buddhist psychology at least since the time of Carl Jung (1939/1992). More modern proponents are Mark Epstein (1995, 1998), Jeffrey Rubin (1996), Anthony Molino (1998), Barry Magid (2002), and Jeremy Safran (2003). Peter Fonagy's (2000) notion of "mentalization," or the capacity to think about one's own mental states or those of others, is a mindfulness skill. Daniel Stern's (2004) recent work on the "present moment in psychotherapy" highlights implicit processes within the intersubjective field, all notions related to Buddhist psychological principles.

It is understandable that psychodynamic psychotherapists discovered mindfulness before their behaviorist colleagues, because psychoanalysis has historically shared common features with mindfulness practice: They are both introspective ventures, they assume that awareness and acceptance precede change, and they both recognize the importance of unconscious processes. Chapter 2 explores commonalities and points of divergence among these three traditions.

Humanistic Psychotherapy

Mindfulness practice was originally intended to alleviate the suffering associated with existential conditions, such as sickness, old age, and death—not clinical conditions, as this category did not exist in the Buddha's time. According to Buddhist psychology, suffering comes from how we relate to these unavoidable challenges.

Mindfulness has much in common with humanistic psychotherapy, which broadly encompasses existential, constructivist, and transpersonal approaches (Schneider & Leitner, 2002). Like Buddhist psychology, the existential approach "emphasizes the person's inherent capacities to become healthy and fully functioning. It concentrates on the present, on achieving consciousness of life as being partially under one's control, on accepting responsibility for decisions, and on learning to tolerate anxiety" (Shahrokh & Hales, 2003, p. 78).

There are other points of concordance. The work of Eugene Gendlin (1996), especially his idea of the preverbal, bodily, "felt sense" of a psychological problem, is strikingly similar to mindfulness-oriented psychotherapy (see Chapter 7). Constructivist psychotherapies, such as narrative therapy (Leiblich, McAdams, & Josselson, 2004), share with mindfulness theory the notion that "reality" is created by the person in interaction with the environment. Transpersonal therapy and Buddhist psychology have the common assumption that the individual is essentially indivisible from the wider universe, a theme that recurs regularly in future chapters.

Brain Science

The convergence of brain science and mindfulness is particularly fertile. It was given an initial boost by the impressive work of James Austin, *Zen and the Brain* (1998). As brain imaging technology advances, such as in the expanded use of functional magnetic resonance imaging (fMRI), we can correlate the first-person reports of experimental subjects with objective images. It is noteworthy that the 2,500-year-old tradition of rigorous Buddhist introspection never revealed *where* in the brain mental events occur. That is now changing, as we shall see in Chapter 11.

"Neuroplasticity," including the ability of the mind to shape the brain, is an exciting field of inquiry. Jeffrey Schwartz (Schwartz & Begley, 2002) and Richard Davidson (2003) are exploring how mindfulness practice may change brain function. Ordinary people trained to meditate for 8 weeks showed left prefrontal activation while they were at rest and in response to an emotional challenge (Davidson et al., 2003). Schwartz (1996) found changes in the brain from mindfulness-based cognitive therapy of obsessive–compulsive disorder that were similar to those from psychoactive medication.

A fascinating bit of brain research by Benjamin Libet (1999) showed experimentally what many meditators have observed about "free will"—that people become aware of the intention to act *after* (350–400 ms, to be exact) the brain has readied itself to act and *before* (200 ms) motor activity. In other words, we can "veto" an action, but our *intention* to act is formulated in the brain before we become aware of it! This kind of research, along with neuroplasticity studies, suggest that we may be able to change the brain itself through mindfulness practice, and that the individual has an opportunity to better control behavior by increasing mindful awareness of brain activity.

Ethics

Buddhist psychology does not distinguish between "good" and "bad" actions, which are often merely social conventions, but rather between "wholesome" and "unwholesome" actions. Wholesome actions are those that diminish suffering for oneself and others, while unwholesome actions increase suffering. Mindful attention allows us to observe carefully the consequences of behavior. This harming–nonharming ethical distinction is entirely consistent with a secular psychotherapeutic agenda.

Within mindfulness and acceptance-based psychotherapy, values have a high priority. ACT, for example, includes exercises for patients to discover their values ("What do you want your life to stand for?") and to identify obstacles to achieving those goals ("Are you willing to openly experience what gets in your way?"). Buddhist psychology also emphasizes how our intentions determine the direction our lives will take.

Spirituality

The integration of spirituality into mindfulness-oriented psychotherapy is a vast subject, beyond the scope of this book. Spirituality often refers to an appreciation of intangible yet meaningful aspects of our lives. The intangibles may be values (love, truth, peace), God, a life force, interpersonal connections, or perhaps a sense of transcendence.

Buddhism is an "immanent" approach to spirituality, suggesting that what we seek is happening right in front of our noses, within the actual experience of day-to-day living. The thrust of spiritual aspiration within the immanent approach is to embrace each moment more wholeheartedly. In contrast, a "transcendental" approach is a "trickle-down" methodology, in which repeated experiences of mystical union (closeness to God) gradually make our daily experience more complete. Although mystical states may occur during mindfulness meditation, they are still considered mental events and, hence, are not accorded special status. Freedom from suffering occurs when no mental events can snag our awareness.

Health Psychology

The health benefits of mindfulness are becoming increasingly apparent (Carlson, Speca, Patel, & Goodey, 2003, 2004; Reibel, Greeson, Brainard, & Rosenzweig, 2001; Roth & Stanley, 2002; Speca, Carlson, Goodey, & Angen, 2000; Williams, Kolar, Reger, & Pearson, 2001). Most benefits seem to derive from a less reactive autonomic nervous system—feeling less stressed. Mindfulness practice may also help patients recognize health needs before they develop into illness. For example, patients with diabetes might be more conscientious taking their insulin, asthma patients may be able to detect sooner the emotional reactions that can trigger attacks, and patients with obesity may be able to identify food cravings before the urges become compulsive behaviors. Mindfulness meditation has also been shown to improve immune function (Davidson et al., 2003) and to help clear psoriasis (Kabat-Zinn et al., 1998).

Positive Psychology

In Buddhist psychology, mental health is complete freedom from suffering, generally referred to as enlightenment. From this perspective, we are all mentally ill.

Western psychology has made remarkable progress in understanding the biological, psychological, and social roots of a troubled mind, but it has neglected positive experiences, such as well-being, contentment, love, courage, spirituality, wisdom, altruism, civility, and tolerance (Seligman & Csikszentmihalyi, 2000). We also do not have a method for cultivating Olympic (i.e., extremely advanced, not competitive!) levels of positive mental health. Buddhist psychology is comprehensive program that cultivates happiness, and mindfulness is the basis of the program. There is a curious paradox in the Buddhist approach to positive psychology: The more fully we can embrace unhappiness, the deeper and more abiding our sense of well-being. A detailed discussion of mindfulness and positive psychology is presented in Chapter 12.

THE WORLDVIEW OF MINDFULNESS

Each of us has a dominant worldview, or inclination to perceive the world in a particular way. Worldviews seem to depend on the personality of the individual (Johnson, Germer, Efran, & Overton, 1988). For example, one parent may want to send a child to a school that emphasizes creative thinking, whereas another might want to send the same child to a school that focuses on reading, writing and arithmetic. People of different worldviews can argue about priorities, but the assumptions of worldviews are so fundamental that they cannot be easily validated, justified, or challenged.

All psychological theories and therapies are embedded in particular worldviews. Worldviews are also known as *paradigms* (Kuhn, 1970); *cosmologies* (Bunge, 1963), or *world hypotheses* (Pepper, 1942). Since the notion of mindfulness has endured for millennia and is currently inspiring clinical researchers and practitioners in diverse areas, we might expect to find a metatheoretical frame of reference for it in Western psychology. That frame is *contextualism* (Hayes, 2002).

Contextualism

The contextual worldview was first articulated by Stephan Pepper (1942). Worldviews explain the nature of reality (ontology), describe how we know reality (epistemology), account for causality, and contain a concept of personhood. The contextual worldview makes the following assumptions:

- *Nature of reality.* Activity and change are fundamental conditions of life. The world is an interconnected web of activity.
- *How we know reality.* All reality is constructed, created by each individual within a particular context. There is no absolute reality that we can know.
- *Causality.* Change is continuous and events are multidetermined. Apparent causality depends on its context. The most accurate causal description of an event is the *universe of causes* at a particular point in time.
- *Personhood.* The person is best described as a single moment of awareness or activity embedded in an unlimited field of interpersonal and impersonal events. A helpful metaphor is a fountain of water that is made up of different drops from one moment to the next but appears to hold its shape over time.

George Kelly's (1955) theory of personal constructs broke ground for psychology within the contextual worldview. Kelly, an early constructivist, said that the human being lives simultaneously in a primary, preconceptual reality, as well as in a world of interpretations about that reality. As we grow into adulthood, we continually "update" our day-to-day, preverbal experience with new personal constructs. Narrative therapy (White & Epston, 1990) is a familiar example of modern constructivist psychotherapy, as are mindfulness- and acceptance-based psychotherapies.

Mindfulness-oriented psychotherapy may differ slightly from other constructivist therapies by emphasizing what the individual is *not* rather than what he or she *is*. Mindfulness guards somewhat against the human tendency to reify—to make something flowing like water into something hard like ice. This extends to our view of symptoms. Efran, Germer, and Lukens (1986) wrote that "the basic insight that contextualism offers to the field of psychotherapy theory is that complaints, problems, or symptoms are not objective *things*—stable entities that are to be diagnosed and then excised" (p. 171).

Buddhist Psychology and Contextualism

The assumptions of Buddhist psychology closely correspond to the contextual worldview. We need only to turn to the "three characteristics of existence"—key insights about life to which intensive mindfulness meditation often leads. The three characteristics are suffering, impermanence, and selflessness. Impermanence, or change, is precisely the ontology of contextualism, and selflessness is the contextual view of personhood. More is said about these subjects in the following chapters. Another key concept in Buddhist philosophy, "dependent co-origination," is a fancy expression for a multidetermined universe—the notion of causality in contextualism.

Buddhist psychology assumes that the way we construct our private realities is mostly delusional; we unconsciously elaborate on events as they emerge, based on our past experience, and this leads to unnecessary suffering. The antidote, mindful attention, allows us to see things more clearly. What we see, however, is not some absolute truth; rather, we see through the delusion of our conceptualizations. We learn to hold our constructions more lightly.

DOES MINDFULNESS MATTER TO THERAPISTS?

It is difficult to predict just what the impact of mindfulness on our profession will be. Padmasambhava, an eighth-century Tibetan teacher, said that "when the iron bird flies, the dharma [Buddhist teachings] will come to the West" (cited in Henley, 1994, p. 51). Although it is now over 100 years since Buddhist psychology made it to our shores (Fields, 1992), it is only fairly recently that the ideas have captured the imagination of the clinical and research communities in psychology. The grand tradition of contemplative psychology in the East and the powerful scientific model of the West are finally meeting.

Scientifically, what we know is preliminary but promising. Clinicians are on the vanguard of exploration, and even marginal success in the consultation room can be an important beginning. We have many more questions than answers: We need to determine which mindfulness-based interventions work, and for whom. We should explore the impact of a meditating therapist on therapy outcome. We may wish to understand better the cognitive, biochemical, neurological, emotional, and behavioral factors that contribute to mindfulness. It may also be fruitful to investigate the outer reaches of mindfulness—what human beings are capable of in terms of attentional control and emotional regulation, and how this translates into the way we live our lives.

To have psychological techniques at our disposal, drawn from a 2,500-year-old tradition, which appear to change the brain, shape our behavior for the better, and offer intuitive insights about how to live life more fully, is an opportunity that may be difficult for psychotherapists to ignore. Only time will tell what we make of it.

The remainder of this book explores how the simple human capacity for mindfulness may be able to enrich our understanding and effectiveness as psychotherapists. Chapter 2 considers commonalities and divergences between the Buddhist tradition of mindfulness and Western psychotherapy. Part II examines how mindfulness may be cultivated by the psychotherapist and its effect on the therapy relationship. Part III explores the application of mindfulness to particular psychological conditions and patient populations. Part IV discusses the historical context and Buddhist teachings on mindfulness, as well as the potential of mindfulness for the future, within the emerging field of positive psychology. Finally, the appendices provide resources for clinicians and a glossary of Buddhist terms.

CHAPTER 2

Buddhist and Western Psychology

Seeking Common Ground

PAUL R. FULTON
RONALD D. SIEGEL

Mindfulness has been practiced deliberately for over 2,500 years, primarily in the form of mindfulness meditation, to alleviate human suffering. While it has been subjected to scientific scrutiny only recently, millions of anecdotal reports from Asian cultures over the centuries attest to its usefulness. Western psychotherapy is quite new by comparison, and originated in a very different time and place.

Can we expect to find parallels between an ancient Asian practice of mind training and modern Western systems of psychological treatment? Are the problems of ancient India and the modern West so different that comparing their systems of healing is misguided? Or is there some universality to human psychology and suffering that both traditions address? How does each tradition understand suffering and its treatment? Only recently have mental health professionals given serious consideration to the healing potential of mindfulness practice. This chapter takes a preliminary look at how these ancient and modern traditions relate to one another.

In approaching the topic, at least two distinct relationships between mindfulness and psychotherapy present themselves. First, mindfulness meditation, a deliberate practice designed to alleviate psychological suffering, can be compared and contrasted with Western psychotherapy. Second, mindfulness itself—awareness of present experience with acceptance— may be seen as a common factor contributing to the efficacy of both Western psychotherapy and formal mindfulness meditation practice.

Of course, many varieties of psychotherapy have developed in its relatively brief history, and many variants of mindfulness meditation have been practiced over the centuries. It would be impossible to review all of these here. Instead, we go back to beginnings, and explore core similarities and differences between mindfulness meditation in its early form, practiced as part of *vipassana* or insight meditation, and the psychodynamic and behavioral traditions out of which most modern psychotherapy has developed. These two psychotherapeutic traditions are chosen with the open-eyed understanding that there are many more forms of treatment. Even the psychodynamic and behavioral psychology traditions are diverse. However, we emphasize these two schools of therapy due to their pervasive influence on our field, and because each has interesting qualities in common with mindfulness practice.

ALLEVIATING PSYCHOLOGICAL SUFFERING

Like Western psychotherapy, mindfulness meditation developed in response to suffering that was understood to have a psychological cause. Also, like psychotherapy, the domain of mindfulness meditation includes thoughts, feelings, perception, intentions, and behavior.

Given this focus, Buddhist psychology naturally shares with its Western counterpart a basic framework for understanding psychological disorders. Both systems (1) identify symptoms, (2) describe their etiology, (3) suggest a prognosis, and (4) prescribe treatment. This formulation is found in the Four Noble Truths, reported to be the Buddha's first formal teaching (see also Appendix B).

Before looking at looking both traditions within this framework, let us consider a clinical example that we use to illustrate subsequent points:

> Richard, a young man of 23, living in New York, had been socially insecure in high school, did not excel at sports, and was often intimidated by other guys. He had several girlfriends throughout high school and college, but until recently had felt uncertain of his attractiveness. He regularly smoked marijuana and experimented with hallucinogens.

During his last year at college, Richard became involved with an unusually attractive and sensual young woman, Jessica, who was a year behind him at school. They began a torrid sexual relationship. It was complicated, however, by the background presence of her previous boyfriend, who had moved away to California.

Jessica was at a crossroads in her life. She invited Richard to live with her. This made him anxious, and he told her that he did not feel ready. After many painful conversations, she announced that she, too, had decided to go to California.

Richard was devastated. His mind alternated between intense longing and wild jealousy as he imagined Jessica passionately making love with her ex-boyfriend. He had trouble sleeping at night and could not concentrate at work. He started smoking marijuana daily and tripping frequently on LSD in an effort to loosen his attachment to Jessica. He could not bear to watch other couples together. Every time he passed someone who looked at all like Jessica, he was overwhelmed with sadness and anger.

Richard found his weekly psychotherapy to be supportive, but he remained miserable. Desperate to do *something*, he signed up for a 2-week intensive mindfulness meditation retreat.

Few psychotherapy patients are like Richard, choosing to try intensive retreat practice when in an emotional crisis. Nonetheless, his experience helps us to compare and contrast how psychotherapy and meditation traditions can address a typical psychological problem. By amplifying the effects of mindfulness, Richard's intensive retreat experience will offer a window into the workings of the practice.

Symptoms

The symptoms that are the focus of Western psychotherapy include both unpleasant subjective states such as anxiety and depression, and patterns of maladaptive behavior such as phobic avoidance and compulsions. Richard's difficulty concentrating, repetitive intrusive thoughts and feelings, sleep disruption, and dependence on illegal drugs are not atypical.

The "symptom" addressed by mindfulness meditation is simply the suffering that is inescapable to all who exist. No state, however pleasant, can be held indefinitely, nor can unpleasant experiences be avoided. However, we are so conditioned to avoid discomfort and seek pleasure that our lives are colored by a sense of "unsatisfactoriness," of something missing. Such suffering may or may not rise to the level of a formal psychiatric diagnosis. Rather, it arises from deep misunderstanding about the nature of our lives and our minds. In this sense, suffering is seen not as a symptom of a medical disorder but as a result of the nature of our relationship to the existential realities of life. As we see throughout this book, clinicians are now attempting to use mindfulness meditation in the treatment of a wide variety of psychiatric disorders. Nonetheless, the practice was originally intended to address more universal, nonclinical, aspects of human suffering.

Interestingly, many of the "symptoms" that mindfulness meditation addresses do not become apparent to an individual until he or she begins mindfulness practice. For example, meditators notice that it is very difficult to sit still and follow the breath; they find that their minds are constantly leaping forward into fantasies of the future or reviewing memories of the past. They begin to notice, in fact, that they are rarely fully present to life experience. They often also notice an array of anxieties and other affects that may not have been apparent before they attempted to be mindful. The realization that we habitually omit so much from ordinary awareness can be quite unsettling.

This unsettled feeling is not unlike what patients entering psychodynamic psychotherapy experience as they begin to feel that they are more neurotic than they had originally thought. They begin to notice themselves defending against all sorts of thoughts and feelings, and enacting neurotic patterns based on past experiences.

There are parallels to this phenomenon in many behavioral treatments also. Procedures such as self-monitoring or completing behavioral inventories can make clients suddenly aware of just how pervasive their symptoms are. Being asked to approach feared activities in the name of treatment can also amplify symptoms dramatically.

> Richard's gross symptoms—his depression and obsessive thoughts of his girlfriend—were initially quite obvious to him and others. When he started meditating intensively on retreat, however, he also noticed that he was frequently awash in intense fears whose object he could not identify. In addition, his mind began to be filled with violent images in which he dismembered Jessica and her ex-boyfriend.

(We return to these images shortly.)

Etiology

Modern mental health clinicians see the complex etiology of psychological disorders as involving biological, psychological, and sociological factors. Nature verses nurture arguments have given way to recognition that both genetics and environment interact in shaping human experience and behavior.

Both psychodynamic and behavioral traditions have concluded that much human suffering is caused by distortions in thoughts, feelings, and behavior. Here, they find common ground with mindfulness meditation traditions, however much they differ on the causes of these distortions.

Psychodynamic psychotherapists generally presume that distortions in thought and feeling, born usually of childhood experience, have created psychological scars that distort our responses to present circumstances. The defenses we develop selectively to avoid some experiences prevent us from seeing current reality clearly, and restrict our range of affect and behavior. For example, in his therapy, it was apparent that intimacy and commitment were highly conflicted for Richard. These difficulties arose from an inflated self-image ("Why should I *settle* on any one woman!") that compensated for his feelings of inadequacy ("I'm not really much of a man"). Both of these ideas had roots in his childhood relationships.

Behaviorism, with its focus on maladaptive external behavior, did not initially address subjective experience. It viewed the mind as a "black box" that did not require investigation. Psychological difficulties were understood as the result of maladaptive reinforcement contingencies (Skinner, 1974).

Nonetheless, behaviorists eventually developed an interest in subjective experience (Beck, 1976; Ellis, 1962). They came to see that the thoughts, feelings, and images associated with maladaptive behaviors were important links in the causal chain leading up to those behaviors. Cognitive-behavioral therapy (CBT) emerged as a technique for capturing or noticing thoughts, feelings, and images as they pass through consciousness, particularly identifying "irrational" thoughts as a cause of suffering. For Richard, the most obvious cognitive distortions involved catastrophizing—thoughts such as "I'll never find another woman like Jessica" and "I'll never enjoy life again."

Mindfulness meditation shares the observation that holding a variety of distorted core beliefs leads to suffering. As we will see, Buddhist psychology identifies false beliefs about who we are to be the most pernicious distortion.

At their roots, behavioral psychology, psychodynamic psychology, and Buddhist mindfulness all rest on the idea of conditioning, though the issue of conditioning is addressed differently by each. Psychodynamic psychology is interested in understanding an individual's unique conditioning and how it informs the present, through the misapplication of early adaptive strategies, and how early experience shapes the sense the individual makes of him- or herself and the world. Behavioral psychology, like mindfulness practice, is less interested in the way an individual constructs meaning than in helping that individual to see the role conditioning plays in present-day life, thereby empowering him or her to modify current conditions to pave the way for more satisfactory outcomes.

What all three traditions share, then, is a recognition that suffering is not random, not a consequence of divine retribution for sin, nor a test for entrance into a future paradise, not a result of moral weakness, but a natural consequence of conditions. This recognition offers hope for relief, because suffering arises from causes that can be understood and often modified. Human suffering is rendered as part of a lawful order.

Prognosis

The prognosis for treatment in psychodynamic and behavioral traditions, of course, varies with the disorder being treated, and the same may be said of mindfulness meditation. While the apparent emphasis on suffering and impermanence in Buddhist psychology may seem excessively gloomy, it is actually remarkably optimistic. Given the pervasiveness of "symptoms" of repeated striving, frequent disappointment, and difficulty being fully present that we initially observe during meditation practice, it can be hard at first to imagine that this method can actually alleviate suffering!

In fact, the prognosis, as described in the Buddhist literature, is radically optimistic. It states that while no one is immune from suffering, there is the potential for its complete alleviation, though this level of freedom is afforded only to fully enlightened beings. However, even in its more modest application, mindfulness offers a surprisingly good prognosis; if we can learn to embrace life as it is, we will not suffer as much. In the case of Richard, he realized at the beginning of his retreat how he was continually absorbed in his thoughts and fantasies. He saw the possibility of grounding himself in the immediate reality of moment-to-moment sensory experience. This realization brought the first ray of hope he had had since Jessica announced she was leaving.

Treatment

All three of the traditions we have discussed involve a combination of introspection and prescribed behavioral changes in their efforts to alleviate suffering. A brief overview reveals several parallels.

Introspection

Psychodynamic psychotherapy, with its historical emphasis on free association, begins by exploring the contents of the mind. Patients are encouraged to say whatever comes into awareness, and this material is examined for patterns that reveal underlying thoughts and feelings. It is through gaining insight into these contents, correcting distortions based on early experience, and healing psychic wounds that reduction of suffering becomes possible.

In CBT, the emphasis has traditionally been on identifying and changing irrational patterns of thought that lead to maladaptive behaviors. Irrational thoughts are labeled, challenged, and replaced with more rational thoughts, leading to more adaptive, satisfying behavior. This approach has been broadened recently with the development of mindfulness-based CBT that borrows from ancient mindfulness practice the idea that learning to *accept* painful experiences, rather than seek to be rid of them, can be transformative.

Mindfulness meditation involves repeatedly observing the mind, moment-by-moment. It differs from the introspection practiced in psychodynamic therapy in the nature of the objects chosen for attention, and in the sort of attention brought to them. This repeated observation eventually leads to insight into the workings of the mind, which, as we will see, brings relief from suffering. It also allows the mindfulness practitioner to increasingly and wholeheartedly embrace the full range of human experience.

Behavior Change

In recent years, many psychoanalysts have recognized the limits of insight, and even "working through," to effect visible change, and have come to value deliberate efforts at behavioral change. Obviously, in behaviorally oriented treatment, deliberate, practiced action assumes a central role.

The mindfulness meditation tradition also includes prescriptions for behavior change. At first glance, these appear to depart radically from Western psychotherapeutic traditions in their emphasis on morality. Both psychoanalysis and behaviorism differentiate themselves from Western religions and other cultural institutions in their relative neutrality around moral issues. By remaining nonjudgmental, therapists seek to allow patients to explore their true feelings, whether or not the feelings are ethical or socially acceptable. In most settings, therapists take a similarly nonjudgmental stance toward their patients' behavior, despite being legally mandated to report certain conduct to outside agencies.

"Treatment" in the Buddhist tradition is described in a group of principles known as the Eightfold Path (see Appendix B). Three of these eight principles—Right Effort, Right Mindfulness, and Right Concentration—describe mental practices, while another three refer explicitly to moral conduct—Right Speech, Right Action, and Right Livelihood. While these ethical guidelines include many of the prohibitions found in Western religions, they are presented somewhat differently in the Buddhist tradition. Practitioners are invited to watch their minds carefully to see the effects that following or not following these guidelines have on the quality of consciousness. The guidelines are thus recommended as a foundation for mindfulness meditation practice, based on the observation that an individual engaged in unethical activities will find peace and tranquility elusive. Conducting oneself in a moral fashion is therefore seen as a practical—even therapeutic—matter. This approach actually parallels what might occur in dynamic or cognitive-behavioral psychotherapy, in which the patient is invited to observe the consequences of his or her behavior in order to make better informed choices.

INSIGHT AND THE DISCOVERY OF TRUTH

Increased awareness is presumed to lead to greater psychological and emotional freedom in *both* the psychodynamic and mindfulness traditions. Neither tradition deliberately seeks to cultivate a particular feeling state, but rather sees deeper states of well-being as a consequence of the freedom won by replacing mental distortions with clear understanding. Insight is both the vehicle and the goal of both practices. While each tradition speaks differently about what constitutes "truth," it is only by moving toward such truth—and not by the cultivation of comforting illusion—that freedom becomes possible.

Insight has both similar and differing meanings across these traditions. In psychodynamic psychotherapy, *insight* refers to recognition of what was formerly hidden, unconscious, distorted, or otherwise defended against. In the meditation tradition, insight is often described as the direct perception of the characteristics of existence, notably, the changing nature of all phenomena, the absence of an essential, enduring nature to things, and the suffering that arises from not seeing all this clearly. Insight into these characteristics is transforming; with direct insight into how suffering arises from our mistaken clinging, we begin a natural and automatic process of letting go, much as one reflexively lets go of a burning object.

In both traditions, insight involves stepping back and seeing the way one has mistakenly come to believe that thoughts and perceptions are more real than they are. This is often described as loosening our "identification" with our thoughts and emotions. With insight, we come to see how what was once taken as a natural and inevitable reflection of our world is actually a construction, and how our adherence to that construction gives rise to suffering. Insight is a process of loosening our grip on rigid beliefs. Experientially, it may be more accurate to say that beliefs loosen their grip on us.

One way that insight leads to diminished suffering is by the light it sheds on the nature of suffering itself. We begin to see the difference between the arising of raw experience and our responses to it. In ordinary, nonmindful awareness, these two dimensions are indistinguishable, and our experience of events is an undifferentiated confounding of event and reaction. With close, mindful attention, we can distinguish the event from the quality of our relationship to it, and in the process see how suffering is in the reaction, not inherent in the raw experience itself. Insight into this source of suffering opens new avenues for freeing ourselves of harmful mental reactions. Chapter 9 illustrates this potential in the realm of physical pain.

Adherence to fixed, mistaken, and unhelpful thoughts is identified as a source of distress in CBT as well. Various techniques used in CBT seek to loosen a patient's identification with a distorted or rigid thought, or to replace a maladaptive idea with one that permits greater flexibility. Insight per se is less the focus of CBT, though it shares with insight meditation and psychodynamic therapy the purpose of loosening the grip of unreflectively held ideas.

Points of Departure: Insight, Thought, and Language

Despite theses similarities, the role and importance of thinking differ in CBT, psychodynamic therapy, and mindfulness meditation. In CBT, erroneous thinking is seen as a cause of distress, and correcting mistaken ideas is a mechanism of relief; that is, tightly held thoughts and ideas cause suffering to the degree to which they are unrealistic.

In psychodynamic psychotherapy, words are a necessary currency for the conduct of treatment; thoughts and feelings must be symbolically represented in language to be communicated. However, language is understood to be an imperfect and often disguised vehicle for communicating subtle subjective experience. The words we speak are assumed to mask underlying meanings that may be hidden from the speaker. It is not the expressed thought per se—accurate or inaccurate—that requires examination, but the underlying motivations, conflicts, and desires lying in disguised form behind the spoken word. While treatment must rely on language, the therapist and patient learn to listen *beyond* the spoken word, "with the third ear" (Reik, 1949) to the unspoken, the avoided, and the accidental—to find the reality that lies imperfectly revealed and imperfectly disguised in thought.

As a method, mindfulness meditation is distinguished from these other traditions by its near total abandonment of thinking. The practice differs from reflection by the continuous effort to set aside thinking—or at least to avoid being caught up in it—in favor of watching the arising and passing of all sensory, perceptual, and cognitive events. In this stance, thoughts are not granted any special status and are observed in their arising and passing, just as one might note an itch or passing sound.

Across its history, Buddhist psychology has been part of a vigorous and sophisticated philosophical tradition, trading in logic and argument. Despite this, it has generally regarded thinking, as a means of knowing or cultivating insight, as suspect. Thinking is shaped and confined by the structure, categories, and lexicon provided by language. For instance, we tend to perceive the world in a manner that reflects the way our language breaks the world up into objects (nouns) that conduct actions (verbs) on other objects. We divide up the world into classes that correspond to the categories in language.

In meditation practice, words are regarded as relatively limited and primitive, and our efforts to understand the world through the intellect and ideas is therefore ultimately superficial. Indeed, thinking actually obscures direct seeing into the nature of things. For individuals new to meditation, the idea that active, alert attention can exist without thought is unimaginable. However, with experience in meditation, it becomes clear that the process of knowing becomes more penetrating, subtle, and direct as thought is set aside; in the absence of discursive thought, a clear and penetrating awareness remains.

The practice of mindfulness (and its distilled expression in mindfulness meditation) involves direct attention unmediated by language. *Content*, or the narrative story as is understood in therapy, is given little weight. Indeed, when we are hijacked by discursive thinking about past or future, we have left the domain of mindfulness practice.

This difference in method is essential to understand where psychotherapy and mindfulness meditation depart. Mindfulness meditation is *not* intended to replace one meaning with another, to reframe experience through interpretation, or to rewrite a personal narrative. By operating at a more fundamental and "refined" level of attention, mindfulness meditation has a more primal and transformative power. It has a quality of deep certainty and insistence that is beyond refutation. As a concept, this is difficult to grasp. The insight that arises through mindfulness practice is not a proposition or syllogistic truth but is experienced as a condition of being, which depends upon the training of consciousness.

While Richard had been struggling in therapy to rewrite his personal narrative, the process was going slowly. What began to give him hope was the direct, felt experience during his meditation retreat that *reality* was not the same as his thoughts. Yes, he was haunted by images of Jessica reunited with her old boyfriend, and by powerful, often painful emotions, but these existed against a backdrop of the more immediate reality of the present moment— sensations in his body, the taste of food, the color of the grass and sky.

Along with this experience came the dawning realization that *all* of his concerns were actually just thoughts and fantasies. While Richard had begun to consider in psychotherapy that his ideas about himself might not be accurate, his experience in mindfulness meditation was beginning to suggest that there was no "final word" on his life or on himself.

GOALS

It is difficult to make general statements about the goals of psychotherapy, in part because they are construed differently by different schools, and because they must necessarily arise from the unique experience of each patient. Nonetheless, some general observations can safely be made.

An important contribution of ethnopsychology to the mental health field over the past half-century has been the realization of how our understanding of psychological health and pathology is highly culture-bound (Barnouw, 1973; Kleinman, Kunstadter, Alexander, Russell, & James, 1978). All systems of psychological healing are embedded in a cultural context and are inevitably expressions of cultural beliefs and values. They all share the goal of helping to restore an individual to "normal" development as it is understood in that culture, or fuller participation in his or her society. It is thus not surprising, given their different origins, that there are significant differences between the goals of modern Western psychotherapy and those of the mindfulness meditation tradition.

The Western View of the Self

One salient quality of the Western concept of the person and the self is its emphasis on separateness. By contrast with non-Western cultures' conceptions of the person that emphasize embeddedness in the clan, in society, and in nature, we have tended to hold a view that is radical in its emphasis on separateness. This quality of separateness has been extensively described by anthropologists. For example:

> In our commonly held unreflective view, the self is a distinct unit, some-
> thing we can name and define. We know what is the self, and what is not
> the self: and the distinction between the two is always the same. . . . Our
> own linguistic usage through the years, reveals a conception of increas-
> ingly assertive, active, and even aggressive self, as well as of an increas-
> ingly delimited self. (Lee, 1959, p. 132)

In Western psychological traditions, healthy development has meant becoming well individuated, not overly dependent on others, knowledgeable of one's own needs, and appropriately respectful of one's own
boundaries, with a clear and stable sense of identity and a sense of self
marked by cohesion and esteem. While this view has been criticized by
contemporary relational theorists (Gilligan, 1982; Miller & Stiver,
1997), it continues to form the backdrop for both psychodynamic and
behavioral therapies.

It is no surprise, then, that the complaints brought into psychotherapy by individuals in the West are often precisely the relative absence of
any of these qualities. Both the course of development toward the ideal
conception of the person and the ways individuals can fall off this developmental pathway are culturally determined. Naturally, psychotherapy
seeks to restore individuals to fuller participation in the culturally normative conception of selfhood.

Written treatment plans often express these cultural ideals. We say
treatment is intended to "improve self-esteem . . . identify one's own
needs in a relationship . . . establish a more cohesive sense of self . . . establish boundaries and learn to maintain them in relationships," and so
on. Our emphasis on the autonomy of the individual (often against evidence from our own social science) has led to a large technical vocabulary to describe disorders of the self and the consequent impairments in
relationships.

In the psychodynamic tradition, volumes have been written about
"the restoration of the self" (Kohut, 1977) and related topics, while behaviorists have studied extensively constructs such as "self-efficacy"
(e.g., Bandura, 1977, 1982). We take these terms to be scientifically
sound, and despite mounting evidence, they are applied with poor results to understanding emotional disorders in non-Western societies
(American Psychiatric Association, 2000).

Since the psychology field has attempted to be less culture bound,
we have begun to speak of behavior that is "adaptive" or "maladaptive," rather than "healthy" or "sick." Still, although the tools of
psychotherapy (honest conversation with a trusted individual) predate
scientific medicine, this vehicle for emotional healing has found its insti-

tutional home in Western medicine. It is now nearly impossible to avoid resting in our assumptions that distress is a matter of health relative to an ideal of selfhood.

> The therapist discussed Richard's difficulties with self-esteem, and how his sense of self had become dependent upon the affections of his girlfriend. He also pointed out Richard's difficulties with assertiveness, and how these had contributed to a variety of insecurities. In therapy, Richard felt that if only his sense of self were stronger, he would not be so affected by Jessica's decision.

The Self in Buddhist Psychology

As much of this volume suggests, mindfulness may be a useful adjunct to the effort to know and become a healthy self. But it is also important to recognize that in its original context, mindfulness was not a technique to help restore a sense of self as we ordinarily understand it. The purpose of mindfulness is not to become someone, but to cultivate insight into "no-self."

The goals of psychotherapy and mindfulness meditation depart significantly on this point. Mindfulness meditation is intended for nothing short of total psychological, emotional, moral, and spiritual emancipation, commonly called "enlightenment." This concept is elusive, because it cannot be described in psychotherapeutic terms. While mindfulness offers benefits conventionally recognized as psychotherapeutic, it also reaches toward a "treatment goal" that lies outside of the culturally constituted conception of the healthy self found in developmental and clinical psychology. In the original context of Buddhist psychology, mindfulness does not seek to restore a sense of self or improve self-esteem. It seeks instead to illuminate the insubstantiality of the self and the consequences of its misapprehension.

The notion of the "insubstantiality of the self" is one of the most challenging for Westerners who delve into mindfulness. However, the idea is not alien in contemporary science. Biology describes the human organism as a collection of cells composed of molecules and atoms. All of these elements are in constant flux, and simple reflection demonstrates that the boundary between the human body and its environment is actually quite arbitrary.

When I hold an apple in my hand, the apple is clearly not part of "me." It remains a separate object as I chew it, and perhaps even in my stomach, when I could still throw it back up. But is the apple "me" when in my intestines? How about when the apple's sugars are circulating in my blood? Or when the energy from those sugars has gone into building new cells?

Biology also points out that the level at which we identify an "organism" is arbitrary. An ant colony or beehive may be seen as a collection of individuals, but the communities are more meaningfully understood as complex organisms, much as our bodies can be seen as a collection of interdependent cells (Thomas, 1995).

The insight into "no-self" that mindfulness meditation is designed to foster involves actually experiencing ourselves in constant flux, a field of movement, always changing. Even our cherished self is seen as an event that arises when supporting conditions exist and passes when they do not; it is more "state" than "trait." As insight into the self-as-process grows, we begin to see the folly of accepting our naive adherence to the idea that the "I" is fixed, enduring, or even truly "mine." This insight greatly reduces our concerns for self-protection or self-aggrandizement and allows us to respond compassionately to others as we perceive our genuine interdependence with all of creation. This positive psychological experience is described further in Chapters 5 and 12.

Ironically, in the formulation offered by Buddhist psychology, the successful effort to establish a more stable sense of identity, self-esteem, self-efficacy, and the like, is often seen as the condition of "pathology," a delusion from which the path of mindfulness meditation begins. The achievement of a sense of self is the problem it addresses.

It is not uncommon for modern writers to suggest that the goals of mindfulness meditation begin where the Western concept of self-development ends (Boorstein, 1994). In this analysis, Western psychotherapy brings a person so far along a path of development, and mindfulness meditation continues the process from that point. "Ordinary human unhappiness," Freud's description of the best expectable outcome of psychoanalysis (Freud & Breuer, 1895/1961) is described as its point of departure.

While these differences between the goals of Western and Buddhist psychological practice are profound, in some ways the gap is not so wide. The contrast between the traditions can appear wider when discussing them conceptually than when observing them in practice. This is because the "no-self" of Buddhist psychology does not involve eliminating adaptive ego functions; rather, it describes an observing ego that is much more objective and much less identified with individual desires than we typically see in Western psychotherapy (Epstein, 1995).

Let us consider what "well adjusted" individuals, each with a well-developed "sense of self," look like in our psychotherapy traditions. They are flexible and open to new experiences. They are resilient, richly feeling the ups and downs of life, while maintaining perspective. They are capable of close, loving relationships and are compassionate toward others. They are able to see things from multiple perspectives. They are productive at work—able to identify goals and pursue them. They are aware of their strengths and weaknesses, and are not compelled to exaggerate the former or deny the latter.

While enlightenment is traditionally understood as the permanent extinction of greed, hatred and delusion, there is no litmus test by which one can positively identify an enlightened person. However, all of the qualities just described would be expected to develop from successful practice in the mindfulness meditation tradition. Whereas intensive meditation practice may lead to profound transformation in ways invisible to an outside observer, in many ways, an "enlightened" person resembles the "healthy" individual described earlier. We see this overlap in Richard's mindfulness meditation experience:

> Because he was practicing intensely, Richard had moments in which his discursive thoughts became quiet. He marveled at small events, such as a flower opening toward the sun and the complex patterns of cracks in a stone wall. Along with these experiences came a profound sense of peace—feeling part of this natural world. Personal fears and desires diminished in importance. Interspersed with sadness and violently jealous images, he felt moments of love and compassion toward Jessica. Richard was experiencing moments of "no-self" that produced effects a lot like those we would expect from the "healthy self" his psychotherapy was cultivating.

Instincts, "Root Causes," and Human Nature

It is not surprising that, as introspective practices, both psychodynamic and mindfulness meditation traditions have noticed that impulses in the human heart give rise to suffering. (Early on, behavioral psychology differentiated itself from psychodynamic schools by declaring that since these impulses were inferred rather than directly observed, they could not be a suitable object of study.)

Freud originally posited two drives—erotic and aggressive—as the source of human motivation. By describing these as instinctual in nature, he was affirming their persistence; they are "hardwired" and immutable. Because they are enduring vestiges from our evolutionary past, the well-adjusted person is ultimately capable only of accommodation to these drives in a socially permissible fashion. The cost of such accommodation is the need for psychological defenses, which enable some gratification of drives, while ideally permitting sufficient sublimation to enable us to get along with others.

The immutability of the instincts sets a limit on human aspirations for freedom; if we are forever tied to this evolutionary inheritance, the best that we can hope for is healthy compromise and the replacement of primitive defenses with mature defenses. From this perspective, human nature can never transcend the aggressive, ignorant, insatiable demands of the id.

Buddhist psychology describes three "root causes"—greed, hatred, and delusion—that give rise to suffering (see Chapter 12 for a fuller description). The similarity of the first two root causes to Freud's instincts is evident: erotic drive = greed, and aggressive drive = hatred. Both psychodynamic and mindfulness meditation traditions describe how these forces wreak havoc on mental life, and both suggest ways to understand and address their influence. Where they depart, however, is the ultimate status of these forces.

Whereas Freud saw them as immovable, Buddhist psychology teaches that they can be uprooted once and for all. In this respect, Buddhist psychology takes the terminus of successful psychoanalytic treatment—ordinary human unhappiness—as the pathological point of departure for meditation practice and reaches beyond symptom reduction, to a condition beyond suffering. Though this is an accomplishment that comes only with "full" enlightenment, in principle, these instinctual forces can be overcome. This goal is surely a stretch, but the idea that the instincts could be eradicated suggests a potential for human perfectibility absent in Western psychological traditions. In the mindfulness meditation tradition, the expressions of these forces in the life of a meditator are seen as hindrances to be recognized, worked with skillfully, and overcome. While the permanent extinction of these drives may be the sole province of a fully enlightened being, as these forces are exposed to awareness through mindfulness, they gradually become weakened, and practitioners grow incrementally in understanding and compassion.

Seeing our work as part of a path to complete psychological freedom can infuse it with a kind of hope and enthusiasm that working toward ordinary human unhappiness, or the adaptive life skills of behavior therapy, may not.

METHODS

Exposure

A noteworthy area of overlap among psychodynamic psychotherapy, behavior therapy, and mindfulness meditation is their emphasis on what behaviorists call *exposure*. In essence, all three traditions identify our propensity to avoid what is unpleasant as a cause of suffering, and work to counteract it.

Behaviorists articulate this clearly in exposure and response prevention treatments for obsessive–compulsive disorder, phobias, and other anxiety disorders (Barlow, 2002; Foa, Franklin, & Kozak, 1998). They describe how we develop conditioned fears of situations that have been unpleasant in the past, avoid them, and consequently miss the opportunity for the fears to be extinguished. For example, a boy who is bitten by a dog may develop a generalized fear of all dogs. If he subsequently avoids contact with dogs, he misses the corrective learning that dogs can be friendly. Out of fear of being bitten, the boy's life becomes unnecessarily restricted.

Treatment for such fear and avoidance involves bringing a person into contact with the feared stimulus, and maintaining that contact until he or she learns through experience that it is actually harmless. In the case of the dog, we bring the child closer and closer to a nonaggressive dog, until finally he can play with it. The "response prevention" component of treatment is the commitment to stay with the unpleasant situation, even if uncomfortable feelings arise, rather than flee, as we normally would.

In psychodynamic psychotherapy, exposure begins with discussion of thoughts, feelings, and memories that have been avoided because they are unpleasant or shameful. It is a kind of implicit, interoceptive exposure. The therapy is the invitation to turn toward formerly forbidden memories or feelings. In the trusting environment of the therapeutic relationship, patients learn that these mental contents are tolerable and come to accept them. In this way, a patient's conscious awareness becomes much freer, and he or she can relax the neurotic defenses associated with symptoms. As mentioned earlier, in current practice, this exposure within the office is often followed by encouragement to pursue more traditional behavioral exposure by facing feared situations outside of the therapy hour.

Insight meditation functions similarly to psychodynamic psychotherapy in this area. As one sits and follows the breath, thoughts, feelings, and images inevitably arise. The practitioner notices the persistent tendency to hold on to pleasant events and to reject unpleasant events— in short, to try to control experience. By following the instruction neither to pursue nor to push away these experiences, meditators learn that they can tolerate unpleasant mental contents and need not fear them. The habit of avoidance is deliberately, tentatively set aside, and all events are invited regardless of our opinions about them.

Through this practice, the meditator becomes comfortable with the contents of his or her mind. In this sense, mindfulness is like exposure therapy, without discriminating among the objects and events to which one is being exposed. Goleman (1988, p. 173) referred to it as "global desensitization." This raises an intriguing question for future research: Is this sort of global desensitization sufficient without the need for directed exposure to particular stimuli?

When the "object" we are exposed to is an emotion, exposure treatment may have an additional benefit. Folk wisdom has long paralleled psychodynamic psychotherapy in emphasizing that it can be helpful to express painful emotions, to "get them out of our system." Experimental literature supports this, suggesting that contact with our emotions can be highly therapeutic (Pennebaker, 1997). Similarly, existential and humanistic psychotherapies espouse the value of "being with" affects in order to reintegrate them (Schneider, 2003). This latter process occurs regularly as part of mindfulness practice. Richard's experience during intensive practice is illustrative:

> While meditating, Richard was visited by intense sadness and fear, as well as by violent images, including the dismembering of Jessica and her ex-boyfriend. Sometimes the emotions would be experienced as intense pain in the body—tightness of the throat, muscle tension everywhere. The images were also disturbing. Hours would pass, with violent scenes playing like a movie before his eyes.
>
> These scenes were difficult to endure, and they persisted on and off throughout the 2 weeks of intensive meditation. Richard nonetheless tried to follow his instructions: He continued to allow the sensations and images to arise, and neither pushed them away nor distracted himself with another activity.
>
> Over time, things began to change. First, through exposure, aversion to these experiences became less prominent. Whereas Richard would ordinarily try to distract himself or take drugs, during the retreat, he practiced staying with whatever arose. Second, the grieving over Jessica's decision seemed to be accelerated by the retreat due to the unflinching exposure to the images and feelings. This seemed to kindle a cathartic experience, even though it occurred in silence. By the end of the 2 weeks, Richard felt more at peace.

Learning to avoid situations associated with pain has adaptive value. Most other animals learn to avoid hazards, such as poisons and fire, through this basic mechanism. In humans, however, with our complex affective and representational capacities, circumventing or skirting potential pain can lead to complex avoidance patterns. We come to block out whole realms of life and learn to substitute a version colored by our fears and desires. It is interesting that behaviorism, psychodynamic psychotherapy, and insight meditation all agree that much human suffering results from the counterproductive habit of avoiding painful situations, and all have evolved treatments involving exposure to counteract the tendency.

The Interpersonal World

A clear difference between psychotherapeutic and mindfulness traditions is in the role of interpersonal relationships. Most psychodynamic and behavioral psychotherapy is dyadic, occurring within a significant interpersonal relationship. Group and family treatments are also quite interpersonally oriented. (There are exceptions; some psychotherapy may include exercises conducted in solitude.) Relationship issues are therefore likely to become stimulated and raised in psychotherapy.

Conversely, the solitary nature of meditation, and its focus on the present moment, may influence what material is *unlikely* to arise. The lore among meditators is replete with stories of individuals who find themselves falling into familiar neurotic interpersonal conflicts despite years of intensive meditation practice. Indeed, the solitary quality of meditation practice makes it vulnerable to misuse as a means of avoiding interpersonal conflicts; solo meditation may be an escape from the troublesome tension stimulated by the world of intimate relationships. While some maintain that meditation is the most complete form of "treatment," for many, it may leave some interpersonal issues unaddressed.

In classical psychodynamic psychotherapy, the analysis of transference is the principal tool of treatment. While mindfulness meditation traditions enlist the relationship between a student and teacher as an essential element of practice, and may use the presence of a group of other meditators for support, meditation is primarily solitary and makes no effort to understand transference. Buddhist psychology lacks the understanding of subtle aspects of transference, often with adverse consequences; the fact that a meditation teacher may make no explicit effort to address transference does nothing to ensure that it does not arise powerfully in the meditation student. Lacking such an understanding, meditation teachers may become ensnared in countertransference. Meditation centers are increasingly turning to clinicians for help on matters of countertransference, group dynamics, and forms of psychopathology that periodically emerge in their communities.

This is an area in which Western psychology has much to offer meditation students and teachers. Buddhist practice was first taught to monastics, and the community of monks and nuns has preserved the teachings in a relatively pure form. While Buddhist practice has become more available to lay practitioners, it has never placed primary emphasis on navigating the ordinary difficulties faced by laypeople in the world of work and love.

Structure and Support

Both meditation and psychotherapy advance by enabling the individual to examine his or her thoughts, feelings, and actions. This examination requires turning toward experience with greater openness, without recourse to habitual avenues of escape and avoidance. Both these traditions provide supports to facilitate this counterintuitive movement toward difficult experience.

Supports in Psychotherapy

Elements of the structure of psychotherapy that support an individual's efforts to face difficulty are well known. The most essential is arguably the quality of the therapeutic relationship. (The way this relationship is enhanced by the therapist's mindfulness practice is described in detail in Part II.) An essential element is the therapist's stance of openness and acceptance. In the face of genuine fearlessness on the part of the therapist, the patient may be emboldened to stand closer to painful or humiliating experiences and memories. Qualities of empathy, sustained interest, and genuine care, tempered by professional neutrality, also establish an environment conducive to a therapeutic alliance. This is the "holding environment" described by D. W. Winnicott (1971).

The trust that is crucial to therapy is supported by the integrity of the therapist. Elements of this trust are codified in the therapist's absolute commitment to confidentiality, and a clear statement of its limits (e.g., in the face of serious, imminent harm). Establishing and maintaining consistent appointment times (both starting and ending) also lends a sense of reliability. Genuine integrity is the basis of trust.

Finally, the mutual trust in the efficacy of the therapy process and methods can enable patients to suspend some of their ordinary caution. Outcome studies point to both the patient's and the therapist's confidence in the process as predictive of a positive outcome; if the therapist is confident in a good outcome, the patient may relax into this confidence (Meyer et al., 2002).

Elements introduced by behavior therapy also lend support. The use of rating scales and inventories help to lend a sense of scientific legitimacy to the work. When "homework" is used in psychotherapy, and almost all therapists do so in some form (Scheel, Hanson, & Razzhavaikina, 2004), the patient can become more confident in his or her ability to continue the therapeutic work independently.

Support in Meditation Practice

Mindfulness meditation is a well-developed practice, refined over centuries. As a result, many "bugs" have been worked out. Meditation practice can be arduous at times, but there are many sources of support for the individual's efforts, including elements of the structure of practice:

• *Traditional teachings as a map.* A student of meditation can turn to a long history of formal teachings for guidance. Though the focus of practice is one's own unique experience, these teachings describe where the practice is headed, what one may expect, and methods suited to different obstacles that may arise. These teachings provide a way to understand difficult or frightening experiences, so that the student need not feel that he or she has "fallen off" the path. The map of these teachings provides a degree of predictability that is fortifying.

• *The community of like-minded people.* Historically, a community of monks and nuns has ensured the continuity of instruction and practice. Today, in the West, a community of like-minded individuals can similarly be enormously supportive. This support is seen at a number of levels. An individual is simply less likely to bolt from a difficult session of meditation if it is conducted in a room full of other silent meditators. Also, this practice can seem unusual or even exotic, because it runs counter to the prevailing ethos of consumerism and materialism; being with others helps us to feel that the practice is legitimate. Through discussion with fellow meditators, one is also reassured to learn that the difficulties encountered are not unique; others endure physical pain, restlessness, doubt, and sleepiness. The practice can seem less daunting when one realizes that others share the same struggles.

• *Others' experience as models.* The example of countless others who have benefited over the course of centuries provides inspiration that can carry us through periods of difficulty. Having firsthand contact with an experienced teacher can be especially inspiring, if that individual evinces the qualities of wisdom and compassion. An experienced teacher may also provide advice on meditation practice at just the right time; such "customized" advice can be very helpful during difficult periods.

• *Success in practice as reinforcement.* As in the acquisition of any skill, having some success in mindfulness practice reinforces one's efforts. The task of paying sustained attention may seem impossible at first. However, the taste of even a little clarity is enormously rewarding and reinforcing. Once a student begins to experience insight, the practice becomes compelling. At a certain stage, mindfulness becomes fascinating, regardless of the contents of awareness. Merely trying to pay attention to the present moment becomes a source of satisfaction.

- *Concentration* helps to contain the tumultuousness that can arise in mindfulness practice. Concentration grows naturally alongside mindfulness in meditation practice and is stabilizing, calming, and fortifying. As one's mind becomes more stable, it becomes better able to allow its attention to rest on difficult experiences without flinching.
- *Physical posture.* Sitting upright with a straight spine supports practice efforts. While traditions differ in their emphasis on a formal meditation posture, many meditation teachers throughout the years have emphasized posture as an aid in developing concentration, remaining alert, and feeling "held" in our capacity to face whatever arises in our awareness (Suzuki, 1973).

As mentioned earlier, one result of mindfulness meditation is enhanced feelings of interconnectedness with the world. As we come to see that our desire for happiness and well-being is shared by all others, such feelings of affinity naturally lead to compassion. Furthermore, while mindfulness does not prevent difficult experiences from arising, *my* suffering eventually leads to an understanding that all beings suffer. Through this shared experience, compassion (empathy for suffering in others) arises, which embraces all living beings, including oneself. Compassion helps us to be less judgmental of our meditation practice, to respect our efforts, and to realize that the benefits of meditation practice extend beyond ourselves.

EPISTEMOLOGY

Another important area of overlap between Western psychotherapeutic and mindfulness meditation traditions involves their methods of discovery. These methods are particularly worthy of attention in modern times, in which clinicians are actively searching for empirically validated treatments.

We saw earlier that psychodynamic, behavioral, and mindfulness traditions all share an interest in seeing reality clearly, though they differ somewhat in their conclusions about that reality. Interestingly, although it predates the Western Renaissance by over two millennia, the Buddhist psychology from which mindfulness practice derives has a surprisingly modern attitude toward discovering "truth."

Mindfulness meditation focuses on direct observation for understanding the workings of the mind. While maps and guidelines based on the observations of others are taught, the tradition strongly emphasizes that one should not accept any principle without first verifying it in one's own experience. The tradition is replete with thousands of pages of extraordinarily detailed descriptions of the workings of consciousness and the mechanisms for its transformation, presented as hypotheses to be tested anew by each individual. Adherence to doctrine is repeatedly criticized as unreliable. While not based on the modern scientific experimental method, mindfulness meditation nonetheless is part of a highly empirical tradition.

Psychoanalysis, from which psychodynamic psychotherapy grew, has historically seen itself as an empirical, scientific discipline. From Freud onward, the enterprise has been interested in finding truth through observation. While Freud believed that the method of psychoanalysis could yield scientific truth, modern critics have pointed out that many psychodynamic postulates cannot readily be tested experimentally, and more recent theorists have moved toward a more hermeneutic approach to meaning and discovered truth.

Of course, both psychodynamic traditions and Buddhist psychology have exhibited the human tendency to create orthodoxies, so that at times each has relied on received teachings in a way that inhibits discovery. But within the Buddhist tradition, the direct apprehension of truth revealed in experience is the most valued; no axioms or dogma, no matter how supported by accumulated data or promulgated by high authority, are to be accepted until tested in the laboratory of one's own experience.

Behavior therapy is a radically empirical tradition in a different sense. Especially in recent years, it has been trying to test all of its postulates experimentally (American Psychological Association, Division 12 Task Force, 1995). It differs from the other two traditions in an important regard: Rather than encouraging each practitioner or client to see whether principles apply to his or her experience, the behavioral tradition looks to replicable peer-reviewed experimentation to identify general principles that can be applied across individuals. Truth is what stands up to the scrutiny of the scientific method.

The scientific method seeks to predict and control phenomena through observation, hypothesis generation, experimentation, and replication. It embodies an underlying belief consistent with the Western rational tradition, that what is true is true, independent of our apprehension of it; truth is objective.

The truth sought in Buddhist meditation is of a different sort. The purpose of systematic investigation in meditation is not to create a replicable model of reality that holds up to scientific scrutiny. Rather, it seeks understanding for a single purpose—to assist the individual practitioner to become psychologically free. In this sense, it does not emphasize the search for objective truths that stand apart from practical application, but it nonetheless remains a highly empirical tradition.

Psychotherapy and mindfulness are both concerned with finding relief from psychological suffering, making the effort to find common ground worthwhile. A respectful appraisal of each illuminates their respective strengths and limitations, helps to avoid reducing one to the other, and alerts us to the dangers of overlooking the integrity of each practice within its own tradition. Having tried to take such precautions, we can now turn to the ways that mindfulness can expand and deepen the practice of psychotherapy.

PART II

The Therapy Relationship

CHAPTER 3

Mindfulness as Clinical Training

PAUL R. FULTON

Avenues for the integration of mindfulness and psychotherapy differ by the degree to which mindfulness is *overtly* introduced into treatment, ranging from the implicit influence of the meditating therapist to theory-guided, mindfulness-informed psychotherapy, to explicit teaching of mindfulness practices to patients (mindfulness-based psychotherapy; see Chapter 1). This chapter is concerned with the most implicit end of this spectrum—mindfulness practice as training for the therapist.

Most current research on mindfulness-based therapy focuses on the effectiveness of various techniques, while the therapist's own meditation practice remains in the background, invisible to the patient. Although the meditating therapist is the least explicit way of integrating mindfulness into therapy, this hidden element may be quite influential. In fact, mindfulness practice may be an untapped resource for training therapists of any theoretical persuasion, because it offers therapists a means to influence those factors that account most for success in treatment.

WHAT MATTERS MOST IN PSYCHOTHERAPY?

In general, psychotherapy works (Seligman, 1995). However, taken as a whole, efforts to establish the efficacy of one method over another have been equivocal (Lambert & Bergin, 1994; Luborsky, Singer, & Luborsky, 1975). The range of treatments, patient types, diagnostic conditions, and other methodological variables makes it difficult to arrive at the kind of certainty the field is called on to provide. Since the mid-1960s, the number of distinct approaches to treatment has increased from 60 to more than 400.

Many new treatments have fared well in empirical research, demonstrating their efficacy compared to other types of treatment, placebos, or no treatment at all. The mental health field must scientifically validate its methods in order to spend limited health care dollars wisely and deliver effective care to patients. The lay public is right to insist that clinicians draw on scientifically proven methods and avoid charlatanism. The effort to identify which treatment methods are effective makes good sense.

Empirically Validated Treatment

Alas, despite the progress made in designing empirically validated treatments, the evidence suggests that they do not entirely deserve the trust we place in them. Meta-analyses of outcome research have suggested that support for the superiority of one method over another is rather weak; most forms of treatment work as well as most other forms of treatment (Luborsky et al., 2002; Wampold et al., 1997). "The model of therapy simply does not make much difference in therapy outcome" (Miller, Duncan, & Hubble, 1997, p. 7).

This is not to say that treatment models are irrelevant. Rather, the model is simply one of a number of variables that influence outcome, and not a terribly important one. The importance of the treatment model and technique is not commensurate with the attention given to them by psychotherapy outcome researchers. Reviews of decades of outcome research and a number of meta-analyses estimate that only about 15% of the variance of treatment outcomes is due to the model and methods of the therapist (Lambert, 1992; Shapiro & Shapiro, 1982).

If the *type* of treatment contributes relatively little to successful therapy, what does matter? The majority of the variance is accounted for by *patient* characteristics unrelated to diagnosis. These characteristics include the strength of a patient's social supports outside of treatment (Mallinckrodt, 1996), level of motivation and other resources the patient brings to the therapy, and situational events in the patient's life (Lambert & Barley, 2002). For example, an individual who presents with depression due to a job loss may receive more relief from finding a new job than from treatment. Such extratherapeutic factors seem to account for approximately 40% of treatment outcome. Placebo factors and the expectancy of change account for another 15% of the outcome, commensurate with the influence of the particular treatment model used. On average, the remaining 30% may be attributable to "common factors" that are present in most successful treatment relationships.

Common Factors and the Therapeutic Alliance

What are the common factors in effective therapy? Many have been studied, but the most potent predictors of a positive treatment outcome are related to qualities of the therapist and the therapeutic relationship. Consequently, researchers have recently turned their attention to empirically validated *relationships* and the therapeutic alliance. Across modalities, "high impact" sessions share the principal quality of a strong alliance (Raue, Golfried, & Barkham, 1997). Needless to say, therapists differ from one another, and these differences are likely to be more important to treatment outcomes than the particular treatment method or theory embraced by the therapist (Luborsky et al., 1986; Wampold, 2001). It is not surprising that the qualities patients attribute to therapists in positive treatment alliances include empathy, warmth, understanding, and acceptance, and are short on behaviors such as blaming, ignoring, or rejecting (Lambert & Barley, 2002). Empathy in particular has received empirical attention, and while it is an elusive factor to measure, "overall, empathy accounts for as much and probably more outcome variance than does specific intervention" (Bohart, Elliott, Greenberg, & Watson, 2002, p. 96). Based on their review of research, Bohart and colleagues suggest that empathy may be even more influential in intervention-based treatment than in relational-based therapy. It might almost be said that the relationship *is* the treatment (Duncan & Miller, 2000).

If the therapeutic alliance is so important in effective treatment, it stands to reason that this should be taught to clinicians. Paradoxically, graduate programs emphasize models of treatment, protocol-driven therapy, and technique over the less tangible qualities of the therapist. This may be simply because it is easier to do so. Indeed, advanced training may correlate little with effectiveness. Bickman (1999) found little empirical support for the idea that effectiveness is improved with experience, continuing education, licensing, professional degree, clinical supervision, or other markers of professionalism. Instruction in therapy skills is essential, but given the greater importance of the therapeutic relationship, the larger challenge is to find a way to help cultivate the qualities shared by excellent therapists. Such qualities may be harder to learn than basic skills and knowledge (Lazarus, 1993; Norcross & Beutler, 1997).

MINDFULNESS AS ADVANCED TRAINING

A therapist attends his first 10-day intensive mindfulness meditation retreat. The felt effects of this retreat seem to remain with him for several weeks, during which time he returns to seeing psychotherapy patients. All of his activities, including working with patients, seem to occur in a space of stillness and openness. He finds that listening is effortless and deep, and he resonates more naturally with each patient during the sessions. The comments he makes seem to arise as spontaneous responses from this stillness, and all seem to hit the mark. Insights flow like water during the sessions. Both the therapist and his patients feel these sessions are special in some way. As weeks pass, the therapy experience seems to return to normal.

In addition to the other benefits amply described throughout this volume, mindfulness cultivates numerous qualities that are highly suited to establishing a strong therapeutic alliance. Some authors have argued for the benefits of meditation that would logically inform psychotherapy skills, such as the cultivation of attention, compassion and empathy, therapeutic presence, and a broader perspective on suffering (e.g., Chung, 1990; Deikman, 2001; Henley, 1994; Thompson, 2000; Tremlow, 2001). Others have sought empirical evidence of the impact of mindfulness training on those qualities of mind that are arguably related to a strong working alliance (Brown & Ryan, 2003; Neff, 2003; Sweet & Johnson, 1990; Valentine & Sweet, 1999). It would be interesting to see research that evaluates the influence of a therapist's meditation practice on these factors that enhance psychotherapy outcome.

Yet even as we await empirical evidence of this nexus, it seems natural to infer that the influence of mindfulness on the mind of the therapist is consistent with the qualities underlying a successful treatment relationship. There is evidence of another sort for this connection, that found in therapists' own experience of meditation, which, for those willing to take the journey, is compelling and self-evident.

The focus of this chapter is not on specific treatment interventions borrowed from my own meditation practice, but rather on the therapist's cultivation of mental qualities, well-described in meditation literature, that relate to the common factors underlying effective treatment. Some of these qualities are described in detail, while those taken up in subsequent chapters are covered more briefly.

Paying Attention

A young trainee in psychotherapy at a major psychiatric teaching hospital was delighted to be invited to attend a supervision group with senior clinicians. On one particular day, a seasoned psychiatrist spoke in a confessional tone about his experience doing psychotherapy. As he stroked his beard, he admitted to having enormous difficulty paying attention to his patients. His mind, he said, wandered off with regularity. The trainee was shocked. Because she had a number of years of meditation experience, she took for granted that therapists could pay sustained, close attention. "How could they do psychotherapy without paying attention?"

Every clinician knows the experience of a wandering mind during therapy. At times, this may be a response to what is—or is not—happening in the therapy hour. An emotionally disengaged patient can leave the therapist similarly disengaged, and bored. The therapist may also be made anxious by the material offered by the patient and may reflexively respond by "tuning out," becoming restless, sleepy, or otherwise partially absent. The therapist may take his or her own inattentiveness as clinical information, inviting the question, "What is happening with this patient that is making it hard to stay interested?" This may or may not be sufficient to shake off the shroud of disinterest.

Experienced therapists may fall victim to inattention more readily than eager novices and can be adept at covering for lapses of attention. It can become second nature to ask a probing question that suggests to both the therapist and patient that things are going apace. We can learn to fake it in the belief that the patient is none the wiser. Ordinary therapy can continue with an ordinary state of mind.

By contrast, genuine interest and close attention are hard to fake. When we are totally alert and focused, the energy is quickened, and both parties are more fully awake to the work at hand. This may be a function of the material presented by the patient when, for example, the patient is emotionally engaged or the account he or she delivers is simply riveting. Close attention is a natural response. But these moments may not characterize long stretches of a course of therapy.

Sustained mindfulness practice is an antidote to a wandering mind. While it falls short of a permanent cure for daydreaming, mindfulness is the exercise of bringing the mind back to the present, sometimes hundreds of times in a single practice session. The mindfulness-oriented therapist may practice "presence" *independently* of the content of the present moment. All events, including boredom or anxiety, are invitations to return to attention. In time, the capacity for attention is strengthened. It is possible to generate interest in the simplest events.

When we are bored in meditation or in life, we may seek excitement or stimulation. It is possible to create an entire lifestyle based on seeking thrills and novelty. For thrill-seeking individuals, "ordinary" life can become aversive in its dullness. Mindfulness meditation takes a different approach to generating interest. In training the mind to be attentive to the smallest details of experience, it is as though we have become sensitive to events ordinarily too trivial to merit interest. Rather than "turn up the volume" of external events through novelty and stimulation, we discover that our lives, as they are, are full of richness. When we are alert, fascination is a natural response. Boredom flees in the face of interest.

Wholehearted attention is surprisingly uncommon. When we meet someone who is interested and utterly undistracted, we come away with a feeling that the contact was unusual. We *know* we have been heard in an uncommon way. To pay genuine, wholehearted attention is a gift we can offer to anyone we encounter. This is as true in our contact with our children, partners, or colleagues as it is with our patients. In clinical encounters, the presence of close attention catalyzes the session. This level of attention can be learned, practiced, and deepened. Chapter 4 describes practical exercises for the cultivation of attention, interest, and other qualities described below.

Affect Tolerance

When we practice mindfulness, strong emotions will be among the invited and uninvited guests. These are welcomed with the same attitude of acceptance and interest as any other mental event or physical sensation. Although the feelings may seem overpowering, when we set aside the fear that we may be overwhelmed, we discover that no emotion is ever final. We may also find that we can tolerate more than we suspected. *Tolerance* may be a poor word to use, because it connotes a clenched-teeth, white-knuckled relationship to the emotion, as though we can muscle our way by sheer strength and willpower. *Mindful* tolerance is marked by softening into and embracing the experience. In this process, powerful emotion loses some of its ability to intimidate. We may experience fear of being overwhelmed, become mindful of this fear, and as a result become less possessed by it. Feelings are not so much endured as known. This is the development of *affect tolerance*, a capacity that was first described in psychoanalytic terms by Elizabeth Zetzel (1970). We might also call it the willingness to face our feelings.

Affect tolerance is enormously important for therapists. It is ordinarily considered a skill to be cultivated by patients (Linehan, 1993a). However, if we cannot tolerate our own difficult emotions, we may find it difficult to sit with our patients' powerful affects. We may find that we have distanced ourselves from our patients and invalidated their experience. Far from providing a safe environment for exploration, our own intolerance of feeling may prematurely eclipse the patient's freedom. Therapy can become arid. This can all happen outside of conscious awareness.

> A young psychology graduate student with a long-term interest in meditation entered psychoanalysis, 5 days a week. The analysis did not go well. He was inhibited and stuck. After more than 2 years, the unfinished analysis ended by common agreement. Some time later, the student had his first 10-day mindfulness meditation retreat, during which he was assailed by all manner of challenging thoughts, sensations, and emotions. In the process, he discovered how a low level of fear had been a constant companion throughout his life, causing him to become subtly avoidant. The ubiquitous effects of the fear were seen in abundance.
>
> Not long after the retreat, the graduate student reentered psychotherapy. The second therapy felt qualitatively different from the first. The fear, which had formerly been lurking quietly, exerting its constricting influence, became, for the first time, fully experienced and conscious. Paradoxically, the more the fear was known in his experience, the less he was controlled by it. He became less defensive, and the therapy progressed rapidly and with greater ease.

What mindfulness teaches in our own experience—that all emotions are transitory, and can be received without fear—extends naturally to our patients. When we are not intimidated, patients are offered the opportunity to bring forward more of their own seemingly intolerable experience. Our receptivity in the face of difficult emotional content reassures patients that they need not censor themselves so much to protect themselves or the therapist. Emotions lose some of their threat.

In mindfulness circles, a metaphor is often used to describe this capacity to receive and hold difficult experience: If a tablespoon of salt is added to a cup of water, the water will taste strongly of the salt. If a tablespoon of salt is added to jug of water, it will taste less salty. If the salt is added to a pond, its taste is further dissipated. Mindfulness practice is likened to becoming this larger container. Difficult emotions (like the salt) remain, but their power to disturb is diffused in the openness of mind. We become larger containers.

The power of this deepened capacity to bear affect is amply illustrated in a number of examples offered in other chapters throughout this volume.

Practicing Acceptance

Mindfulness is acceptance in action, not as a single act or decision, but repeated each time attention is returned to the primary object of aware-

ness. The act of returning with full attention is performed without regard for the pleasant or unpleasant qualities of the object. Everything is
welcomed equally.

Judgment is so deeply rooted in the human mind that the practice of
mindful awareness itself is subject to self-criticism. As any practitioner
knows, this seemingly simple practice is difficult; in the beginning, it
seems impossible. It is all too common for mindfulness practitioners to
compound the natural frustration of learning to train attention with
judgments about one's ability to do the practice. Self-criticism easily
arises with dismay at what seems like an endless stream of failures to
stay present.

As one's mindfulness practice matures, the tendency toward self-
criticism is mitigated by several developments. First, one begins to have
moments, albeit temporary, of relatively steady, uninterrupted awareness. This is one of the first rewards of consistent effort, and it is positively reinforcing. A second shift occurs when thoughts arise but are
taken simply as more objects to be aware of, neither to be pursued nor
rejected. When this happens, it is possible to witness *self-judgment* as
just another thought, arising and passing. Judgment begins to lose its
sting when seen in this impersonal light. We identify less with the message and do not get lost in believing it. By identifying self-judgment and
allowing it to pass, we cease to add fuel to the fire by engaging it and can
avoid a protracted litany of self-criticism.

Turning again and again toward all that arises, including familiar
patterns of self-criticism, is the practice of self-acceptance. Like anything
that is repeated, self-acceptance becomes stronger over time. This practice, which may originate in meditation, can be carried into the therapy
room. Therapists have ample opportunities to watch the pendulum
of self-congratulation and self-doubt swing during the practice of psychotherapy.

Therapists are familiar with how our judgments of others arise in
direct proportion to self-judgments, although the close connection may
be outside of awareness. Conversely, people at peace with themselves are
less likely to find fault with others.

Clinicians are taught the importance of being accepting of patients
to cultivate a therapeutic alliance. However, judgment is pernicious; we
can harbor many prejudices, while flattering ourselves that we do not.
We are often unaware of how the views we hold remain unexamined.
Such unexamined views, however, lower the headroom of the patient's
freedom as they subtly find their way into psychotherapy. An attuned
patient may know well before the therapist that the therapist's ostensible
acceptance is paper-thin.

Mindfulness practice is a vehicle for the ongoing and ever-deepening training of acceptance. It is a method to forge what we *know* to be valuable into something real. The safety of genuine acceptance is spontaneously extended to our patients and may provide some patients their first truly trustworthy relationship.

Empathy and Compassion

Despite the importance of empathy in the therapeutic relationship, there is a dearth of compelling evidence that it can be taught. In psychotherapy literature, one can find recommendations to teach communication styles and the ability to tailor therapists' relational stance to different patients (Lambert & Barley, 2002). Even if these skills are teachable, they may fall short of true empathy. Mindfulness practice may be the most potent method for its cultivation.

Most forms of meditation employ their own unique mix of mindfulness and concentration practices (Goleman, 1977). What distinguishes Buddhist mindfulness practice is the explicit intent to develop insight and compassion. Empathy toward others is a natural extension of the compassion toward oneself that is cultured in mindfulness practice.

How does mindfulness generate empathy and compassion? Compassion for ourselves arises in the practice of opening to our own suffering. The mere presence of suffering is not enough. Consider how easy it is to become hardened by devastating loss or hardship. Mindfulness offers a way to change our relationship to suffering by surrendering our need to reject it. This is an act of kindness to oneself. Our own suffering offers an opportunity to become openhearted rather than merely oppressed.

Compassion for others arises from the recognition that no one is exempt from suffering and that everyone wishes to be safe from it. In addition, as mindfulness begins to dissolve the artificial boundaries that define our separateness, we begin to experience our innate affinity with all beings. Compassion toward others becomes a natural expression of this growing perception of our interdependence. Finally, the tradition of mindfulness meditation contains a number of practices deliberately intended to enable compassion to grow. Several of these exercises are described in Chapter 4.

Equanimity and the Limits of Helpfulness

We can develop compassion and empathy toward our patients and at the same time recognize that it may not make a big difference in the quality of their lives per se. The quality of compassion developed in mindfulness practice is balanced by the cultivation of equanimity. In the mindfulness tradition, *equanimity* has a number of meanings. It describes an attitude of nondiscriminating, open receptivity in which all experience is welcomed. It has a narrower meaning as well; it is the recognition that despite our best efforts and our most heartfelt wish for the welfare of others, there are real limits to what we can do to help. Therefore, even as the therapist's mindfulness practice begets empathy for the suffering of a patient, the wish to be of assistance to others is tempered by the sober recognition of patients' ultimate responsibility for themselves.

The following example illustrates the limits of helpfulness.

> Colleagues of mine opened a residential treatment center some years ago. I had the chance to visit the center and had a conversation with one of the staff members, an art therapist. She described a very difficult patient who demanded help but rejected everything offered to her. The patient's stance engaged the entire residential staff in finding new ways to approach her, variously including greater limits, greater leniency, different primary therapists, and so on. The patient's behavior toward the staff was hostile, belittling, and challenging. The worse the patient behaved, the more committed the art therapist and others became to finding something that worked.
>
> Eventually the therapist ran out of ideas and patience; she was frustrated and angry. The art therapist described to me how one day, looking across an activity room at the patient, she had the thought that there was nothing left to offer and the patient was going to have to figure it out for herself. At that very moment, the patient looked at her, walked across the room, and apologized for her horrible conduct.

Accepting our limits may be a prerequisite for patients to assume greater responsibility for their own growth and well-being.

If therapists and patients subscribe to the fantasy of therapy's unlimited reach, it can only lead to disillusionment and anger. It may also lead to unnecessarily prolonged treatment as a substitute for effective treatment. Mindfulness meditation practice helps illuminate the way our own conduct creates the conditions by which we live, and gives life to the direct understanding of personal accountability. It helps cultivate respect for the integrity of another person's experience. This perspective provides a useful balance to our sense of efficacy as therapists. Giving our very best efforts to our patients out of compassion is balanced by the sober recognition of the absolute and genuine limits of our ability to change anybody. Holding this paradox of compassion and equanimity, familiar to therapists, is well described by T. S. Eliot in "Ash Wednesday" (1930), when he writes,

Teach us to care and not to care
Teach us to sit still

Patients come to therapy for help, and therapists are trained to help. One predictor of successful treatment is the therapist's confidence in the efficacy of his or her methods (Frank, 1961; Garfield, 1981; Kirsch, 1990). Consequently, the therapist's feeling of helplessness in the face of an intractable problem can undermine treatment. Therapists are armed with many techniques that can be used to mask this helplessness, waving the next new treatment technique to distract both him- or herself and the patient from the dread that the limits of therapy have been reached. Consider, for example, how reassured we are to have a stage model of death and dying to guide us in dealing professionally with death or catastrophic loss (Kübler-Ross, 1997).

Therapists and patients sometimes collude to get busy, endlessly examining a problem to avoid an unexamined truth that some problems cannot be fixed. Being busy becomes a defense perpetuated by both patient and therapist. We need to distinguish what is not fixable from what is. In running from inescapable suffering toward an imagined cure, an opportunity to turn toward the truth of the situation is squandered. The chance for the therapist to offer what is most called for in the moment— standing fully and simply with the patient in the full flame of suffering— is missed. Far from signifying surrender, these moments may be the most transformative in therapy.

> By his own description, Gerald's "lights are on, but nobody's home." His life was orderly but flat. He was rarely excited about anything and felt little to persuade him he was alive. The treatment—one of many for Gerald—was nearly intolerable for the therapist, who circled persistently, seeking an unsecured door or window into Gerald's inner life. The therapist became despondent about the prospects for any success. He sought supervision, and to his supervisor described feeling dead in the water, alone in a small boat with Gerald in flat seas. The therapist was out of ideas, feeling genuinely helpless and useless. To Gerald the therapist simply observed their mutual helplessness. Gerald brightened. Though he had little real expectation that another round of therapy with another therapist would change anything, for now, he felt less alone in his helplessness than he had in months.

Equanimity allows us to stop trying to fix things long enough to see what *is*. We learn to distinguish neurotic suffering from existential suffering. Unburdened by the need to help the therapist feel effective, this still point offers the patient the freedom to move, or the freedom to stand.

Our patients may attribute to us the power to change their lives. This attribution can sometimes be very useful; a positive transference is not a problem unless it becomes an obstacle to treatment. The danger arises when therapists begin to "buy their own press" and believe they are omnipotent and endlessly wise. In helping us recognize the limits of our powers as therapists, the equanimity cultivated in mindfulness practice helps teach us humility.

Learning to See

One of the great, unheralded assets therapists possess is that they are not their patients; that is, whatever therapists' struggles or difficulties may be, they are unlikely to be identical to those of their patients. This distance permits a degree of perspective. The availability of perspective is supported by training, which exposes the clinician to multiple models of treatment, each with its own unique approach to the problem. Having this knowledge enables the therapist to have some flexibility in finding a formulation that accords with the patient's understanding, yet permits new pathways for a solution.

A problem may seem intractable to a patient because of the way he or she formulates it. For example, an individual might dread work because he or she feels disliked by a supervisor, and is left feeling that the only alternatives are to suffer or quit the job. In such a situation, the therapist opens new avenues for consideration. "Is it true the supervisor dislikes you?" "How do you know?" "If it is so, is there a way to address the source of tension between you?" The therapist offers potential solutions that formerly lay outside the patient's consideration. Frequently, the problem is redefined entirely. For example, closer examination may reveal that the problem is a powerful and unexamined negative transference directed toward the supervisor. In this instance, the patient's limited and inflexible formulation was itself the problem to be addressed.

> Todd comes to therapy with a legacy of work inhibition; he has been unable to finish his college degree, work to his level of talent and intelligence, or overcome crippling procrastination. He believes it is too late for him, because he has failed to achieve several goals, including attending a prestigious university and other achievements he believes are essential gateways to full membership in the society of adequate citizens. He feels doomed. On further exploration, it becomes clear how he unquestioningly imagined that the rest of the

world was watching, and worse, that the world shared this harshly critical judgment.

One key insight was the dawning understanding that there was no one watching as closely as he was, and surely no one was nearly so judgmental. Todd was free to succeed, free to fail, free to enjoy himself; he was not doomed to some imagined eternal debt that could never be repaid. Gradually, the energy his inhibition required was made available to him. He discovered that he loved work when unhindered by shame. Within months of joining a large business firm, he was winning awards for his initiative.

In this case, the young man constructed a scowling world populated by disapproving figures. This belief was so convincing that the therapist's suggestions to the contrary were considered preposterous. It was liberating to see how what was once taken as real ("The world is watching and knows I'm inadequate") was a mental construction and could be abandoned.

Mindfulness practice augments the therapist's access to such alternate avenues of explanation and growth. As we gain insight into the ways we construct our world, we recover the freedom that is available when we loosen our grip on those constructions. We discover the ways our bondage was self-created and arbitrary—we see that it is ultimately workable. This process of insight in mindfulness practice is not fundamentally different from the insight gained in insight-oriented psychotherapy, but it can go further, because it reaches beyond awareness of personal mental content (see the discussion of insight in Chapter 2).

By learning to set aside discursive thinking and to see the products of cognition as events with no special reality, we become familiar with the tendency of our own minds to build imaginary scenarios, which we inhabit as if they are real. As this capacity deepens, we simultaneously enhance our ability to see how our patients (and others as well) engage in the same process of construction. We become more acute in our ability to see *their* minds. This makes us better therapists.

Exposing Our Narcissistic Needs

One uncomfortable aspect of our own minds, as revealed in mindfulness practice, is our incessant concern with self-esteem and self-image. Our desire to be effective therapists is laudable, but it subtly becomes intertwined with the need to see ourselves as "good" therapists. Our professional self-esteem is being perpetually renegotiated and may vary with the quality of our most recent session. This becomes a hindrance when we blur our own narcissistic needs with the therapeutic needs of the patient. This tendency is not easily stopped, but it can be seen and handled wisely.

Like a good psychoanalysis, mindfulness can help us to root out the ingenious ways our sense of self intrudes on the therapy. Mindfulness also has the potential to take this examination to a more profound level, exposing the self as constructed and illusory. Direct insight into this aspect of the experience of self reveals our insidious and incessant efforts to bolster our sense of self. Chapters 2 and 12 take up this issue in greater detail.

Overcoming Our Infatuation with Theory

Life is like music; it must be composed by ear, feeling and instinct, not by rule. Nevertheless, one had better know the rules, for they sometimes guide in doubtful cases, though not often.
                                                           —SAMUEL BUTLER

The Problem

Much professional training emphasizes theory and its application to practice. In the course of this training, we learn categories of diagnoses, personality types, and treatment models. Possession of this knowledge becomes a hallmark of professionalism and specialization, and we come to treasure our mastery of this proprietary knowledge. It is appropriate that we embrace the accumulated knowledge of our field. Unfortunately, we may confuse our models and theories for the "truth" of what we are looking at, taking our constructions as something more real and deserving of our trust than they merit.

Models of psychopathology and treatment are a fundamental element of our efforts to be effective healers. For example, borderline personality disorder would be even more difficult to understand and treat without the contributions of researchers who have helped to illuminate the social and biochemical etiology of the disorder and how it manifests in interpersonal relationships. Our diagnostic categories reduce staggering human variability in order to find underlying consistencies. Our psychological models also protect us from uncertainty and anxiety in our clinical work; even an inaccurate map is more reassuring than no map at all. Our training and accumulation of knowledge remind us that we are entitled to practice psychotherapy. Furthermore, as mentioned earlier, our confidence in the efficacy of our methods correlates to positive outcomes in therapy; our patients need to feel that we know what we are doing.

However, our psychological models should not be overvalued. Unlike some medical conditions that can be reliably diagnosed with lab tests or imaging techniques, most psychiatric conditions are harder to nail down, typically resting on statistical analyses of prevalence, cultural standards, maladaptive behavior, or personal reports of distress. These parameters are notoriously changeable over time, shifting with prevailing trends in the field. The original *Diagnostic and Statistical Manual of Mental Disorders* (American Psychiatric Association, 1952) listed 112 mental disorders; by 1994, the number of diagnoses in the manual (DSM-IV) had grown to over 400 (American Psychiatric Association, 1994).

Either human beings have recently evolved new and unique mental disorders, or we have to regard our diagnostic categories as metaphors-in-progress, more or less helpful, subject to refinement or abandonment over time. While earlier diagnostic categories often described institutionalized patients, the newer categories largely address less serious disorders more commonly found in ambulatory populations. The line between a bona fide disorder and the difficulties of daily living is becoming blurred. We can now find a diagnostic term for most forms of human suffering; the *International Classification of Diseases* (ICD-9; World Health Association, 2003) even contains a diagnostic code for "misery and unhappiness disorder."

Problems arise when we take our descriptive clinical categories to be natural representations of an objective world of disorders, conveniently provided in a manual. Despite all the well-known reasons that a diagnosis and treatment philosophy are important, unreflective attachment to our models and categories poses concealed risks. A diagnostic label used as a kind of shorthand can come to replace a more nuanced appraisal of the whole person. In the process, we stop looking, convinced that we know enough. It becomes a cover for our ignorance, masquerading as knowledge and certainty.

One example of this danger is found in the concept of "theory countertransference" (Duncan, Hubble, & Miller, 1997), which describes clinicians' excess loyalty to their theories. The therapist unconsciously imposes his or her theoretical predispositions on the patient. The result is psychotherapy that conforms to and confirms the therapist's assumptions. As Abraham Maslow (1966) said, "If you only have a hammer, you tend to see every problem as a nail." That which convinces us we understand the patient's problem becomes a barrier to that understanding. When treatment stalls, we try more of the same, or chalk the failure up to the patient's resistance.

Our clinical categories may be helpful when they provide an alternative—a more auspicious account to a patient for his or her distress.

For example, a man suffering from a fixed paranoid delusion (e.g., that he is being pursued by enemies) may not consider antipsychotic medication an appropriate solution to his problem. Psychotherapy at this stage may include helping to substitute his delusional explanation for his distress with another explanation, namely, that he is suffering from an illness. The latter idea permits a more constructive course of action (i.e., medication rather than defensive violence). However, the misuse of easily available diagnostic terms to describe a person's distress may actually be subtly harmful.

> Adele presents for psychotherapy with distress about being bypassed for a promotion and ultimately squeezed out of her current position when a new boss is hired over her. She is angry and humiliated, feeling that her reputation has suffered. A veteran of several long-term psychodynamic psychotherapies, she starts a new therapy, convinced that her rage at the unfortunate turn of events is evidence of old, unresolved personal conflicts. She believes that her pain reflects excessive sensitivity that a "healthy" person would not suffer. Furthermore, she expects her therapist to agree that her anger must be pathological.

In this example, even a moderately skilled therapist may take the opportunity to suggest that being angry at an injustice does not necessarily reflect unresolved personal problems; it is natural to be angry in such circumstances. While we may recognize that there are persistent maladaptive patterns in this woman's history (e.g., her conviction that anger is evidence of weakness), the process of clinical hand wringing by a therapist too embedded in a literature of disorders can inadvertently add the weight of a clinical condition to the patient's burden. The subtle—or not so subtle—practice of pathologizing may be harmful. In this instance, Adele's painful loss of a job becomes compounded by self-blame, even if it is wrapped in "objective" clinical terms. A bad situation is unnecessarily made worse.

Learning to Not Know

How does mindfulness help us hold our models more lightly? By returning to the present moment and loosening the grip of thinking, we practice setting aside thoughts of past and future. By allowing ourselves to be attentive to the present moment, we tacitly allow that we simply do not know what the next moment will bring. We surrender—albeit temporarily—our wish to know and control. We allow ourselves to not know.

This attitude of *not knowing* is not alien to psychotherapy. Consider psychoanalyst W. R. Bion's (1967) now classical admonition to rid oneself of preconceptions about a patient, cast off the bondage of memory and desire, and abandon even the desire to cure. There is evidence to suggest that therapists become more flexible and eclectic in orientation as they grow in professional experience (Auerbach & Johnson, 1977; Schacht, 1991).

Mindfulness practice facilitates the process and extends it beyond an intellectual intention to "keep an open mind." This is possible, because the practice of mindfulness—the exercise of setting aside discursive thought—operates at a level of awareness that enables insight into the way we identify with products of thought. Particularly in mindfulness meditation, we perceive the unbridgeable gap between life as it is and our *ideas* about it. As one man said of his experience during an intensive mindfulness retreat, "It felt as though I had jumped out of an airplane without a parachute, which was terrifying until I realized there was no ground!"

Not knowing is valuable because it may not only enable therapy but it is also ultimately the truth of the matter; we actually know so little about our mysterious and complex lives. The following account by an elderly man illustrates the wisdom of not knowing:

> I have a friend, a woman I know already many years. One day she's mad at me—from nowhere it comes. I have insulted her, she tells me. How? I don't know. Why don't I know? Because I don't know her. She surprised me. That's good. That's how it should be. You cannot tell someone, "I know you." People jump around. They're like a ball; rubbery, they bounce. The ball cannot be long in one place. Rubbery, it must jump. So what do you do to keep a person from jumping? The same as with a ball; make a little hole, and it goes flat. When you tell someone, "I know you," you put a little pin in. So what should you do? Leave them be. Don't try to make them stand still for your convenience. You don't ever know them. Let people surprise you. This, likewise, you could do concerning yourself.

To hold any fixed view, including a fixed view of our patients or ourselves, leads to suffering. Fixed positions are snapshots, arrested moments sampled from an unfolding flux, instantly out of date. The desire to find something stable is natural; we seek certainty to bind the anxiety of the unknown. Once we take up a position, we begin to defend it and attempt to shape our view of reality to fit our concepts.

The invitation of mindfulness to "not know" should not be taken as license to abandon all our clinical training; it would be irresponsible and dangerous to reinvent everything de novo. Rather, it is a process of learning to cling less firmly to imagined certainty, and to trust that an open and attuned mind (fortified by firm clinical training) will be far more responsive to the demands of the moment than one resting on concepts alone. It grants us access to all the tools at our disposal, based on the genuine needs of the present, and allows us the freedom to jettison them when they are unhelpful.

The Possibility of Happiness

Mindfulness practice helps to cultivate joy. Most feelings, both positive and difficult, begin to lose some of their apparent solidity when beheld in mindful awareness, and there is a measure of calm joy that arises with mindful awareness that is not easily disturbed by changing conditions. While I am unaware of research that correlates the therapist's own personal happiness to positive outcomes in therapy, I suspect it is a factor. When I am deciding to whom to send a prospective patient, I generally consider the therapist's personal happiness. Mindfulness offers the possibility of serenity that is not won by avoidance of tough challenges or complacency. Therapists who have tasted such calm joy implicitly extend to patients the idea that happiness may emerge *in spite* of the conditions of our lives. By example, therapists can inspire their patients to start to live more fully, right now, in the midst of all their difficulties.

Mindfulness practice can develop many beneficial qualities of mind, only a few of which have been described here. Implicit mental qualities of the therapist invariably influence whatever the therapist says or does. In Chapters 4 and 5, the authors discuss ways that a therapist's personal mindfulness practice, including the cultivation of beneficial mental qualities, can be intentionally engaged while doing the relational work of psychotherapy.

CHAPTER 4

Cultivating Attention and Empathy

WILLIAM D. MORGAN
SUSAN T. MORGAN

In Chapter 3, Paul R. Fulton identified a number of personal qualities engendered in the therapist by mindfulness practice that may positively affect therapy outcome. This chapter takes up two of the most important of these qualities: attention and empathy. Therapists receive little or no formal training in the cultivation of attention or empathy. We seem to understand their importance as therapeutic skills, and perhaps we pick up a few tricks through supervision and trial and error. Beyond this, it is assumed that these skills will naturally manifest in the treatment room. Can psychotherapists use mindfulness techniques to enhance attention and empathy in the therapeutic encounter? We explore this question and offer exercises designed to strengthen these mental faculties.

ATTENTION

Sigmund Freud wrote that the analyst should have "evenly hovering attention" during the therapy hour (1912/1961a). Was Freud suggesting that this state of mind would somehow naturally arise? Was it something to strive for? We propose in this chapter that an increased capacity to invite evenly hovering attention into the office deepens and enriches the techniques and approaches we currently use as therapists. We often ask therapists, "Given the choice, would you rather be 20% more attentive during your therapy hours, or would you rather have 20% more techniques at your disposal?" Most clinicians choose more attention.

Mindfulness as Attention Training

While training attention may initially seem like a chore (particularly when it requires turning away from some pleasant fantasy, or turning toward some unpleasantness), as it is strengthened, there is satisfaction in the practice of awareness itself. Events that were previously too insignificant or mundane to merit our attention may become vivid and rich in detail. The ordinary can become revelatory; getting dressed, packing a lunch, or parking a car can become full experiences in themselves, rather than obstacles on the way to something better. The pleasure of living each moment more fully makes mindfulness training self-reinforcing.

Mindfulness practice enhances the capacity for evenly hovering attention both directly and indirectly. Directly, mindfulness strengthens the capacity of the mind to remain with any mental object in a sustained and concentrated manner (Reiman, 1985; Valentine & Sweet, 1999). Mindfulness training may also improve attention indirectly via intuitive *insights* that can emerge within the therapist. These insights, such as the ubiquity of mental suffering and the passing nature of all experience, can make the thoughts and feelings that threaten to ensnare our attention less compelling, or "sticky."

Insight into Mental Suffering and Impermanence as a Support to Attention

Insight into mental suffering refers to an individual's awareness of the self-defeating ways in which the mind reacts to our impermanent, rapidly changing experience. We observe that the habitual and prevailing tendencies of the mind are to hold on to and embellish pleasant experience, to push away unpleasant experience, to identify with certain states while disowning others, and to attempt to manipulate the world in order to make ourselves feel better. In other words, the mind of everyday awareness, when left to its own devices, is seldom in a state of evenly hovering attention. Rather, our relationship with present experience is defined by either wanting things to be different or wanting them to continue as they are. Because neither of these positions is tenable in an ever-changing field of experience, mental suffering becomes an integral part of our existential and psychological landscape. In this context, mental suffering can be understood as the low-grade, chronic stress and insecurity associated with futilely resisting our current experience, or attempting to make the impermanent permanent. It is the opposite of mindful awareness of the present moment with acceptance.

Insight into this restless mental activity progressively results in letting go, or stated differently, a gradual increase in "nonattachment." We learn how holding on tightly to something desirable is both ineffective and self-defeating. This does not imply that pleasant moments are not appreciated. It is the posture of clinging or craving, now seen as central in the creation of mental suffering, that relaxes. As William Blake (in Stevenson & Erdman, 1971, p. 162) suggests:

> He who binds to himself a joy
> Does the winged life destroy.
> But he who kisses the joy as it flies
> Lives in eternity's sunrise.

We can kiss the *joy* as it flies, and we can also kiss the *pain* as it comes and goes. For example, in Kabat-Zinn's mindfulness-based stress reduction (MBSR) program for chronic pain patients (1990), participants reported that the mental effort expended to avoid painful sensations accounted for a significant proportion of their suffering. The subjective experience of pain diminished as the unpleasant aspects of experience were increasingly accepted.

Nonattachment to both joy and pain enhances attention. As less energy is expended in manipulating and avoiding unpleasant aspects of experience, as we grow in our ability to accept our moment-to-moment experience, the mind begins to rest more comfortably within a wider range of events and becomes less easily ruffled or agitated. Energy that was formerly deployed to control or defend becomes available in a conflict-free realm. A word that captures this economy of functioning, which comes from Morita therapy (originally practiced in Japan), combines Buddhist and cognitive-behavioral principles. The word is *aru ga mama* (Doi, cited in Molino, 1998, p. 89), which means "the state in which the mind in not unduly arrested by anything and runs smoothly." Attention is then naturally drawn to what is before us, such as to our patients and their difficulties.

Limitations of Attention Alone

The focus of this book is on mindfulness, but in Buddhist psychology, mindfulness is only one of seven interdependent "factors of awakening" or qualities of mind that facilitate increased awareness. The privileged position of mindfulness is not an accident, however. A firm foundation in mindfulness provides a vantage point from which one can see whether the other six factors (described below) are strong or weak, and mindfulness practice supports the development of these factors. All the factors of awakening can really be thought of as arising from mindfulness and part of the full expression of mindfulness in our lives. Together, the seven qualities of mind form a recipe for optimal psychotherapeutic presence.

Partial Attention

Everyday attention often involves tepid, vague, or nondirected awareness. Mindfulness practice focuses attention; it is like a firm handshake with one object at a time in the field of experience. Mindfulness neither squeezes the object nor is casual in its grip, but the object is distinctly perceived. For example, we are generally alert when we drive, but we focus our attention more intensively when driving in the passing lane or parallel parking. Similarly, we are vaguely aware when reaching for vegetables in the refrigerator but pay great attention when slicing a tomato, particularly as the knife nears our fingers. While our ordinary activities all involve some attention to the present moment, we would not characterize them as states of full mindfulness.

Partial attention is combined with, and affected by, other qualities of mind. We could liken this kind of attention to a boat headlight that, while clearly noticing objects in front of and on either side of the boat, will not notice barnacles which attach to the hull. We have all had the experience (not generally reported to our clinical supervisors) of being somewhat present with a patient, while unconsciously reflecting on something with which we are personally wrestling—our barnacles.

What is missing when we have partial attention during psychotherapy? What do compelling events, such as watching a beautiful sunset or empathizing with a grieving patient, contain that our less attentive moments lack? Buddhist psychology maintains that what separates moments of uninspired or partial awareness from those which are full and sublime is the presence or absence of the additional six "factors of awakening": (1) investigation, (2) energy, (3) joy, (4) tranquility, (5) concentration, and (6) equanimity (see also Appendix B). We can say we are truly mindful while doing psychotherapy if all these factors are present.

Optimal Presence

Both patients and therapists experience delight when they are fully present in the therapy relationship. *Optimal presence* refers to the combined working of the seven factors of awakening, including the foundational factor of mindfulness.

Optimal presence may be imagined as being like seven acrobats standing on a pole. (The bottom acrobat is "mindfulness.") Each must do his or her part, or else they will all fall. In other words, to maintain optimal presence, each mental factor needs to be present and in balance with the others. We now examine each of these factors.

Investigation

Investigation functions to keep our thoughts appropriately focused on the object at hand. Our attention is like a searchlight. For example, while sitting with a patient, investigation will keep the mind of the therapist actively engaged in trying to understand the patient better: "What does he or she mean by that?" "Why does the patient think this?" "What is happening here?" Investigation enriches therapy by constantly probing for deeper layers of understanding.

Energy

Too much agitation or anxiety interferes with optimal presence, as does sluggishness or indifference. Neither of these states is conducive to effective therapeutic responses. This is illustrated by Hans Selye's (1956) well-known bell-shaped stress response curve that depicts how performance increases up to a certain point of arousal. Performance drops as arousal continues to increase. Caffeine can sharpen attention up to a point, beyond which it creates agitation. To have optimal presence in therapy, we need calm energy: alert yet relaxed, neither restless nor drowsy. Balanced energy is at the peak of the bell-shaped curve.

Joy

Joy is animated delight in what is happening in the moment. It is that quality of presence in which we would not prefer to be anywhere else, which sees the present field of experience as an embarrassment of riches. In therapy, genuine interest and affection are the manifestation of this joy. Genuine interest cannot be faked; it is evident to both the patient and the therapist.

Tranquility

Tranquility is being pleasantly unruffled by the flow of moment-to-moment experience. It is peace of mind not based on the absence of thoughts and feelings, but on the acceptance of whatever is arising. Patients generally admire when their therapists take hardship in stride and are role models for calmness. Therapists require tranquility to act wisely and avoid the mistakes we make when we feel compelled to say or do something in the therapy hour.

Concentration

Concentration is the sustained quality of nondistraction, cultivated through the willing and repeated return of attention to the present moment. It is the "backbone" of optimal presence. When concentration is insufficiently developed, mindfulness wavers and is easily distracted. In therapy, concentration means remaining undistracted by any concerns outside of the session.

Equanimity

Equanimity is the "even" in evenly hovering attention. It is the attentional rudder that keeps mindfulness smooth and steady. This is a subtle matter, as the mind is continuously steering toward that which is interesting, and turning away from, or holding at arm's length, that which is less appealing. Equanimity encourages a posture of equal nearness to each moment within the therapeutic process.

Training in Evenly Hovering Attention

In 1952, psychoanalyst Karen Horney suggested that the quality of *wholehearted attention* was of central importance in psychotherapy. Her study of Zen Buddhism led her to wonder about its applicability to psychotherapy. After observing the performance of an unusually mindful headwaiter at a restaurant, she spoke to colleagues about the value of attention training:

> Well, there you have a description of wholeheartedness and of a person who, in this particular performance, was entirely absorbed in what he was doing. . . . This is commonplace in Zen because it is the very essence of Zen. But you know, of course, that such wholeheartedness is a rare attainment. Still, as a goal or an ideal it is good to keep wholeheartedness in mind so we can know how far away from, or how close we are, in approximating it. Sometimes we need to ask ourselves what factors might frustrate wholehearted attention. I will add one thing. The headwaiter could not have performed in this way without training, skill and experience. Without training, such effectiveness is impossible. But then, with training and experience, this degree of absorption in what one is doing becomes possible, at least. (1952/1998, p. 36)

Horney was alluding to the idea that evenly hovering attention could be learned, and although the blueprint for such learning was absent from psychotherapy training, there might be attention practices within the Buddhist tradition that could be helpful. We now know that highly sophisticated techniques for training attention can be found in the mindfulness tradition.

Therapist Exercises

Exercises 1 and 2 cultivate *concentration* and *mindfulness*, which serve as a foundation for the remaining five factors, culminating in optimal presence. They can be practiced in two ways: (1) in a sustained manner during longer formal practice periods, and (2) during the workday as an *intermezzo* between patients (informal practice). In the first approach, it is helpful to set aside a time and place where you are unlikely to be interrupted or distracted for however long you choose to practice. A timer is useful to avoid the need to interrupt the practice to check the time. In the beginning, practice periods should not be so long as to become tedious; 10 or 20 minutes are enough. When practicing in the office between patients, 3–5 minutes can suffice.

When attention is repeatedly returned to a single object, the factor of concentration is strengthened. Once the mind is able to settle down with one object, it is less likely to be distracted when attending to a continually changing series of sensory or mental impressions.

Exercise 1: Concentration

1. Find a comfortable posture. Close your eyes. Allow your body to be held, supported by the chair. Notice directly the sensation of your body in contact with the chair.

2. Notice that your breath is already moving on its own.

3. Narrow your attention to the flow of the breath at the tip of your nose, as it contacts the nostrils.

4. Whenever your attention wanders, and you notice that it has wandered, return your attention to the flow the breath at the tip of your nose.

5. Allow yourself a few more breaths before slowly opening your eyes.

Exercise 2: Mindfulness

1. Find a comfortable posture. Close your eyes. Allow your body to be held, supported by the chair. Notice directly the sensation of your body in contact with the chair.

2. Allow whatever arises in your field of experience—visual images, sounds, physical sensations, feelings, thought formations—to come and go, to move freely.

3. Next bring attention to whatever becomes predominant in the field of experience. Mentally notice and give a word label to the type of thoughts that may arise, such as *analyzing, planning, remembering, hearing,* and so on.

4. Take a few more breaths before slowly opening your eyes.

The point of Exercise 2 is to bring attention to whatever predominates in the field of your awareness. This is the cornerstone of mindfulness practice, and it is what makes mindfulness not merely skill training but a psychologically rich endeavor. We may notice impatience, boredom, or feelings of inadequacy as they arise, neither suppressing them nor shifting attention to something more desirable. When the mind tries to avoid what is difficult and replace it with, for example, a pleasing series of thoughts, this, too, is simply to be noticed.

The reader is encouraged to experiment with these twin strategies—concentration and mindfulness—for regulating attention. Additionally, the creative therapist can explore his or her options when the other five factors of awakening need strengthening. For example, nervous (not calm) energy may mean that the therapist needs some physical exercise, loss of equanimity may mean the therapist needs clinical support or supervision, lack of interest may mean the motivation for the patient being in therapy is not clear to the therapist, and so forth. We find that keeping a "shopping list" of the factors of awakening nearby helps to galvanize one's intention to be optimally present in the therapy room and provides a map for finding one's way back to present-centered awareness once it is lost.

EMPATHY

Mindfulness is often mistaken to be a cognitive pursuit—the cultivation of attention—rather than a feeling enterprise. In this section, we discuss the *attitude* or feeling of mindfulness-oriented psychotherapy. In Buddhist psychology, mindfulness and compassion are likened to two wings of a bird; both are essential for awakening to take flight. *Compassion* refers to awareness and feeling for the suffering of others. A broader term familiar to the clinical audience, *empathy*, encompasses *all* the feelings of others, not just their struggles. Compassion may be understood as "unflinching empathy" for the suffering of others (Marotta, 2003). Although words for the therapeutic attitude—empathy and compassion—may differ somewhat in meaning, they both fit under the umbrella of kindness. We now explore the use of mindfulness exercises for the cultivation of this therapeutic attitude and issues posed by these practices for the psychotherapist.

As we grow in mindful awareness of our own struggles in life, and in awareness of our psychological landscape and mental processes, we can more readily identify with and understand the same in our patients. Consider the following example:

> A psychotherapist goes on an intensive meditation retreat and, predictably, after many hours of sitting in a half-lotus posture, his back muscles tighten and soon spasm. This familiar malady threatens to dominate much of his experience, at times overwhelming his ability to concentrate on anything else. After days of seeking ways to block out or to surrender to this pain, an image of an individual with cerebral palsy spontaneously comes to his mind. Individuals with cerebral palsy, he realizes, suffer muscle spasms most of the time, in many parts of their bodies, and are unable to relieve the spasm by a simple change of posture. They can expect no relief at the end of a retreat. Having given little previous thought to those with cerebral palsy, he is surprised to find himself filled with compassion for them, and is paradoxically grateful for these muscle spasms for opening his heart in this way.

Although we all experience difficulties, the sense of deep fellow feeling may not occur in the Sturm und Drang of daily life. Mindfulness meditation practice may create a "time-out" for us to open to our own suffering and, thereby, to the struggles of others.

Empathy has received considerable attention in the clinical literature. It is classically understood as an "accurate understanding of the [patient's] world as seen from the inside. To sense the [patient's] private world as if it were your own, but without losing the 'as if' quality—this is empathy" (Rogers, 1961, p. 284). Self psychology pioneer Heinz Kohut stretched the definition and role of empathic understanding. For him, it is an observational tool, a bond, a curative factor and a necessity for psychological health (Lee & Martin, 1991). Empathy requires a particular sort of attention. Rollo May (1967, p. 97) noted that empathy calls for "learning to relax, mentally and spiritually, as well as physically, learning to let one's self go into the other person with a willingness to be changed in the process."

It is assumed that therapists are able to affectively tune in to patients' feelings hour after hour. But empathy is a "relative potential" (Jordan, 1991, p. 74), arising as a multitude of professional and personal variables are brought into delicate balance. Professional variables include clinical training and experience, the complexity of the patient population, the number of patients seen in a given day, and the work environment. Personal variables include the quality of primary relationships, current life stressors and one's ability to manage them, the quality of sleep, physical and mental health, and the stress of that day's demands. Our capacity for empathy fluctuates from day to day and moment to moment.

Although the importance of empathy for the psychotherapy relationship is well established (Norcross, 2001), there is relatively little evidence that it can be taught to psychotherapists to improve their performance (see Chapter 3). There is, however, a growing corpus of literature on the use of meditation and mindfulness to cultivate empathy (Lesh, 1970; Newman, 1994; Pearl & Carlozzi, 1994; Reiman, 1985; Riedesel, 1983; Shapiro, Schwartz, & Bonner, 1998; Stile, Lerner, Rhatigan, Plumb, & Orsillo, 2003; Sweet & Johnson, 1990). To date, there appears to be no research *directly* linking empathy cultivated in the therapist's mindfulness practice to what actually happens in the therapy hour, or to treatment outcomes (Fritz & Mierzwa, 1983). However, it stands to reason that any method that develops empathy in the therapist would support a positive treatment relationship and, therefore, improve treatment outcome. In a field generally lacking in systematic methods to cultivate empathy or evenly hovering attention, mindfulness training may have great potential.

Empathy Arising from Insight

In Buddhist psychology, empathy is understood to arise with deepening insight into impermanence, mental suffering, and the constructed nature of self: We tend to believe that things are stable from one day to the next, we create suffering for ourselves with grasping and avoidance, and we misperceive the "self" as separate from the world around us. As these illusions soften in the practice of mindfulness, by watching how the mind creates illusions, our sense of self as separate, in need of special protection, gives way to an appreciation of our affinity with all beings. Compassion and empathy are natural products of this deep, intuitive understanding.

Empathy Cultivated in Dedicated Practices

Mindfulness is ordinarily practiced as "choiceless awareness," attention to whatever arises in our experience without discrimination. Practices that deliberately aim to cultivate particular mental qualities are not choiceless, but they balance and stabilize mindfulness, and are practiced as a deliberate antidote to harmful mental states such as anger and hatred. In Buddhist psychology, some such practices relate to the four *brahma viharas* ("limitless qualities of heart") and include lovingkindness, compassion, sympathetic joy, and equanimity. These mind training techniques are described more fully in Chapter 5. As training for psychotherapists, we emphasize the practice of *lovingkindness*.

While lovingkindness is often taught as a unique practice, it is merely the expansion of the ordinary human capacity for friendliness. Its basis is the recognition that, just like us, others wish for happiness and well-being. More an attitude than a feeling, lovingkindness is naturally expressed as compassion toward another's suffering and empathic joy for another's happiness. It does not necessarily lead to being "nice," nor need one feel any special affection for another person to practice it. Lovingkindness is an *intention*. It is an ideal that gives direction to our endeavors, not an opportunity to evaluate our value or merit. Merely the intention to be kind is a practice in and of itself.

The teaching of lovingkindness as an antidote to harmful mental states is based on two psychological tenets from Buddhist psychology. First, only one state or condition exists at a time, however rapidly one state may replace another. In a single moment, two affectively contradictory states cannot coexist. It is also based on the understanding that any action that is repeated becomes stronger, while behaviors that are no longer practiced are gradually extinguished. Therefore, the practice of lovingkindness is intended to weaken harmful habits and replace them with those more conducive to happiness. These wholesome mental states further reinforce concentration, fearlessness, and factors supportive of wisdom.

Empathy toward Oneself and Others

In Buddhist psychology, empathy is a "cohesive factor" (Salzberg, 1995, p. 28), because it connects us to our own experiences and to those of others. It cuts through notions of a separate self and speaks to our interconnection with others. Empathy relies on the interplay of cognitive and affective skills, and a high level of ego functioning (Jordan, 1991). When turned toward oneself, empathy requires that one be interested, willing, and able to revisit or experience an event and its corresponding affect without judgment. Self-acceptance leads to the ability to "step into another's shoes." This development alters our view of others from a position of separateness and difference to one of connectedness and understanding.

> Searching all directions with one's awareness,
> One finds no one dearer than oneself.
> In the same way, others are fiercely dear to themselves.
> So one should not hurt others if one loves oneself.
> —THE BUDDHA (Bhikkhu, 2004a)

Traditional lovingkindness practice begins by offering kindness to oneself, since it has been considered easiest to generate positive feelings in this manner. But Western teachers drew a different conclusion from their own meditation experiences. Joseph Goldstein (2002), a prominent meditation teacher, observes that Western students struggle in their meditation practices with feelings of low self-esteem and disconnection. Indeed, even the Dalai Lama (1997) was confused by the prevalence of low self-esteem among Western meditation students, because this particular malady is generally absent among his Eastern pupils. The problem may be due to the emphasis on individuality in Western culture, discussed in Chapter 2, which places an impossible burden of achieving happiness on the efforts of the self. By contrast, people in some Asian societies experience the self as part of the whole of life and subject to the laws of nature (Keown, 2000). Unhappiness is not viewed a personal failure or a source of guilt.

The tendency toward low self-esteem among Western meditation students has led meditation instructors to teach lovingkindness practice to beginning students, along with mindfulness practice. This helps counter what Tara Brach (2003) calls "the trance of unworthiness." Furthermore, they have modified the lovingkindness practice by starting with images of *others* for whom we have positive feelings, because it is sometimes easier to generate warm feelings for people we love and admire than toward ourselves. This sequence differs from the traditional lovingkindness practices in which we begin by extending lovingkindness to *ourselves*, then to a benefactor, then a good friend, then a neutral person, then to a difficult person, and finally, to all beings without discrimination. Difficulties are almost certain to arise in generating and or maintaining positive feelings toward some people. However, with practice, a path is being cleared that will enable the practitioner to access kindness toward an increasingly broad range of individuals.

Exercises

The following exercises are intended for therapists to expand their natural empathy, particularly toward their patients. The exercises are adapted from traditional Buddhist practices. A description often used in teaching these exercises is how a mother feels upon first seeing her newborn child. The practitioner seeks to summon these tender feelings, while calling up an image or felt sense of a selected person to whom the feelings are then directed. Throughout the exercises, various images are offered to help evoke empathy.

Find the images that best suit you. The goal is to cultivate the intention to extend these feelings, not to manufacture a glaze of sentimentality or suppress how you naturally feel. Concentrate on your *intention* to open your heart more fully. Trust that by planting seeds (intention) and attending to them (practice), the harvest (empathy) will follow organically.

It is suggested that you spend a few minutes on each category and repeat any or all of the exercises at least once a week. Regular practice sets the stage for continuity of empathy over time.

Empathy toward a Benefactor or Good Friend

The benefactor is someone who embodies and inspires the quality of lovingkindness. The person may be someone from your life, such as a parent or a trusted clinical supervisor, or a figure such as Jesus, the Dalai Lama, or Mother Teresa. Sometimes simply a good friend stimulates this feeling most naturally. We may feel a sense of appreciation for this person's presence in our life and/or feel inspired to offer our best.

Exercise 3: Empathy toward the Benefactor/Good Friend

1. Find a comfortable seated position. Close your eyes. Allow the body to be held by the chair. Notice the bodily sensation of contact with the chair.

2. Relax your abdomen. Notice that the breath is already moving on its own. Follow the breath for a few moments.

3. Bring to mind a visual image or a felt sense of someone who embodies the quality of lovingkindness. Imagine that this person is sitting across from you.

4. Now imagine that you are emanating feelings of gratitude or love toward your benefactor.

5. When your attention wanders, simply return to this image or felt sense of the person and begin again.

Despite the simplicity of the exercise, the cultivation of positive affect is often not easy. While positive thoughts associated with this person may be present, the actual feeling of warmth may only be sporadically available, if at all. Though feelings of warmth may be weak or absent at first, subtle shifts occur with repeated effort. Returning again and again to the object of meditation trains the mind to strengthen lovingkindness.

Focusing attention on the breath in the heart area can serve as a reminder that you are arousing the heart's emotions. Over time, you may notice subtle changes, such as a slowing of your breath, warmth in the heart area, a softening of tension, and feelings of ease and openness.

Empathy toward the Neutral Patient

In this next category, bring to mind a patient with whom you struggle to stay emotionally engaged. The neutral patient is one for whom you have neither a strong positive nor a negative affinity. It may be a person who tells you the same story week after week, or someone with a monotonous voice. His or her story fails to hold your attention. Although this lack of interest may initially go undetected by the patient (who may not find this level of engagement unusual), the challenge for the therapist is to remain connected.

Exercise 4: Empathy toward the Neutral Patient

1. Find a comfortable seated position. Close your eyes. Allow the body to be held by the chair. Notice the bodily sensation of contact with the chair.

2. Relax your abdomen. Notice that the breath is already moving on its own. Follow the breath for a few moments.

3. Bring to mind a visual image or a felt sense of a patient for whom you lack strong positive or negative feelings. Imagine that this person is sitting across from you.

4. Now imagine that you are emanating friendly feelings toward the neutral patient. [*Note: If you are having trouble generating this feeling, imagine that your benefactor is sitting next to this neutral patient and direct friendly warmth to both of them.*]

5. When your attention wanders, simply return to this image or felt sense of the neutral patient and begin again.

The challenge most commonly faced with this patient is that of boredom. The mind tends to wander when it is not sufficiently stimulated. As an antidote to this tendency, the benefactor is used to arouse positive, friendly feelings toward the neutral patient.

Empathy toward Oneself

In one way or another, we often encourage patients to "go easy" on themselves. Can we extend this generosity to ourselves? Some therapists find that it is easier to offer love and care to their patients and loved ones. Without attention to ourselves, however, we run the risk of burnout. The growth of workshops on "caring for the caregiver" attests to this problem. "Burnout is the index of the dislocation between what people are and what they have to do. It represents an erosion in values, dignity, spirit, and will—an erosion of the human soul" (Maslach & Leiter, 1997, p. 24). Offering love and care to ourselves replenishes the physical and emotional reservoirs that are necessary to care for others. "Unless the joy of living is within me, I would be offering myself to others with an empty hand. This special kind of selfishness, that I should want a good life for myself, is to me a primary hallmark of the mature person" (Warkentin, 1972, p. 254). Empathy toward oneself is the practice of mindful acceptance.

Exercise 5: Empathy toward Oneself

1. Find a comfortable seated position. Close your eyes. Allow the body to be held by the chair. Notice the bodily sensation of contact with the chair.

2. Relax your abdomen. Notice that the breath is already moving on its own. Follow the breath for a few moments.

3. Bring to mind a visual image or memory that evokes a feeling of friendliness toward yourself.

4. Now imagine sending friendly warmth toward this image or representation of yourself. [Note: If you are having trouble generating this feeling, imagine your benefactor sitting next to this image of yourself and offer warmth to both of you. Or imagine your benefactor offering friendly warmth to you.]

5. When your attention wanders, simply return to this image of yourself and begin again.

The mind may get pulled into revisiting pleasant and painful memories, recalling unskillful actions, or leaning forward into planning for the day. You may notice that particular patterns of thought arise with regularity. Without judgment or criticism, redirect your attention to the object of meditation—yourself. As the muscle of empathy strengthens, we open to and feel compassion for our pain and appreciation for our joy. The strong, tender heart of compassion that emerges from self-empathy is better prepared for holding another in its care.

Empathy toward the Difficult Patient

We all have patients who test the limits of our empathy. For example, fear about suicidal behavior may cause us to pull away from a patient, or anger at demands for between-session phone calls may obscure the emotional hunger in the patient's heart. Difficult patients may require deeper attention than we are willing to give.

Sending warm feelings to the difficult patient is challenging. Though it may be challenging to put aside their unpleasant traits, try to get in

---

Exercise 6: Empathy toward the Difficult Patient

1. Find a comfortable seated position. Close your eyes. Allow the body to be held by the chair. Notice the bodily sensation of contact with the chair.

2. Relax your abdomen. Notice that the breath is already moving on its own. Follow the breath for a few moments.

3. Bring to mind a visual image or a felt sense of a patient for whom you have strong negative reactions. Imagine that this person is sitting across from you.

4. Now, imagine that you are emanating friendly warmth toward the difficult patient. [*Note: If you are having trouble generating this feeling, imagine your benefactor is sitting next to this difficult patient, and send warmth to both of them. Consider what makes this person unhappy, what motivates this person's actions.*]

5. When your attention wanders, simply return to the image and begin again.

---

touch with the part of the patient that desires to be happy, cared for, and loved. This will take time. Once again, the benefactor can support the empathic connection.

The following metaphor may help generate compassion for the difficult patient or other difficult people in our lives. Imagine walking in the forest and coming across a small dog. You reach out your hand to pet the dog, and the dog responds by snarling and biting you. Your first reaction to the dog may be uncharitable at best. Imagine instead that on coming across the dog you discovered that its leg is caught in a trap buried beneath a pile of leaves. Your reaction to its ill temper is quite different; you are likely to harbor only compassion toward the dog. You understand that it is aggressive because its leg is in a trap. It is helpful to remember that anyone who is hostile to others also has a leg in some trap; a person who is *not* in pain has no need to strike out. When we recognize that others' harmful actions are a reflection of their own suffering, it becomes easier to extend compassion to them.

The Greeting Exercise

There are innumerable practice opportunities in our work as therapists. This final exercise is another *intermezzo* we can practice on the hour, every hour.

Whether it be a patient you have never met or one you have seen many times, all patients come with the hope that you will care about their suffering and walk with them as they gain their own footing in this uncertain world.

Exercise 7: The Greeting

1. Take a moment and feel the rise and fall of your breath before rising to meet your next patient.

2. As you walk to the door, imagine that on the other side of the door, another human being is waiting. This human being is someone who is suffering, who has hopes and dreams, who has tried to be happy and only partially succeeded, and who is coming to you, believing that you can relieve his or her suffering.

3. Now open the door and say "hello."

Paradoxical Reactions to Attention and Empathy Exercises

If you have tried these exercises, there is a good chance that your experience was not what you sought or expected. It is very common to experience a sort of backlash to them, such as negativity, anger, or aggression. Consequently, we may redouble our efforts only to discover that our negative emotions grow stronger, as if to restore the balance of our ambivalence. This result can be humbling and discouraging. However, such a reaction is not evidence of failure, and it is not unlike resistance encountered in psychotherapy. Can we receive these uninvited reactions with a quality of interest and equanimity?

While these exercises are not intended as an opportunity to examine this negativity, negative emotions that arise should not be rejected or become an occasion for further self-recrimination. We do not get to choose what arises, but we can work skillfully with these feelings when they present themselves. In the moment when difficult emotions emerge, we acknowledge and greet them with kindness before gently returning our attention to the exercise at hand. The purpose of this practice is not to force a particular emotion to arise; rather, it is to establish the conditions that allow empathy and lovingkindness to develop. It is not necessary to do the practice and make it work; it is only necessary to do the practice and trust that you are planting seeds that in time will take root.

> The bud
> stands for all things,
> even for those things that don't flower,
> for everything flowers, from within, of self-blessing;
> though sometimes it is necessary
> to reteach a thing its loveliness. . . .
> —KINNELL (1980, p. 9)

CHAPTER 5

Relational Psychotherapy, Relational Mindfulness

JANET L. SURREY

Freeing ourselves from the illusion of separateness allows us
to live in a natural freedom.
—SHARON SALZBERG (1995, p. 1)

We believe that all relationships . . . can be renewed by
restoring the pathways to connection.
—JEAN BAKER MILLER AND
IRENE PIERCE STIVER (1997, pp. 22–23)

Mindfulness meditation is ordinarily considered an individual enterprise, although it is frequently practiced with the support of a community. The fruits of meditation may include a growing experience of deep interconnection with others, and with the larger world. When this perspective is carried into the treatment setting by the therapist, the stage is set for a fertile therapy relationship.

Unlike some medical remedies whose effectiveness may require little effort or intention by the patient, psychotherapy requires mental presence; treatment cannot occur among passive participants. In this sense, some degree of mindfulness by the patient and the therapist is present in any effective therapy. Mindfulness practice is learning to become *more* present, and relational psychotherapy may be understood as a process whereby both the therapist and patient are working with the intention to deepen awareness of the present relational experience, with acceptance. While the therapist may be the only person in the room to carry this intention at first, over time, the therapist and patient discover healing together in shared moments of mindfulness.

In Chapter 3, we saw that the qualities of the therapy relationship are of central importance to the success of treatment, independent of the treatment model. Some clinical approaches regard the relationship as an intervention itself, rather than seeing it solely as a context or support for the therapeutic work. This chapter will explore one such approach, relational–cultural theory (RCT; Jordan, Kaplan, Miller, Stiver, & Surrey, 1991), and its attention to "movement-in-relationship," and will explore how RCT and mindfulness contribute powerfully to one another. Following an introduction to RCT and a discussion of areas of commonality with mindfulness, I discuss other elements of Buddhist psychology as they contribute to a relational perspective and illustrate the contribution of this approach through a clinical case study. The chapter concludes with meditative exercises that therapists can use to enhance treatment within this model.

RELATIONAL–CULTURAL THEORY AND PRACTICE

Since 1978, I have been part of a community of clinicians and theorists at the Stone Center at Wellesley College, who have been developing RCT and practice. From the lens of women's experience as the "carriers" of the work of connection in this culture (Miller, 1976), relational theorists have described psychological development and healing in a manner that challenges cultural and professional ideals of "self" and "separation" as the cornerstones of health, well-being, and optimal development. Authentic connection is described as the core of psychological well-being and is the essential quality of growth-fostering and healing relationships. In such relationships, each participant feels able to *be* and *be seen* empathically. Each feels held, enlarged, and often stretched by the presence of the other and the challenge of mutuality. The invitation to meet this challenge exists in intimate dyads, families, or groups of all sizes.

From a relational perspective, psychological suffering results from being cut off or prevented from engaging in mutually authentic, empathic, and empowering relationships. Healing and therapy are described as the practice of recognizing and honoring the ways people have struggled in nonmutual relationships and the strategies of disconnection they have evolved as protection. Nonmutuality has many forms, such as relationships that are abusive, oppressive, violating, violent, distant, superficial, impassable, enmeshed, or undifferentiated. Miller and Stiver (1997) describe how the state of chronic disconnection leads to the experience of "condemned isolation," in which the child or adult begins to feel that something about him- or herself is wrong and must be responsible for the disconnection. Chronic disconnection results in loss of energy, immobilization, lack of clarity, and negative self-images. For example, a child, Laura, learns that when she shows her fear or sadness, she upsets her parents. She develops an image of relationships that does not include the open expression of painful feelings. She becomes increasingly disconnected from her own painful feelings and from relationships. At a stressful time of life, she is unable to know her feelings or how to find and utilize relational power and support.

The intention of therapy is to work through the effects of isolation and disconnection, as they play out in life and in therapy, toward the goal of reconnection and restoration of growth-fostering relationships. Miller and Stiver (1997) describe five desired psychological outcomes of the restoration of mutual connection: (1) new energy and vitality; (2) greater capacity to act; (3) increased clarity; (4) enhanced self-worth; and (5) the desire and capacity for more connection.

Theorists and practitioners of RCT have described the healing dynamic of the therapy relationship as a collaborative search for authentic engagement and mutuality. The qualities of relational presence that are described as most fundamental for the therapist are sustained empathic attentiveness, responsiveness, and openness to joining and to being moved in the relationship, as well as an attitude of respect, inquiry, care, and humility (Jordan, 2003). In contrast to the early psychoanalytic emphasis on objectivity, neutrality, and accurate interpretation, or the use of specifiable interventions in many protocol-oriented treatments, RCT stresses the centrality of the therapeutic relationship. The task of the therapist is to maintain professional focus, intention, expertise, and integrity, while remaining present and accessible in his or her shared humanity in the face of whatever material the patient presents.

THE INTERSECTION OF RELATIONAL
THERAPY AND MINDFULNESS

The intersection of RCT and mindfulness is particularly fertile, because their goals and methods merge in many respects. This volume describes a variety of ways mindfulness practice contributes to psychotherapy. Indeed, mindfulness practice supports the capacity of the therapist to attend to connection and, in the process, repair its breaches. RCT also offers a view of how psychotherapy, conversely, can become an opportunity for mindfulness practice. Deeper still, as therapist and patient are mutually engaged in this process, RCT can be understood as a potent form of "co-meditation," harnessed as a method to further mindfulness training itself. These reciprocal contributions of mindfulness and relational psychotherapy to each other are described below.

Connection as the Object of Mindfulness

Connection, whether to our own experience or to others, is never static. It is a process of successive moments of turning toward, turning away, and returning. Mindfulness cultivates awareness of this movement, informed by the intention to return to connection again and again. In mindfulness, the object of our investigation is our connection to whatever arises in awareness. For the committed practitioner, there is no experience—including doing psychotherapy—that falls outside of this practice.

In a session of mindfulness-informed relational therapy, the therapist remains attentive to moment-to-moment changes in *his or her own sensations*, feelings, thoughts, and memories. While the patient is describing his or her own feelings, thoughts, perceptions, and body sensations, the therapist is also paying attention and registering *experiences of the patient* as the object of awareness, using these perceptions to facilitate the movement of the relationship. This is moment-to-moment attention to the living reality of the other—his or her words, voice, feelings, expressions, body language, breathing, and so on. In addition, the therapist is attending to the *flow of the relationship* and the shifting qualities of connection and disconnection, including their energetic, textural, and emotional qualities. This tripartite awareness (self, other, and the movement or flow of relationship) best describes the therapist's use of mindfulness in the relational approach to psychotherapy.

Relational Therapy as Co-Meditation Practice

Mindfulness does not end with the therapist. While the therapist's focus remains on the experience of the patient, *both* patient and therapist are engaging in a collaborative process of mutual attentiveness and mindfulness in and through relational joining. Patterns of mistrust, terror, doubt, connection, and disconnection become the focus of this shared investigation. This view of therapy as *co-meditation* offers new possibilities for the therapeutic enterprise.

Through the relationship, the therapist offers the patient the possibility of staying emotionally present with the therapist, perhaps staying with difficult feelings for "one more moment," thus enhancing the patient's capacity for mindful awareness of self-in-connection. The therapist's empathic attunement helps to draw out the truth of the present moment without flooding or shaming the patient—with acceptance. Psychotherapy becomes mindfulness practice, and mindfulness becomes a collaborative process, even without labeling it as such. Mindfulness and the attuned relationship seem to support each other.

Because both therapist and patient are called on to be present to the best of their abilities (to themselves, to the other, and to the movement of the relationship into and out of connection), the therapy process is deepened and enlarged. It begins to show a quality of growth consistent with the broader goals of mindfulness.

For example, authentic relationships always offer challenges for stretching and releasing images and ideas of who we are or should be, who the other is, and how the relationship should be. Learning to rest in the truth of the moment begins to free us from the grip of limiting self or relational images. "I guess I am not 25 years old anymore. I guess my partner is not either! We are *all* aging. Perhaps that is natural and all right." Our fixed ideas of self and other begin to loosen their tight grip on us. We learn to accept "what is." The moments when this occurs can be healing.

In addition, in moments of deep connection in relationship, we break out of isolation and contraction into a more whole and spacious state of mind and heart. This is difficult to grasp intellectually. Through the doorway of connection, we come to heightened awareness of our own and the other's reality, and importantly, the interdependent nature of our existence is intuitively experienced. These moments of deep connection go beyond the nature of relationship as customarily described in object relations, relational, or intersubjective psychology literature. This point deserves further explanation.

Intersubjectivity to Interbeing

Recent work in intersubjectivity helps to illuminate how our inner world is constituted through interaction in the interpersonal world, both in the course of early development and in ongoing, real-time contact with others. The early development of self, subjectively experienced as separate, depends on contact with others for differentiation to occur (Thompson, 2001). Psychoanalytic theorists have drawn on this observation to help describe the complex interplay between subjects and how we draw conclusions from within the "intersubjective field" (Atwood & Stolorow, 1984, p. 41). Others have sought the basis of our experience of others in brain physiology (Gallese, 2001; Rissolatti, Fadiga, Fogassi, & Gallese, 1996).

The experience of connection suggested by mindfulness-informed RCT deepens our understanding of intersubjectivity and may be better described in terms found in Buddhist psychology. In the relational model, openness to relationship in our daily life expands to a felt connection to the global community. Healing our personal wounds becomes a first step in a process that gradually widens to include compassion for the suffering of everyone and everything, potentially including the intent, described in ecopsychology, to heal planetary wounds (Conn, 1998). In Evan Thompson's (2001) words, we move from "intersubjectivity to interbeing." *Interbeing* is a term given by Thich Nhat Hanh (1992) to describe the interconnectedness of all beings. The uncommon experience of this level of interdependence is regarded as direct insight into our original concordance with all of nature.

This is described in Hindu metaphor of the "jeweled web of Indra," in which each being is seen as a jeweled node of a web that reflects all others. The implication is that the phenomenal world is interwoven in a deeply holistic and holographic way, in which each node can be an entrance or doorway to the whole. This interplay of part and whole is a metaphor for how moments in the therapy relationship may become doorways to profound connection and realization of interdependence; the relationship (deep and sustained care and attention) to a particular Other can open the heart to awareness of the whole. The therapist's practice could be described as tending to and mending the net of Indra (Kabat-Zinn, 2000), through overcoming the psychological obstacles to realizing our fundamental connectedness. When the obstacles become known and skillfully addressed, we experience ourselves as part of the web.

Our patients are deeply influenced by their personal, familial, and cultural locations. The particular American context of suffering has been described as a fundamental crisis of connection, a loss of a sense of rootedness, belonging, community, and continuity of care. There is great longing for connection and for relational and spiritual renewal. Mindfulness, as a practice that opens and deepens our capacities for connection, seems therefore to have particular relevance in this culture.

To summarize, mindfulness practice cultivates an expansive awareness in the therapist, which is implicitly or explicitly extended to the patient. For the patient and the therapist, the work of psychotherapy becomes an exercise of mindful awareness of relationship directed toward the movement of connection and disconnection, and toward the creation of a new, more empathically connected culture within which healing occurs. In this way, mindfulness supports psychotherapy. Psychotherapy practiced with an expanded view can also become a vehicle for personal development of the therapist. When qualities of openheartedness, fearlessness, close attention, and empathy take root in this collaborative psychotherapy, growth occurs. Both parties find in the practice of opening wholeheartedly to the present reality—of themselves, of each other, and of their connection—an expanded receptivity that goes beyond the particularity of *this* relationship, or *this* setting. Therapy, practiced in this way, has a distinctly spiritual dimension to it, although it may not be described in religious terms.

ADDITIONAL BUDDHIST CONTRIBUTIONS TO RELATIONAL PRACTICE

While RCT was not originally based on concepts derived from Buddhist psychology, many Buddhist concepts are particularly congenial to relational psychotherapy, because they incline the therapist toward awareness of our inherent interconnectedness.

Vow to Alleviate Suffering

Some schools of Buddhist psychology (described as "middle period" teachings in Chapter 13) emphasize the importance of cultivating good intentions, especially vowing to work throughout our lives for freedom from suffering for all beings, thereby being a beneficial presence in the lives of others. This is also an essential aspect of moment-to-moment, relational practice—extending to others what we want for ourselves. Our deep and sustained attention to another person in therapy is a reflection of our intent to extend compassion and connection to an ever-widening circle that excludes no one.

The commitment to healing and liberation of all beings, as an ideal, can enliven professional study and practice. While clinical psychology holds us accountable to recognize our neurotic, unwholesome, or narcissistic intentions while doing clinical practice, Buddhist psychology offers a touchstone in moments of profound doubt, despair, or professional burnout. Commitments such as the vow to alleviate suffering can be a source of meaning and energy for psychotherapists.

Qualities of Heart

In addition to mindfulness practice, Buddhist psychology contains practices deliberately intended to cultivate four particular qualities of heart (briefly mentioned in Chapter 4). These four *brahma viharas* are lovingkindness (basic human friendliness), compassion (kindness in response to another's sorrow), sympathetic joy (happiness in the good fortune of others), and equanimity (allowing success and failure to occur, without attaching our self-worth to such outcomes). While these are considered essential qualities in human nature that are renewable and can never be fully extinguished by the circumstances of life, they can also be cultivated deliberately. *Brahma vihara* practice "uncovers the radiant, joyful heart within each of us and manifests this radiance to the world" (Salzberg, 1995).

As suggested in Chapter 4, *brahma vihara* practice is a concentration practice rather than a mindfulness practice, insofar as we are attending exclusively to a particular object (typically a phrase or an image of a person), rather than attending to the changing contents of awareness. One may identify the images of a particular person who is easy to love, a "neutral" person, a difficult person, and oneself. The basic technique was illustrated in the lovingkindness exercise in Chapter 4, which consisted of generating a feeling of kindness through an image of a beloved person, then sending that feeling to oneself and to difficult persons. This practice is sometimes accompanied by phrases such as "May I (you) be well, may I (you) be happy, may I (you) be free from suffering." Repetition of these phrases retrains the mind and heart in new mental and emotional habits. In *brahma vihara* practice outside of the clinical hour, it can be helpful to include patients, with particular focus on those undergoing extreme suffering, or those with whom the relationship is difficult. Adaptations of these practices are found in Chapter 4 and at the end of this chapter.

This meditative relational practice can be adapted for use in the midst of psychotherapy, with or without direct verbal acknowledgment. For example, in a moment of great confusion, unhappiness, or extreme suffering, we may become aware of our desire to escape. Recognizable thoughts arise: "I need to get out of this work"; "What's my problem?"; "Dr. X would definitely be doing this better"; or even "I wonder what's for dinner?" Such moments often occur in the face of strong unpleasant emotions, such as rage or blame directed toward the therapist. Sometimes the best response is to recite silently simple lovingkindness or compassion phrases (e.g., "May we find happiness" or "May we be free from suffering") or equanimity practice ("Things are just as they are" or "We will get through this"). This can keep us emotionally available.

The naming and practice of these qualities of heart allow clinicians to reclaim the use of the word *love*, without overly sentimental, romantic, or sexual overtones. Psychotherapy is an expression of love—love as compassion, joy, equanimity, and kindness. It gives our profession a chance to renew and reclaim the deepest elements of our own practice, and the deepest elements of connection and healing. It reminds us that not only compassion but also joy, equanimity, and basic kindness are within us and within our patients at all times, however hidden. This is helpful as an antidote to "compassion fatigue" or "secondary trauma," which are professional liabilities for psychotherapists (Sussman, 1992).

The First Noble Truth and Being with Suffering

The First Noble Truth of the inevitability of suffering in life and relationships helps the clinician maintain equanimity and faith while being with suffering. Suffering is unavoidable, and just because a patient comes to our office does not automatically mean we have the capacity to remove it, nor that it is anyone's fault ("If I am hurting, there must be something bad, deficient or crazy about me"). Much isolation and additional suffering can arise from objectification, personalization, and diagnostic labeling. The freedom inherent in the practice of the First Noble Truth, the acceptance of the simple truth of suffering, is at the core of healing relational practice. Even in suffering (perhaps *especially* in suffering), we can deeply join one another in our common human vulnerability.

The story of the mustard seed illustrates this point. It depicts the Buddha as a skilled relational healer:

> The young son of a poor woman named Gotami died suddenly while playing. Gotami was afflicted with "sorrow-to-the point of madness" (Olendzki, 2002, p. 40) (psychotic grief), and she carried her son's body from house to house pleading for medicine to cure him. The people reviled her saying, "What good is medicine?" But she could not accept the reality of his death. A wise man sent Gotami to the Buddha. She asked him for medicine to heal her son. In exchange for the medicine, the Buddha asked her to first bring him back a mustard seed (which would have been very common in India at the time) from a village household that had never experienced death. Hopeful, Gotami set off on her quest.

The Buddha had prescribed a relational practice that led Gotami to tell her story over and over again in the hope of finding such a household. We can imagine her earnestly searching, telling her story, evoking compassion from the villagers, then listening to their own stories of death, evoking compassion in Gotami.

> Despite visiting every household in her village, Gotami was unable to find a single one that had never experienced death. After her search, she returned to the Buddha without a mustard seed and said, "Thank you, I understand." She was able to bury her child. Gotami was moved to join the community of nuns around the Buddha and, it is said, eventually became enlightened.

Gotami had found common ground with her community, moving out of isolation and denial, and realizing the truth of impermanence. She no longer experienced herself as a reviled "outcast" or less valuable person, but as "human among humans." When pity or sympathy becomes true empathy, a sense of shared humanity can take hold. This story suggests that connection in the face of death and unbearable suffering can lead to the deepest healing insight and liberation.

The capacity to suffer with another person, or the "shared heart of compassion," is at the core of the relational practices of parenting, marriage, friendship, ministry, and medicine. As all parents and therapists know, it is often most difficult to be with the suffering of someone you love or for whom you feel responsible, and almost unbearable to stay with this when you are seen as the source of the problem. Solitary meditation practice alone does not prepare us to be with suffering in a face-to-face encounter. Training in meditation *plus* the cultivation of mindfulness in individual, group, and intimate dyadic contexts is perhaps the most optimal training for mindfulness-oriented psychotherapy. Some dyadic mindfulness exercises are presented at the end of this chapter.

Relational Root Causes: Greed, Hatred, and Delusion

From a relational perspective, the "root causes" of greed, hatred, and delusion (mentioned in Chapter 2 and described more fully in Chapter 11) can be understood as habitual psychological or behavioral patterns that lead to disconnection. Karen Horney (1945) described three similar movements in relationship that impede or distort the healthy flow of connection: moving toward, moving against, and moving away from relationships. The Buddhist description of the three root causes can be seen in these relational strategies:

1. *Greed as movement toward relationship:* a pattern of anxious clinging to or grasping on to fixed patterns, fear that change will bring isolation or abandonment; inability to tolerate and work skillfully with small disconnections.
2. *Hatred as movement against relationship:* a pattern of criticism or negative judgment; anger, blame, or even violence in the face of frustration; attempts to control the other and uphold one's narcissistic image.
3. *Delusion as movement away from relationship:* a pattern of intellectualization, withdrawal, detachment, or dissociation; excessive independence, denial, or flooding in the face of vulnerability or yearnings for connection.

Mindfulness practice entails being vigilant to the influence of these root causes. Similarly, engaged relational therapy can be described as working with these root causes, because they are enlisted as strategies of disconnection. Therapists have their own personal and professional patterns of disconnection, such as objectification and distancing, which are often triggered by difficult moments in therapy. A mindfulness-trained relational therapist will be alert to the relational root causes in his or her own experience, identifying strategies of disconnection as they arise.

Speech and Silence

While therapists have traditionally focused on verbal interaction, the experience of being together in the present moment may be felt more deeply in the silence, in the space between words. Psychologists have written both of preverbal silence, before we have words for our experience, and of emerging into a fuller sense of oneself through finding an authentic voice in relationship (Gilligan, 1982). Mindfulness practice suggests a third option—conscious silence that envelopes an inexpressible, direct perception of the intangible, all-encompassing relational world in which we are all connected. Some people find that solitary mindfulness meditation provides the only experience of silence in their busy lives, but genuine connection in relationship can do that as well.

THE ANATOMY OF HEALING MOMENTS

> Where there is true attentiveness, receptivity and
> responsivity, there can be interaction of creative energies in
> the relationship.
> —VIMALA THAKAR (1993, pp. 16–17)

There is new interest in describing the moment-to-moment flow in relational psychotherapy. Daniel Stern (2004) has written that working in the here and now has the greatest potential to bring about therapeutic change. He adds, "It is remarkable how little we know of the experience that is happening right now while we know or have theorized so much more about the past" (Stern, 2003, p. 52).

Stern describes therapy as a "moving along" process, the product of two minds working together. "Sloppiness" is inherent in the process and can lead to eruptions of *now moments*—new states coming into being or threatening to come into being. This refers to a mounting emotional charge in the consultation room when the usual way of being with each other is implicitly called into question. Such moments can be extremely positive when used well. Stern describes "now" moments as calling for a "moment of meeting," when the therapist is required to make a creative, authentic response to resolve the challenge of the moment, and when both treatment partners then share in the "now experience," knowing it implicitly. During these heightened moments of attentiveness and receptivity, something shifts in a dramatic way. This is actually quite similar to the prior description of psychotherapy as a relational practice, in which every moment can be described as a potential "now" moment of mindfulness.

Relational practitioners also focus on individual moments as the place of tangible change in therapy (Stiver, Rosen, Surrey, & Miller, 2001). These are moments when something new is jointly created, built on the interplay of the movements of both persons. These are creative, growth-fostering occasions; that is, the relationship is propelled in a healing and enlarging direction, leading to "movement-in-relationship" (p. 1).

Moments of tangible change are built on what has come before. They may be initiated by an action of the patient or the therapist, but their essence is that both move the relationship forward toward a new experience of connection in the present. In such moments, both patient and therapist open to a deeper connection to self, other, and the relational flow. They can be very simple moments, when an unexpected, spontaneous opening (a smile, a mutual gaze, a pause in saying good-bye) takes the relationship to a new place. The relationship grows; it can be said to enlarge and grow in spaciousness, aliveness, freedom, spontaneity, resilience, and creative power. The intentional direction of change remains focused on the patient's growth, but both participants create and are moved by the momentum of the new connection.

Clinical Example

Most change and movement in therapy occurs gradually, winding in and out, back and forth; but this was an exceptional moment—powerful, instantaneous, and unforgettable. Although rare, it is the kind of moment that keeps us alive and resilient, and gives depth and meaning to the difficult work of psychotherapy. For Kirk, the patient with whom I shared this moment, it was pivotal and transformational.

Kirk actually asked me many times to find a way to speak or write about his therapy. He wanted me to give his name and saw no reason for confidentiality. As a journalist and newspaper editor, he felt that something important like this ought to be reported publicly.

Kirk originally came to see me at the age of 46, in the context of the breakup of his second marriage. In the first session, he described himself as a "recovering white male. I've benefited from every privilege; I'm white, male, affluent, educated, and tall. I don't have any right to be here. You're wasting your time." He was sardonic, sarcastic, and skeptical about this first experience of therapy. Kirk was a very successful newspaper editor, political commentator, and activist. He was a rising star in his work but could not feel much gratification, joy, or sense of worth in it.

In his relationships with women and his three young children, he felt enormous shame and deficiency: a "true failure." He felt that "something is just missing." Kirk was chronically, not clinically, depressed; emotionally constricted; very judgmental; bristly; and quick to anger. He used his wry humor to maintain distance and control, and to circumvent any possibility of connection or surrendering to the relational moment where something new might happen.

Kirk felt responsible for the problems in his marriages. He knew he had great difficulty accepting vulnerability or empathizing with others, particularly women. He recognized his unwillingness to show any depth of feeling except anger or disdain. His incisive and biting humor, coupled with great intelligence, contributed to his success as a political analyst. At first quite hostile, he began to soften. The anger turned to teasing. We often laughed together, because this was his primary way of connecting.

In the first year of our work, I listened to his story and began to feel some empathy. He desperately wanted me to help him learn to be a father. We talked in the greatest detail about his children, in the process building attentiveness, interest, curiosity, and understanding. He tried to learn how to ask them questions that might open the relationships. Through this work, he began to touch on his own sadness and loneliness as a young boy, growing up in an isolated rural area as an only child. His mother had diabetes, and from the time he was 8, her health had deteriorated; she eventually became totally blind and bedridden. She died when he was 22. While she was alive, his mother never left the house. He remembered coming home from school daily and sitting with her, telling her all about his day. He felt he had to be "her light" and bring interesting news from the outside world. But they could never acknowledge together any of the difficult feelings of grief or loss. His father was a good and reliable caretaker but also could not express or share his emotions.

Even in talking about the past, Kirk continued to avoid any sustained relational connection that might evoke sadness. We wondered what it was like for his mother and imagined that she tried to protect him from her grief. He imagined that he, too, might have been trying to protect her, as well as himself, by staying away from his painful feelings.

Weekly sessions with Kirk were difficult and not something to which I looked forward. I often felt frustrated and exhausted, and had to work extremely hard to maintain any emotional connection or relational continuity. Although I knew some part of Kirk desired connection, his relational "dread" (Bergman, 1990) and his strategies of disconnection—humor, anger, sarcasm, and especially self-denigration—were well developed and very controlling. Kirk continued to keep gender issues present between us. "I'm just a man; what do you expect?" But he did begin to be curious about my work and about therapy. He began to understand that he was not simply "empty" and not simply cut off from feeling his sadness and loneliness. He was deeply ashamed and desperately afraid of being alone with these feelings. He had no experience or images of relationships in which feelings moved between and connected people. He did, however, have images of relationships in which feelings of vulnerability were associated with humiliation (part of his socialization in an all-boys private school) and also relationships in which any emotional exposure led to feelings of shame and deficiency.

One year into therapy, Kirk was at a routine medical appointment to investigate a chronic cough and was diagnosed with fast-growing metastatic lung cancer. He lived for 13 months after his diagnosis. Kirk called me between sessions to tell me the news. I remember that when he came in to my office the next time, I changed my seat and moved my chair to sit next to him. I was startled to observe how much more open and willing I was to be with him in the face of his illness and possible death. What a lesson about my own personal and professional strategies of disconnection!

At first, Kirk's bitterness, anger, sense of loss of his future, and, particularly, mourning the chance to grow were stunning. He struggled against his own depression and resignation. And then he began to work earnestly on trying to be open and present to complete the work he needed to do in all of his relationships. Often he felt empty, blocked, and helpless. I referred him for bodywork, to a men's cancer support group, and to a meditation group. We began to start our sessions with silence. He began to talk about his life as a mosaic of moments, with each one having its own completeness and beauty.

Halfway through his last year, as he became physically symptomatic, he asked me to work with him on a visualization exercise. He was trying to locate a safe, peaceful, place in himself where he could find refuge, a place to go in the face of fear and pain and, ultimately, as I look back, in the face of death. He was describing a scene close to his childhood home, actually very close to where I too grew up. I felt very connected to the scene that he described: sitting on a porch of an old abandoned house, looking out at a soft green meadow, listening to the sound of a brook in the background. I said to Kirk, probably with some frustration, but mostly with a kind of wistful sadness softened by acceptance: "I'm still not sure if you want me or anyone else there *with you.*"

Although I had been speaking to this particular scene, I realized this touched a core question for him.

He stopped and answered softly with feeling, "I'm still not sure either."

He was clear, direct, authentic, at one with his thoughts and words in the relationship.

We sat in silence. I sensed something happening. Finally, he looked at me with tears in his eyes and said, "I can feel how hard it is for you—when you're trying to be with me and I don't know what I want."

Another silence. I began to worry about whether I had revealed too much of myself. I felt concern about his focus on me. But the meaning for him was obviously significant, and I did not let my therapist strategies of disconnection—especially the trick of turning the focus back on him—get in the way of letting him be with his depth of feeling.

He began to talk about feeling something grow between us. He noticed that he could just stay with what was happening, without worrying about how it reflected on him, or how *he* had failed again. He described a feeling of love and compassion for the others in his life who struggled to relate to him.

Kirk then described feeling a sense of expansiveness and buoyancy, feeling a new energy surging through his body, particularly through his hands.

Our eyes met, and he held the gaze with me for a long time. I knew we each felt a deep appreciation for where we had been and where we were now. This "being" and "seeing" together reverberated between us as shared insight and understanding were born and realized in the relationship.

After that, Kirk described a growing capacity to be with others, which brought him great joy. He let friends be with him in new ways as he died, although some important relationships remained very difficult and unmovable.

Our relationship remained immensely important to both of us, and I saw him up to the day before his death. I promised him I would write about his experience—although I have not yet found a journalist interested in writing this story for his newspaper.

I have pondered the memory of this moment many, many times. It still remains a mystery, an experience of hard work *and* grace. As a therapist, the moment was as much about what I did as what I knew *not* to do. What mattered was where I was willing to go with him, and where we could go together. We came to this very alive "now" moment of healing connection, of mutual presence together. Clearly, this moment grew out of all the relational moments that came before. It grew out of both of our personal meditation practices. Its meaning was heightened by the closeness of death, which moved both of us beyond our protective and habitual patterns of disconnection. Facing death often helps us to let go of past wounds.

A connected relational moment like this contains and expresses in microcosm the *whole* relationship. Its texture was built on shared experience, pain, understanding, trust, and love. Through the work of weaving authentic and empathic connections between us, we also touched the larger cultural disconnection and the struggle for mutual relationship between men and women. Both of us were deeply aware of the larger gendered meaning of the moment: coming to this moment of mutuality through the particulars of who we are, therapist–patient, woman–man, I and Thou (Buber, 1970), touching deeply into our most fundamental human connection.

Reflections on the Healing Moment

In this moment, Kirk came to compassion and a radical acceptance of his truth: not knowing what he truly wanted and the profound ambivalence that plagued him in all his relationships. Paradoxically, through this acceptance and compassion for himself (arising in the relationship with mine for him) he was also able to experience compassion for me, and through this, compassion for other people, especially the women, in his life. Staying present in the relationship, not stopping this flow of mutual empathy, he came to a place of profound mutuality we may very rightly call love.

Such a moment has a vivid sense of grounding in the actuality and particularity of time, place, and persons. All my senses felt heightened. I can remember the exact slant of the sunshine coming through the window, the crimson color and texture of the couch, the reverberating feeling of tenderness and sadness, the slowing down of time, and the sense of coming to and opening deeply to this moment together. There was no doubt in either of us of the momentous nature of this shared moment, its beauty, its clarity, its power, and its preciousness, in the face of death.

Relational Insight

While psychotherapy focuses on the unique suffering of the patient, it is through our human capacity for mutual empathy and compassion that the deepest experiences of insight may arise. While the relational interplay in therapy usually occurs at a less profound level, there are moments when deep connection offers the opportunity for insight into the "three characteristics of existence" (the universality of suffering, the impermanent nature of all phenomena, and the absence of an essential, enduring essence to things). In relational practice, these truths or insights are mutually experienced in the moment of authentic connection. It can be said that these insights arise through and in relationships.

The truth of suffering that is an unavoidable aspect of human existence manifests particularly within our human relationships. Indeed, it is interpersonal suffering that commonly brings people to psychotherapy. Relationships are the place of *common ground*, the shared heart of compassion, or "suffering with." Opening to suffering opens the heart of compassion, which then invites kindness, care, joy, and equanimity. For Kirk, allowing his sadness to resonate between us and open directly to the suffering of others brought us both to a deep awareness of human suffering, in the present moment, with acceptance.

The truth of impermanence becomes evident as we open to the reality of being with another. Being fully present challenges us to let go of what has been. In the face of death, we are often more able to let go of our images of self and relationships, and to surrender to the living truth of the moment. Surrendering to the truth of impermanence, Kirk opened to the flow and pulse of life and relationship in a totally new way.

The truth of the emptiness of self and our profound interdependence is realized through the dropping or burning away of images and patterns of disconnection we hold so tightly. As Jordan (1997, p. 31) writes, this results in a "shift from a psychology of entities to a psychology of movement and dialogue. Self, other and the relationship are no longer clearly separated entities but mutually forming processes." In these moments, we may glimpse—or simply be in the truth of—our interconnectedness. As Kirk let go of fixed, self-centered images of himself as "deficient," he experienced the simplicity and power of authentic connection in the moment. I, too, had to let go of ideas of what would be healing and accept his ambivalence fully. This moment of surrender was deeply mutual.

Such profound moments—moments of connection that capture universal qualities of the human condition—may be the fruits of sustained practice in meditation and in relationship. They can occur every day when not obscured by inattention. It is my hope that they may encourage us to go more deeply and wholeheartedly into healing practices that lead to greater mindfulness and connection with our clients, ourselves, our profession, and our world.

CO-MEDITATION EXERCISES FOR THERAPISTS

Practicing mindfulness in relationship has been described as fundamental for healing in relational psychotherapy. The following are exercises that may deepen a therapist's capacity for mindfulness and sustained connection in relationship. They are best undertaken in groups in which the atmosphere is relaxed and intimate, and a group leader can provide guidance and support.

Breathing With

1. In dyads, one person is attending (the "therapist") and following the breathing of the other. The therapist attunes his or her breathing to the partner's breathing and silently follows in words, "breathing in . . . breathing out . . . breathing in . . . breathing out" for a number of breaths.

2. As the breath slows down, the therapist may simply say "Letting go" on the outbreath, or make the universal sound of letting go, "Ahhhhhhh" (5–10 minutes).

3. Sit in silence together.

4. Switch roles.

5. Discuss the experience together.

6. Discuss in the large group.

Adapted from Bastis (2000).

Breathing Together

1. Sitting face to face with a partner at a comfortable distance, both partners close their eyes and begin to focus on their own breathing (5 minutes).

2. Then say, "Open your eyes and, staying attuned to your breath, slowly open the field of attention to include the presence of the other, with a soft, respectful focus on their embodied breathing. Allow the flow of attention to self and other to be as it is. It may alternate or may at times become part of an enlarged field of attention."

3. "Notice all the thoughts and feelings that arise, but stay with the actuality of being and breathing together in this moment" (5–10 minutes).

4. Discuss this experience together.

5. Discuss in the large group.

Co-Meditation on the Flow of Connection and Disconnection

1. Sitting face to face with a partner at a comfortable distance, both partners close their eyes and begin to focus on their own breathing (5 minutes).

2. "Open your eyes and stay anchored in the breath, and make soft and respectful eye contact for a few minutes" (3–10 minutes, depending on the leader's assessment of the comfort level in the group). "When the eyes move away, gently return to the shared gaze."

3. "Expand the field of attention to the flow of connection and disconnection, especially uneasiness, self-consciousness, or emotional reactions. Allow these feelings to simply occur as you continue to hold your gaze" (3–5 minutes).

4. "Without words, acknowledge your partner for sharing this time with you."

5. "Gently release your open eye focus and close your eyes."

6. "Attend to your own breathing for five minutes."

7. Discuss this exercise together.

8. Discuss in the large group.

Learning to See Each Other

1. This exercise builds upon the prior exercises. At step 4 above, after holding the gaze, the leader introduces the instruction.

2. "Look into your partner's eyes and allow the words to form in your heart: 'May you be happy.' 'May you be free from suffering.' 'May you touch the deepest joys of life.' 'May you dwell in peace.' 'Notice what it feels like to see and to be seen, to send and to receive.' "

3. "Without words, honor your partner and acknowledge him or her for sharing this moment with you."

4. Discuss the exercise together.

5. Discuss in the large group.

Adapted from Macy and Brown (1998).

Deep Listening and Authentic Speaking

1. This is an exercise to practice informally throughout a meeting of colleagues. Establish a common intention with the group participants to practice deep listening and authentic speaking, even when not participating in exercises.

2. "While others are speaking, practice letting go of your own thoughts, judgments and analyzing, and return to listening receptively. Let your listening be wholehearted and attentive. Bring mindfulness to the comings and goings of your own attention."

3. "Speak from the heart without preparing or rehearsing. Allow the words to be connected to the stream of the unfolding present moment. Speak slowly enough to stay connected to your body and heart."

4. "Pause to listen to yourself and others. With each pause, relax your body and mind. Pause when another is done speaking. After pausing, ask yourself, 'What is true now? What am I feeling? What might this person be experiencing?' The inquiry is both active and receptive. Use this cycle of pausing, relaxing the body and mind, and directing attention to the experience of the contact with the other, whenever you remember to, as a means to return to full presence."

5. "Practice compassion for yourself and others when difficulty inevitably arises in staying present at this level."

6. After a large group discussion, ask people to notice what they have learned about deep listening and authentic speaking.

Adapted from Brach (2003).

PART III

Clinical Applications

CHAPTER 6

Teaching Mindfulness
in Therapy

CHRISTOPHER K. GERMER

Previous authors have discussed how the therapist's mindful-ness practice may enhance the therapy relationship. Now I explore how to teach mindfulness exercises in psychotherapy.

The bulk of the chapter focuses on mindfulness practiced in every-day life. Any person can disengage from automatic thinking by watching a breath for a full inhalation and exhalation, or can become more aware of inner experience by stopping activity for a few minutes and asking, "What am I feeling? What is occurring at this moment?" In contrast, formal mindfulness meditation (perhaps 45 minutes daily) can be a tough challenge for patients who do not come to therapy specifically for mindfulness training. Whereas only 39% of patients in a mindfulness-based stress reduction (MBSR) program practiced sitting meditation regularly or sporadically after 3 years, 83% still used breath awareness, at least sometimes, in their daily lives (Miller, Fletcher, & Kabat-Zinn, 1995). Informal, everyday mindfulness exercises are most easily inte-grated into psychotherapy.

BEGINNING TO PRACTICE

Remembering to *Be*

Slowing down is difficult in our fast-paced society. We are *doing* activities most of our waking hours, striving to reach one goal or another. The simple instruction to slow down and notice what is occurring in the present moment involves *being* rather than doing. We often resist slowing down, or being, because we fear we will not accomplish our tasks for the day. Also, some people do not want to stop striving, because it threatens to open the door to uninvited thoughts, memories, or unfinished emotional business that constant activity keeps out of awareness.

While striving may allow us to acquire physical comforts, living in the present enables us to live more fully. Everyone feels stress to one degree or another. The conditions of our lives never seem quite right, because our inner experience of them is unsatisfactory. We find ourselves either running headlong toward the future for relief or dwelling in the past, or both. A changed relationship to our experience is needed to find lasting peace.

Getting Motivated

Before beginning mindfulness practice, the patient must understand its purpose and be willing to make it a priority. Therapy usually starts at a time of "creative hopelessness" (Hayes, Strosahl, & Wilson, 1999), in which the futility of striving is becoming evident. For example, in the case of panic disorder, a patient may come to realize that fighting panic makes it worse. Motivational interviewing is usually necessary at the outset of treatment. Is the patient willing to suspend feeling calmer— perhaps even initially feeling *worse*, while exploring his or her experience more intimately—to eventually feel better? Can the patient entertain the notion that an ingrained habit of tightening up to reduce discomfort is the root of his or her problem? Is the patient willing to explore whether the feelings pass more easily if allowed to be just as they are? Openness to such ideas is needed before mindfulness practice can begin.

Practicing

A paradox of mindfulness practice is that we never get it right, and we never get it wrong. The notion of "practicing" suggests that we can steadily improve, but lifelong repetition is part of practice. A "skill" implies that we can do it well, perhaps with little need for additional practice. Although our awareness can become more precise and continuous, when we think we have achieved true mindfulness, we have probably become attached to that pleasing thought and are advised, in that moment, to practice more. Like recovery from alcoholism, practicing mindfulness is a lifelong endeavor, since the propensity to get caught in conditioned thought is ever-present. Mindfulness practice may help catch a "lapse" early, before it becomes a full "relapse" (Breslin, Zack, & McMain, 2002; Witkiewitz & Marlatt, 2004).

Therapist Credentials

This is currently a controversial subject, because mindfulness practice is being discovered by a wide range of clinicians. In the Buddhist tradition, many years of practice are required before a person is ready to teach mindfulness. The aspiring teacher needs wisdom and personal experience to help another meditator overcome the varied obstacles in the path of mindful awareness.

Many people believe that the need for personal, practical experience with mindfulness is not very important, if we are teaching mindfulness within the context of psychotherapy. A possible rule of thumb is that we need to have experienced what we teach. Along those lines, dialectical behavior therapy (DBT) trainees are not required to practice sitting meditation, since it is not part of the DBT program. Mindfulness-based cognitive therapy (MBCT) and MBSR therapists, in contrast, are encouraged to meditate, because those programs may include 30–45 minutes of daily sitting meditation.

For mindfulness to have a pervasive influence on the therapist's therapeutic approach—to shape understanding, demeanor, words, and recommendations—the therapist probably has to have spent a lot of time in formal meditation practice. The therapist will have learned to work, alongside a skilled teacher, with the obstacles to mindfulness that inevitably arise during intensive practice. Such committed practice generally leads to firsthand understanding of mind described in Buddhist psychology and philosophy, ("why" we do this, "how" it works, "what" this may mean, etc.). The therapist develops great faith in being able to use mindfulness to work with any experience. This faith keeps the therapist calm during difficult times and naturally guides interventions.

On the other hand, to introduce mindfulness-based techniques such as watching the breath or labeling emotions into therapy, we need only to have had suitable instruction and supervision and to have tried these techniques ourselves. In summary, the question about the need for therapists to practice mindfulness may depend on how much mindfulness we intend to bring into therapy. Resources for meditation training are given in Appendix A.

KEY ELEMENTS OF MINDFULNESS TECHNIQUES

There are countless mindfulness strategies that can be designed to fit the unique needs of a given patient or practitioner. We can cultivate mindfulness by sitting quietly, washing the dishes, doing psychotherapy; just about any activity can be done mindfully. The MBSR program, for example, cultivates mindfulness while lying down, sitting, doing yoga exercises, walking, standing, and eating. What do mindfulness exercises have in common? They cultivate the three key interdependent elements of mindfulness: (1) *awareness,* (2) *of present experience,* (3) *with acceptance.*

Awareness

After establishing the intention to be mindfully aware, the typical components found in most techniques are (1) *stop,* (2) *observe,* and (3) *return.*

Stop

Stopping our activity is a way of preparing for mindful awareness. Our attention is normally directed by our efforts to achieve desired goals and to avoid unpleasant experiences. We can, however, disengage from the accompanying automatic trains of thought by stopping our automatic behaviors. For example, we can stop arguing on the telephone by taking a deep, conscious breath. Sometimes our lives are stopped by external events, such as a snowstorm, an illness, or a delayed train. Barring these events, we usually need a strong intention to create a sufficient momentary interruption for mindfulness to take root.

We may also slow down to enhance mindfulness. Any activity done more slowly can be observed in greater detail. We can explore the wonder of walking, if we do it slowly; we can actually taste a raisin, if we eat it unhurriedly. Our attention stabilizes when it is not jumping from one object to another—when there is less to attend to in each moment. A slow walk allows us to notice details that we cannot see when running down a mountain path. The luxury of eating a meal slowly allows us to taste every morsel. Even our own speech can distract us throughout the day. Remaining silent significantly restricts the amount of information we need to monitor and thereby helps to focus the mind. If we further restrict the flow of sensory information by sitting still and closing our eyes, we create an environment in which we can begin to allow our minds to settle.

Observe

In mindfulness practice, we are not actually "observing" our experience in an objective, detached manner. Rather, we are "calmly abiding" with it as "participant observers."

We need to have an object of focus for our attention. For example, if I am stressing about a fight I just had with my boss, it usually does not work just to tell myself, "Don't worry, your boss still likes you." It is more effective to turn attention away from ruminations altogether by focusing attention on a particular object. The most common object of attention in mindfulness exercises is the breath, but any sensory experience can serve this purpose. We can feel the pressure of our buttocks on the chair, notice the weight of a hand resting in the lap, or listen to ambient sounds in our environment. Intentionally anchoring our attention like this helps us to *find* our attention. This is the "concentration" part of mindfulness practice.

As we become more aware of where our attention is located, we can begin to note sensations, thoughts, and feelings that naturally arise within us. This is what distinguishes mindfulness from concentration practice. We are not "telling" attention where to go; we are observing where it goes naturally. For example, we may notice that the heart is pounding, that it is raining outside, that we forgot to make dinner reservations, and so forth. Each mental event is there to be experienced without judging, analyzing, indulging, or suppressing. We simply want to note what takes our attention away from the breath (or other chosen object of focus). This can be facilitated, particularly in the beginning, by *labeling* experience, such as "thinking," "feeling," "fear," "anger," and so on. With practice, it becomes easier to notice moment-to-moment experience without naming it.

Return

When we notice that we have become distracted or absorbed in a thought, when we "wake up," we can make a mental note of what captured our attention, gently *return awareness* to its original focal object, and then watch where the mind wanders next. Waking up is a moment of mindfulness. If we are immersed in daily activity, we may want to slow down or stop again. If we are quiet, such as in sitting meditation, we obviously do not need to stop activity; we calmly abide with either the primary object of focus or another mental event, depending on how stable our attention is and what is arising within us. Whenever necessary, we can return to the focal object to "find" and anchor our attention.

Present Moment

Sometimes we are so absorbed in our activities that to stop and "be mindful" is actually counterproductive. Imagine the awkwardness of "stopping" to be mindful while having the best ski run of your life on a double-diamond slope? One goal of the whole mindfulness enterprise is to be unified with our activities. In such moments, we are alert, energetic, joyful, creative, calm, concentrated—in the "flow" of the present moment (Csikszentmihalyi, 1991). Intentional mindfulness practice is only necessary when we hit an obstacle in the flow of our awareness.

Even if we are not in a "flow" moment, sometimes we need to focus on our goals to avoid making errors. For example, if we are feeling angry while operating heavy machinery, we may not have the luxury of attending to our emotion. In that situation, the prescription for mindfulness is to pour our attention completely, without reservation, into the most important task at hand—operating the machinery. Hence, *wise* direction of attention to an activity in the present moment is a core mindfulness exercise.

All mindfulness exercises bring attention to the present. The breath or some other focal object of awareness is always available in the present moment, and the distractions that pull our attention away likewise occur in the here and now. Everything happens in the present. When our attention is hijacked by strong sensation or feeling, we lose the moment. That does not mean that the present is actually lost; our *experience* of the present is lost. The only reason to return to the breath or another object is to *find* our attention again, to collect it by focusing on something tangible. Mindfulness practice is therefore training attention to focus on present experience.

When attention is strong, we can simply do what we are doing, moment to moment. If we are peeling an orange, we may notice the stickiness of the juice, the smell of the orange oil, and a host of other sensations. If the mind wanders, the instruction is, "Bring your attention back here!" Sometimes we continue to think about other things. The question is then, "Do you know where your attention is now?" In summary, any instructions that bring the practitioner back to awareness of the present moment of experience—where attention is located—is a mindfulness exercise.

Acceptance

The present moment is colored by *how* we receive it—by our attitude. Acceptance means to receive our experience without judgment or preference, with curiosity and kindness. Full awareness of the present moment depends enormously on wholehearted acceptance of our experience. Sadly, our acceptance, and hence our awareness, is always incomplete; we never stop judging.

Acceptance is soft, gentle, and relaxed. It can be cultivated. Sometimes a patient can be successfully encouraged to "relax into" or "soften into" an experience to cultivate acceptance. Another instruction is to "breath into" aversive experiences, such as physical pain. Goldstein (1993) suggests using a mantra to cultivate a "soft and spacious mind," such as "Its okay, just let me feel this," or "Let it be" (pp. 39–40). We can also diminish the judging habit by practicing lovingkindness exercises presented in Chapters 3 and 4.

DESIGNING EXERCISES FOR PATIENTS

The reader may have noticed how easy it is to design a mindfulness exercise: Simply prescribe momentary breaks from activities, anchor attention in the breath or some other object of awareness, and notice the sensations, thoughts, and feelings that arise. This can be done any time. It can be challenging, however, to develop exercises that both fit a patient's needs and that he or she will actually practice. Fortunately, exercises need not be finished or fixed upon delivery; they can be reshaped as therapy progresses.

The exercises listed in Table 6.1 can be adapted for use in psychotherapy. The techniques were selected to be representative of different ways that mindfulness exercises are traditionally constructed and presented. The list is by no means exhaustive. The exercises are organized according to the element of mindfulness that predominates in each one. For example, "mindfulness of fear" is a skill that emphasizes *awareness*, "mindful eating" favors *present experience*, and "lovingkindness" exercises foster *acceptance*. However, each exercise includes all three elements of mindfulness.

The reader is encouraged to consult the original sources for a full description, usually including guided meditations, of each exercise. Similar exercises are included in chapters throughout this book and in resource materials found in Appendix A.

Selecting Exercises

At this point, choosing or adapting exercises for patients is more art than science. The technique has to fit in the patient's life. The therapist might identify experiences the patient is avoiding, rejecting, or disregarding, such as feelings of sadness, fear, or anger; or unwanted physical pain

TABLE 6.1. Mindfulness Exercises

Awareness	Present experience	Acceptance
Breath	*Awareness*	Lovingkindness: (8) 211–215; (6) 162–169
Breath: (7) 150–151; (4) 8–9	Stopping: (1) 71	
Breath and body: (7) 164–165	Wonderful moment: (4) 9–10	Trance of unworthiness: (1) 22–23
Breathing space: (7) 174	Bell of mindfulness: (4) 18–20	Power of yes: (1) 87–88
Conscious breathing: (4) 8–9	This is it: (6) 14–16	Compassion: (1) 243–245; (3) 93–94
Counting breaths: (2) 53–55	*Action*	Generosity: (6) 61–64
	All activities: (2) 166–168; (6) 201–203	Half-smile: (1) 91–92; (3) 79–80
Other objects	Walking: (7) 179–180; (8) 173–176; (2) 159–162	Parents: (4) 70–73
Body scan: (7) 112–113	Considered action: (7) 286–287	
Embodied presence: (1) 123–125	Washing: (3) 85–86	*Visualization*
Sound: (8) 196–197	Eating: (8) 183–185; (4) 23–26	Mountain meditation: (6) 135–140
Sounds and thoughts: (7) 196–197	Raisin eating: (7) 103–104	Lake meditation: (6) 141–144
Thoughts and feelings: (5) 73–74	Driving: (4) 31–34	Pebble sinking to rest: (3) 87
	Yoga: (5) 103–105	
Posture		
Sitting (Vipassana): (8) 166–120; (1) 46–48; (5) 58		
Standing: (6) 149–150.		
Lying down: (6) 151–156		
Feeling		
Fear: (1) 195–197		
Pain: (1) 126–127		
Anger: (4) 56–59		
Wanting: (1) 157–158		
Longing: (1) 159–160		

Note. Sources: (1) Brach (2003); (2) Gunaratana (2002); (3) Hanh (1976); (4) Hanh (1992); (5) Kabat-Zinn (1990); (6) Kabat-Zinn (1994); (7) Segal, Williams, and Teasdale (2002); (8) Smith (1998).

or arousal. Alternatively, the focus could be problematic thoughts, such as self-criticism or catastrophic ideation; or compulsive problematic behaviors, such as rejecting help or overworking. A mindfulness exercise can be created that brings the patient into a closer, more aware relationship to any experience. The technique should be negotiated with the patient and progress monitored, and misunderstandings that cause the patient to discontinue practice should be addressed. To illustrate, four examples of mindfulness exercises applied to clinical conditions are presented here. Others can be found throughout the following chapters.

Three-Minute Breathing Space

Neil was a 25-year-old man with a history of alcohol abuse. It was becoming obvious to him that he would never leave his parents' home and realize his life goals if he did not quit drinking. Most of his friends were also alcoholics, and he automatically stopped at the package store on the way home from work to pick up the evening's supplies. He sporadically attended Alcoholics Anonymous, but this was not changing his behavior.

We decided that a Three-Minute Breathing Space (Segal, Williams, & Teasdale, 2002) might help him discover the feelings that were behind his urge to drink. Neil agreed to try the exercise for a few minutes whenever he felt upset, up to five times per day.

Three-Minute Breathing Space

1. AWARENESS

   Bring yourself into the present moment by deliberately adopting an erect and dignified posture. If possible, close your eyes. Then ask:

   "What is my experience right now . . . in thoughts . . . in feeling . . . and in bodily sensations?"

   Acknowledge and register your experience, even if it is unwanted.

2. GATHERING

   Then, gently redirect full attention to breathing, to each inbreath and to each outbreath as they follow, one after the other:

   Your breath can function as an anchor to bring you into the present and help you tune into a state of awareness and stillness.

3. EXPANDING

   Expand the field of your awareness around your breathing, so that it includes a sense of the body as a whole, your posture, and facial expression.

From Segal, Williams, and Teasdale (2002, p. 184). Copyright 2002 by The Guilford Press. Reprinted by permission.

Neil noticed during the breathing space that when his boss criticized him, he would automatically plan to get a drink after work. He recognized that he was so conditioned that merely *thinking* of drinking made him feel better when he was stressed out. Neil further realized that feelings of anger or frustration would diminish somewhat if he simply let them come and go. He learned to "urge surf" (Marlatt, 2002). Neil also started to plan alternative ways of managing his distressing feelings the moment they arose, such as mountain biking after work. Eventually, Neil enrolled in college in a different city to find new friends and start building a career.

Measurement of Emotion

Liza, a middle-aged nurse with a severe abuse history, suffered from recurrent depression, resulting in multiple hospitalizations. When concerns about her performance were raised at work, she would often decompensate. She would quit her medications, lose her appetite, withdraw socially, and hear command hallucinations to kill herself. Despite good job performance overall, Liza was terrified of being fired. It appeared that fear of losing her job was more disabling than depression per se, because it meant to Liza that she was a worthless person. We created a Terror Alert Scale, based on the one used by the U.S. Department of Homeland Security, to break the spell of Liza's fear. She rated her fear as red (severe), orange (high), yellow (elevated), and green (low). Liza's mindfulness task was to report her fear level whenever she found herself scared for some reason. She used the scale 8–15 times per day in the first week.

After 1 month of working with the Terror Alert Scale, Liza could readily identify her fear as it arose. She became more accepting of her fear, and this averted the cascade of events that formerly had led to hospitalization. We discussed how she generally feels more fear than the average person, perhaps because her brain was conditioned to fear in childhood, and that fear is not necessarily a reflection of actual danger. Liza's depression subsided as her pervasive fear came increasingly into mindful awareness. The rating scale added precision and interest to her efforts to become aware of her difficult emotion and label it.

Mountain Meditation

Maria was a 43-year-old mother of an adult son with paranoid schizophrenia and substance abuse. Her son was living at home, and the stress of caring for him caused Maria to lose her job and become clinically depressed. She broke out in hives when her son went through a difficult period.

Medication did not improve Maria's ability to weather the storms of her son's mental illness. We decided that she could benefit from a mindful approach to the catastrophe of having a psychotic son living at home. Maria was given a compact disc of Jon Kabat-Zinn's (2002c) mountain meditation. Maria loved nature, and she liked the image of being like an immovable mountain, strong and enduring as harsh weather comes and goes. Maria found 20 minutes per day to sit with the stillness of a mountain in the face of adversity. She was amazed to find stillness within herself despite her son's behavior. Whenever she felt upset during the day, she would "remember the mountain." Maria's hives substantially diminished over a few weeks.

Awareness of Intention

Joel, a 30-year-old engineer with a history of obsessive–compulsive disorder (OCD), was renovating his home and often found himself on the roof of the house. He became terrified that he might jump, which forced him to discontinue the project.

His fear appeared to be an OCD symptom exacerbated by having seen his father plummet from a roof 20 years earlier. Joel was confusing his fear of falling with an *intention* to jump. The mindfulness exercise we devised was to recognize how often in the day he genuinely wanted to jump from the roof. The following week, he announced that that number was zero, and he starting saying to himself, "It's just fear—I don't actually *want* to do it." Joel was able to continue his renovation project without additional medication or psychotherapy. He learned to discern between his wishes and his fears, resulting in greater emotional self-control.

These examples demonstrate the versatility of mindfulness-building techniques. What exercises are our patients most likely to practice between therapy sessions? A student once asked his meditation teacher, Thich Nhat Hanh, how to be more mindful during the day. "Do you want to know my secret?" his teacher asked with a smile. "I try to find a way to do things that is most pleasurable. There are many ways to perform a given task—but the one that holds my attention best is the one that is most pleasant" (cited in Murphy, 2002, p. 85). Since the number of mindfulness techniques is vast and can be as simple as attending to whatever is occurring in the present moment, therapists can collaborate with patients to find exercises that are both easy and pleasant to implement.

Multicomponent Treatment Programs

The four main treatment programs that deliberately attempt to teach mindfulness are MBSR (Kabat-Zinn, 1990); MBCT (Segal, Williams, et al., 2002); DBT (Linehan, 1993a, 1993b); and acceptance and commitment therapy (ACT; Hayes, Strosahl, et al., 1999; Hayes et al., 2005). These programs are all empirically validated. The reader is referred to Appendix A for resources related to these programs, especially websites, because the research literature is expanding so rapidly.

Each program has a different origin in terms of the populations treated and the theoretical inspiration. For example, MBSR was started by Jon Kabat-Zinn for treating chronically ill patients at a university hospital, MBCT was developed to alleviate chronic depression using the MBSR model, DBT was conceived to help patients with borderline personality disorder who have difficulty regulating emotions, and ACT arose out of behavior analysis as it related to the contextual worldview (see Chapter 1) and the use of language. The MBSR, MBCT, and DBT programs were all inspired by mindfulness meditation. Although MBSR and MBCT are organized around the central notion of mindfulness, DBT and ACT each have a substantial mindfulness component as well. In practice, the degree of mindfulness in the treatment might depend more on the persons involved than on the program, but that remains an empirical question.

The MBSR and MBCT programs are in a group format; typically eight weekly 2.5-hour sessions. MBSR adds a daylong mindfulness intensive session at the end of the program. DBT is primarily weekly individual therapy, with specific kinds of telephone contacts allowed between sessions, as well as weekly, 2.5-hour DBT skills training group sessions. DBT clinicians are in regular therapist consultation groups for mutual support in the method. ACT may be implemented in either an individual or group format. All the multicomponent treatment programs include homework. MBSR requires 45 minutes per day, 6 days per week of mindfulness practice. Each program has a plethora of interesting skills to encourage mindfulness, especially the quality of acceptance within mindfulness.

Mindfulness-Based Stress Reduction

All the skills taught in the MBSR program are specifically to cultivate mindfulness. Nonspecific treatment factors may be involved, such as group support, but the focus of MBSR on mindfulness is unique. The main practices taught are sitting meditation (formal mindfulness meditation) and mindful yoga. The program also includes a body scan meditation, in which patients lie down and observe sensations throughout the body, and mindfulness in everyday life, including walking, standing, and eating.

Mindfulness-Based Cognitive Therapy

MBCT is a manualized treatment that teaches the mindfulness practices of MBSR, without the yoga, and with the Three-Minute Breathing Space (discussed earlier) as a core skill. MBCT adds a cognitive therapy component of discovering one's thoughts and feelings. The mindfulness aspect in MBCT is learning to see that "thoughts are not facts" and that we can let them come and go, rather than trying to argue them out of existence, as we might do in traditional CBT.

Dialectical Behavior Therapy

Mindfulness skills in DBT (module 1) are considered core skills for success in the other three modules: interpersonal effectiveness, emotion regulation, and distress tolerance. Mindfulness skills are taught over two or three group sessions and reviewed again when new modules are introduced. Many skills in DBT are derived from the Zen tradition and the practices of Thich Nhat Hanh (1976). Skills related to mindfulness practice within all four modules include counting the breath; adopting a serene, half-smile; focusing awareness on present activity; labeling feelings; letting thoughts slip in and out (practicing "Teflon-mind"); practicing nonjudgment; doing one thing at a time; practicing radical acceptance of feelings; and imagining that the mind is like a big sky, where thoughts and feelings pass by like clouds. The focus of DBT is on helping patients live a more successful life, particularly interpersonally, in spite of how they may feel.

Acceptance and Commitment Therapy

There are well over 100 ACT skills to choose from, and they are individualized for each patient. Many of the "techniques" of ACT are teaching metaphors, such as the Chinese Handcuffs Metaphor (Hayes, Strosahl, et al., 1999, p. 123): The more you pull, the tighter they become. The main components of ACT are (1) creative helplessness (the futility of current efforts to feel better), (2) cognitive diffusion (our thoughts are just thoughts, not what we interpret them to be), (3) acceptance (allow experience to be what it is while effectively engaged), (4) self as context (identify with the observer of thoughts), and (5) valuing (rededicate one's life to what gives life meaning) (Gifford, Hayes, & Strosahl, 2004).

ACT techniques correspond to these general components. Experiential exercises that develop mindfulness include saying your thoughts very, very slowly, or singing your thoughts; saying "I am having a *thought that* . . . (I am stupid)," rather than "I am stupid!"; writing difficult thoughts on 3″ × 5″ cards and carrying them around; and doing something different and paying attention to what happens. Acceptance exercises include the Serenity Prayer ("change what we can, accept what we can't change"); journaling about painful events; and sitting eye-to-eye with another person, allowing the experience just to happen. The focus of ACT is to let experience come and go while pursuing a meaningful life.

The clinician is encouraged to explore the four multicomponent treatment programs for how well they may apply to specific patients and conditions. For example, DBT skill training may be the most powerful mindfulness-based approach to managing self-destructive behavior or highly reactive couples. MBSR may be especially effective with stress-related disorders. ACT, with its "valued life" component, may be uniquely helpful to patients trying to overcome substance abuse.

Similarly, different psychological processes *within* mindfulness practice may apply better to some conditions than others. The practice of "focusing on a single object" may be the best method for patients to interrupt ruminative thinking in depression and panic, "opening the field of awareness" in meditation could help broaden and enrich the lives of chronic pain patients, and the "self-acceptance" component of mindfulness practice may specifically counteract the influence of a patient's invalidating family of origin. These kinds of questions are fertile ground for future research.

Working with Trauma

Since an estimated 50% of adults in the United States have had a traumatic experience (Kessler, Sonnega, Bromet, Hughes, & Nelson, 1995), one of the compelling questions at the interface of mindfulness practice and psychotherapy is how to work with trauma. Bringing awareness to traumatic experience can either decrease or increase suffering. Recent evidence suggests that the exposure of critical stress debriefing may be harmful, because some people initially need to distance themselves from traumatic events (Ehlers et al., 2003; Groopman, 2004). Also, Teasdale and colleagues (Ma & Teasdale, 2004; Teasdale et al., 2000) found that a group of depressed patients with two previous episodes of depression had a nonsignificantly *greater* tendency than the more chronic patients to relapse after their mindfulness-based treatment, suggesting that MBCT did not help these particular patients manage stressful life events. While this study did not deal with trauma per se, it alerts us to the idea that one method cannot be applied as a panacea.

Prescription of mindfulness practices should be guided by clinical judgment. Timing and safety are important. When our attention is overwhelmed by traumatic memories and destabilized, mindful exposure loses its usefulness. It is more helpful to direct our attention *away* from the trauma, until attention is stabilized, and then try again. In some instances, supportive psychotherapy to help the patient establish resilience and ego strength may be a necessary precursor to mindfulness practice.

When dealing with strong emotions, *external* sensory awareness is an effective way to gather our attention and be less overwhelmed. For example, an aggressive, mentally retarded adult learned to shift his attention from an anger-producing situation to the soles of his feet, which eventually enabled him to transition to the community (Singh, Wahler, Adkins, & Myers, 2003). Feeling the earth under our feet or a cool breeze on the cheek can return us to the present moment.

Internal focus generally brings patients closer to traumatic memories and emotions. This can be introduced incrementally when a patient is ready. The patient can mindfully attend to inner experiences associated with trauma, until they threaten to disrupt attention. When the experience becomes too intense, the patient can take refuge in the breath or a comfortable place in the body. If still feeling overwhelmed, the patient can focus attention on the boundary of the body with the world—touch sensations. External awareness is available for safety. Once stability returns, the patient can gently return attention to what is occurring within. Sometimes simply labeling experiences ("hot skin," "tight stomach," "intense fear") provides enough distance from traumatic material, without losing the healing power of attention. A mindfulness-based therapist can work flexibly with focused and open awareness, directed both internally and externally, to create a new relationship to traumatic memories (Miller, 1993; Urbanowski & Miller, 1996).

Psychoactive medication may be necessary when a patient is overwhelmed with affect. The debate about meditation versus medication hinges upon attention. If a patient cannot regulate his or her attention sufficiently to perform activities of daily life—cannot concentrate adequately—then medication may be indicated.

The Special Case of Formal Meditation

Most clinicians will probably introduce informal, everyday mindfulness exercises into psychotherapy more often than they will suggest formal meditation practice. Nonetheless, for some patients, formal meditation can serve as a useful adjunct to psychotherapy. A large body of psychological literature on the subject, beginning in the 1970s, indicates that meditation can be effectively used as an autonomic self-regulation strategy, or to promote self-awareness (Bogart, 1991; Burnard, 1987; Craven, 1989; Deatherage, 1975; Delmonte, 1986, 1988; Engler, 1986; Epstein & Lieff, 1981; Kutz et al., 1985; Kutz, Borysenko, & Benson, 1985; Miller, 1993; Shapiro, 1992; Smith, 1975; Urbanowski & Miller, 1996; VanderKooi, 1997).

Which patients should be encouraged to meditate? Meditation requires regular practice to be effective. Unfortunately, patients often do not stick with it. Delmonte (1988) found that among outpatients who learned to practice concentration meditation for 10–20 minutes twice daily, 54% stopped after 24 months. Those who were extroverted and less neurotic were more likely to continue. Patients were more likely to persevere than nonpatients, suggesting that distress or expectation of benefit enhances motivation. This may help to explain why 75% of chronic pain patients in an MBSR program still practiced meditation up to 4 years later (Kabat-Zinn, Lipworth, Burney, & Sellers, 1987). Therapists should therefore evaluate a patient's motivation.

Boredom and the resulting wish to quit are common obstacles at the beginning of meditation practice. When these arise, patients are instructed to make "boredom" or "wanting to quit" the object of awareness. Paradoxically, this can help make the practice more interesting. Another obstacle is self-judgment—"I am not doing this right." Self-judgment can also be made an object of awareness, perhaps by counting how many times in a given period of time self-judging thoughts appear.

Another important variable when considering formal meditation for a patient is ego strength, or emotional resilience. Meditation practice can lead to adverse effects. Patients who decompensate when cognitive controls are loosened should generally not do formal sitting meditation. For example, destabilizing traumatic memories, including body memories, may rise to the surface, or mild states of depersonalization could trigger panic attacks. In a study by Shapiro (1992), at least one adverse effect was reported by 62.9% of long-term mindfulness meditators either before or after a meditation retreat. Many of these effects were merely expectable negative mind states, such as irritability, hypersensitivity to city life, or awareness of negative personal qualities. Profound adverse effects were, however, reported by two of the 27 individuals studied (7.4%). These included depression, confusion, and severe shaking. Interestingly, 88% of the meditators in the study reported *positive* effects of meditation before the retreat, and among the 13 people who completed a 3-month follow-up, 12 (92%) listed positive effects. A few participants felt the negative effects had a positive aspect, such as helping them to learn patience. One meditator said that "in order to reach a deeper stability, one becomes fundamentally destabilized" (Shapiro, 1992, p. 65).

A competent meditation teacher can help distinguish between temporary discomfort and fragmentation of the sense of self, which may manifest as dissociation, grandiosity, terror, or delusions. Some patients assume that they need more meditation to get through such difficult experiences (a recommendation occasionally supported by meditation teachers with limited psychological understanding). This can cause further deterioration. Meditators who experience personality fragmentation should discontinue formal meditation and, perhaps, switch attentional training to externally focused activities, such as mindful physical exercise, *hatha* yoga, or work.

People with fragile personalities *may* benefit from sitting meditation to develop attentional stability or safe exposure to inner experience, but the period of meditation should be time-limited—perhaps as short as a few minutes (Schmidt & Miller, 2004). It is helpful to apprise patients about the possibility of painful memories surfacing, particularly during intensive mindfulness meditation.

What type of meditation should be suggested? Concentration stabilizes attention and creates calmness, whereas open awareness generates insight into how the mind works and tends to uncover repressed mental content. Concentration meditation alone is generally better suited to fostering short-term relaxation, since mindful awareness of disturbing, distracting thoughts can be anything but relaxing.

Nonetheless, as discussed earlier, mindfulness meditation may be a useful adjunct to psychotherapy, and has the potential to lead to profound awareness and freedom extending beyond the symptom relief generally sought in psychotherapy. An experienced mindfulness meditation teacher, Joseph Goldstein, writes:

> On a more subtle level, as we refine the quality of our mindfulness, we begin to recognize that which knows the pain; we explore *the nature of consciousness itself.* One of the most startling aspects of meditation practice is that whatever the object of our attention might be, the nature of knowing—that open, empty, aware nature of the mind—remains the same. It is completely unaffected by what is known. (2004, p. 12; emphasis added)

Meditation may be recommended at the end of therapy both to support the gains made in psychotherapy and to promote deeper self-exploration.

CHAPTER 7

Depression

Turning toward Life

STEPHANIE P. MORGAN

> . . . to live life as if each moment is important, as if each
> moment counted and could be worked with, even if it is a
> moment of pain, sadness, despair, or fear.
> —JON KABAT-ZINN (1990, p. 11)

"It's a desert—desolate, lifeless. I can't even see you on the horizon. The thing is, I'm not fully here either." This patient's words capture the pain, isolation, and withdrawal that are central elements of depressive experience. Depression involves turning away from experience to avoid emotional pain. This withdrawal deprives the depressed person of the life that can only be found in direct experience. Mindfulness is the practice of turning *toward* the experience at hand, and thereby challenges the depressive stance. In this chapter, I look at how mindfulness can bring the therapist and patient to the heart of the patient's pain. Mindfulness enables the therapist to provide intimate company in this territory, thereby helping the patient turn toward the life at hand.

Depression is pervasive within our culture. It is estimated that 19 million adults in the United States suffer from a depressive disorder (Narrow, 1998). Current research suggests that depression is a complex disorder with biological, psychological, and social components (National Institute of Mental Health, 2001). While psychopharmacology targets biology through brain chemistry, psychotherapy addresses the social and psychological dimensions of depression. The three main psychotherapeutic approaches are (1) cognitive-behavioral treatments, which work by changing maladaptive and distorted patterns of thinking and feeling (Beck, Rush, Shaw, & Emery, 1987); (2) interpersonal therapies, which focus on troubled relationships (Markowitz, 2002); and (3) psychodynamic treatments, which explore personal, historical events as they impact on present experience (Blatt, 2004). Ironically, when therapists treat depressed people, there is often a Greek chorus of competing approaches in their heads that may make it difficult to actually "be with" the patient in a therapeutic way.

Because depression is a complicated biopsychosocial problem, it challenges any narrow theoretical or procedural stance. For example, many psychodynamic therapists are generally no longer shy about suggesting behavioral changes, such as physical exercise or reducing isolation in order to improve mood. Conversely, newer cognitive-behavioral therapies are addressing issues of meaning (Westen, 2000) and transference (McCullough, 2000). Research also supports treating depressed patients with a combination of biological and psychotherapeutic approaches (Arnow & Constantino, 2003; Segal, Vincent, & Levitt, 2002). Mindfulness theory and practice have the potential to contribute to *diverse* schools of therapy by enhancing a therapist's ability to respond therapeutically to depressed patients—to join the patient where he or she is suffering—and to serve as a model for designing specific intervention strategies, such as those we find in mindfulness-based therapies.

MINDFULNESS-BASED TREATMENTS

Mindfulness is a key component of dialectical behavior therapy (DBT; Linehan, 1993a), which was developed to help patients regulate emotion, including the emotions and behaviors associated with depression. DBT is a paradoxical treatment applied by clinicians to help patients to *accept* their emotions, as well as to *change* their emotional experience. Mindfulness is on the acceptance side of the paradox and may work by reducing avoidance of negative emotions through exposure. In terms of research, DBT is a compelling treatment modality for borderline personality disorder, especially parasuicidal behavior (Bohus et al., 2004; Robins & Chapman, 2004). One study specifically on depression indicates that DBT is an effective treatment for older adults (Lynch, Morse, Mendelson, & Robins, 2003).

Another mindfulness-based approach, acceptance and commitment therapy (ACT; Hayes, Strosahl, & Wilson, 1999), focuses on full acceptance of present experience and mindfully letting go of obstacles as patients identify and pursue their life goals. Randomized, controlled trials show preliminary evidence for the effectiveness of ACT in treating depression (Zettle & Hayes, 1986; Zettle & Raines, 1989). Results indicate that the efficacy of ACT is attributable to a reduction in the believability, rather than the frequency, of negative thoughts (Zettle & Hayes, 1986).

Mindfulness-based cognitive therapy (MBCT) is a comprehensive integration of mindfulness in the treatment of depression (Segal, Williams, & Teasdale, 2002). It is an 8-week group treatment adapted from Kabat-Zinn's mindfulness-based stress reduction (MBSR) program (Kabat-Zinn et al., 1990) and includes components of cognitive-behavioral therapy. Segal, Williams, et al. were motivated by earlier research findings that mindfulness decreased overgeneralized memories and ruminative thinking, two common features in chronic depression (Teasdale et al., 2000, 2002; Williams, Teasdale, Segal, & Soulsby, 2000). MBCT explicitly trains depressed patients to become aware of their thoughts and feelings, without considering them to be objective facts, which is referred to as "decentering." Through the process of decentering, patients become less avoidant and reactive to their thoughts and feelings. The treatment reduced relapse by 44% in a group of patients with three or more episodes of depression a full 60 weeks after the 8-week program had ended, compared to a treatment-as-usual control group (Segal, Williams, et al., 2002). Similar patterns of success were found when the study was replicated (Ma & Teasdale, 2004). Segal, Williams, et al. (2002) recommend that to be most effective, the clinician should have a personal mindfulness practice. The therapist's practice of mindfulness, in both daily life and within the therapy hour, is the cornerstone of the approach described in this chapter.

A MINDFULNESS-INFORMED
APPROACH TO DEPRESSION

As clinicians sitting with patients suffering from unremitting depression, we have all had the experience of wracking our brains and opening our hearts to try to discover something helpful. We are moved by our patients' pain. Our treatment plans and protocols often do not work quickly enough, or do not work at all. Our sense of urgency may further increase with the awareness that each depressive episode increases the likelihood of further episodes (McIntyre & O'Donovan, 2004). A growing number of clinicians are noticing that mindfulness may help us stay with and flexibly respond to the complexities and pain of our patients' experience (Brach, 2003; Epstein, 1998; Magid, 2002; Martin, 1999; McQuaid & Carmona, 2004).

The approach described in this chapter is mindfulness-informed; it rests upon the foundation of the psychotherapist's own mindfulness practice and usually does not include explicit teaching of mindfulness skills. It is an individual psychotherapy that may vary in length depending on patient needs. Rather than a planned, sequential protocol, it calls for flexibility based on the understanding that depression manifests in myriad ways and has multiple causes, and each patient's path to wellness is therefore unique. As William Styron (1990) wrote in *Darkness Visible*, his memoir of his depression, "One person's panacea might be another's trap" (p. 72).

The approach illustrated here integrates insights derived from mindfulness practice, with clinical training that is primarily psychodynamic. Appreciation of the primacy of the treatment relationship, strong therapeutic boundaries, and attention to transference reflect its psychodynamic roots. Nonetheless, this approach also integrates cognitive and behavioral interventions, and includes elements of existential–humanistic psychotherapy, with its emphasis on therapeutic presence and attention to experience in the here and now (Schneider, 2003).

ALIVENESS VERSUS TURNING-AWAY

Let us enter the treatment room. A patient sits down, sighs, and says, "I'm depressed." We ask some probing questions, seeking to discover for ourselves and for the patient what, essentially, does "depressed" mean for this person? The primary lens through which we view depression is one of *aliveness*. Regardless of etiology and manifestation, it is likely that our patient will experience a lack of vitality—feeling out of touch with life in an essential way.

We try to make contact. The depressed patient, regardless of the form of the depression, is turning away from his or her experience. "Turning-away" is a less technical expression than "experiential avoidance" (Hayes, Strosahl, et al., 1999), and it is used here for two reasons. First, it is experience-near. It conveys a posture vis-à-vis one's experience that a person can sense. Second, it suggests abandonment, a common feeling in depression. The treatment involves finding where there has been a turning-away. We attempt to foster safety and emotional intimacy with our depressed patients, such that the posture of turning-away, with its consequent lack of aliveness, can be challenged. In therapy, we offer an invitation to *turn toward* and *be with* the experience at hand.

MINDFULNESS AND ALIVENESS

When we are mindful, we feel alive. In the words of the meditation teacher Bhante Gunaratana (2002), "You become sensitive to the actual experience of living, to how things actually feel. You do not sit around developing sublime thoughts about living. You live" (p. 38). In mindfully drinking a cup of coffee, we feel the texture of the cup in our hands, take in the warmth, smell the aroma, notice the thickness of the rim on our lips, experience the liquid swirling in our mouths, and taste the unique flavor as we swallow. We are engaged in a multisensory experience and are awakened to its many dimensions. This is enlivening.

As therapists, mindfulness enables us better to incline our ears and our hearts to the absence of aliveness in someone who is depressed. It refines our attunement to the moment when a patient turns away. Conversely, mindfulness practitioners can also sense signs of life when they emerge in the clinical encounter. There is an awareness of the potential of each new moment. In therapy, we are trying to find the pulse of someone's experience, beat by beat, and provide deep company in whatever challenges arise in experiencing the pulse more directly.

Pain and suffering are always involved in treatment of depression. Pain is inevitable and suffering is what occurs when we elaborate on pain with our fears and regrets. The details of the suffering are crucial; depression is a uniquely *personal* matter in which history and narrative are important. As discussed in Chapter 1, people come into treatment wanting to "feel better." In working with depression, some pain can be alleviated. But it is the changed relationship to pain that ultimately alleviates suffering. With mindful awareness, it is possible for anyone, regardless of the circumstances, to be in more direct contact with his or her life experience and to feel more alive.

This chapter explores the utility of mindfulness when brought to bear on four focal areas of treatment for depression: (1) co-exploration of the patient's experience; (2) the challenges of suicidality, boredom, and hostility; (3) the therapy relationship; and (4) fostering behavior change. In each of these areas, mindfulness can increase the immediacy of contact between the therapist and patient, as well as between the patient and his or her own experience, thereby revitalizing the patient's life.

MINDFUL CO-EXPLORATION

Mindful attention is characterized by awareness, present-centeredness and acceptance. Although it is impossible to fully operationalize mindful exploration, the following questions convey the spirit of mindfulness-informed therapeutic inquiry:

- "What is happening right now?"
- "Can you stay with what is happening?"
- "Can you breathe *into* what is happening, or can you breathe *with* what is happening right now?"

Mindful inquiry is open-ended, without foreclosure or presumption about the patient's experience. It focuses on *what* rather than *why*. It is a stance that is unabashed in attending to whatever is occurring. Like Gendlin's (1996) technique of focusing on bodily "felt-sense," mindful attention fosters access to the area in which therapeutic movement arises.

Philip Aranow (1998) coined the expression *meditative move* to describe any intervention, including an interpretation or a simple "Aha," that "helps [a patient] toward the development of a compassionate, clear-seeing stance toward all of our mental experience and emotions." Gendlin's "felt-sense" of the body is but one domain of mindful attention. Attention can be brought to multiple arenas of experience, including the physical, rational, emotional, intuitive, behavioral, and interpersonal dimensions.

Loving Attention

We shy away from the word *love* in our training as clinicians, perhaps with good reason. Nonetheless, psychotherapy can be a very intimate, loving encounter. In the words of the therapist Paul Russell (1996), "Therapy is a love relationship. . . . It does not work to try to somehow 'be' loving. The only thing that can work is to feel the love that is already there" (p. 13). Russell's words aptly convey that love is not something that we generate; it is found in the activity of intimately attending.

Constancy and care in attention have a quality of love. We try to sit with a patient much as we would attend to the breathing of a newborn child or of someone dying. There is refinement and subtlety to such attention, as well as genuine warmth and interest. As clinicians, and simply as human beings, we all have attended to people in this way. It arises naturally. As discussed in Part II of this book, this quality of attention can be cultivated. We can learn to bring wholehearted attention to more of what occurs, more of the time.

Acceptance of Pain

When a patient enters our office for the first time, we may ask, "What brings you?" Frequently, someone who is depressed will respond, "I just want to feel better." Already the problem I referred to earlier has arisen; in wanting to feel differently, the patient turns away from his or her actual experience. We abandon ourselves as we suffer. Sometimes it can be helpful to address this explicitly by asking the following questions:

- "What do you experience in your mind and your body?"
- "What is the quality of the relationship that you have with your pain?"
- "Do you have compassion or understanding for yourself in how you are feeling?"

Usually these questions will be puzzling. Because the pain is unpleasant, the patient is trying to feel something different. We ask about the pain in a bid for patients to stay with their experience.

It is helpful to observe *with* the patient when he or she self-abandons by noting that his or her voice has dropped off in describing some aspect of experience, or by observing an attitude of self-dismissal. One patient habitually looked down and spoke more rapidly when asked about his sadness. When I observed that he seemed to be trying just to "get through" his response to my inquiry, he acknowledged, "I don't think there's anything to be gained by what we're looking at." This enabled us to challenge his unexamined assumption that his pain was to be avoided.

Value of the Narrative

The story, the narrative history of someone struggling with depression, can be critically important. What happened in our patients' past always bears on their present pain. Sometimes it is more pointedly *who* happened, meaning the central characters in patients' lives, that shapes their pain. People who are depressed are often disinterested in their stories. This is one manifestation of turning away, a form of self-abandonment. It is their unexamined sense that there is no life to be found in the history. They tell us about their past with an air of dutiful compliance. Observing this brings their *relationship to their lives* into awareness. We can begin to explore together the roots of this stance, and shine the light of mindfulness on the territory that has been abandoned.

> Years ago, a man came into treatment complaining of having lost interest in his life. A few weeks later, he mentioned that the sabotage and crash of the passenger jetliner over Lockerbie, Scotland, had hit him very hard. I assumed that the toll of human loss had exacerbated his personal losses. Nonetheless, I asked him what it was about the crash that had hit him so hard. He explained that he felt the terrorism was an indictment of well-intentioned efforts to bring educational initiatives to the third world. It made him question the meaningfulness of his lifelong commitment to education as a means to foster development in other cultures. We had almost neglected the central meaning of the disaster for him.

When we are mindfully attentive, there is subtlety and openness that does not prematurely foreclose on what something means to the patient. We engage someone with the genuine attitude of "What have we here?" We enlist our patient as a researcher of past and present experience.

Thoughts Are Not Truths

The wisdom that thoughts are not irrefutable facts, and the role of negative thinking in depression, are cornerstones of cognitive therapy (Beck et al., 1987). As discussed in Chapter 2, an understanding of the conditioned nature of thought is shared by Buddhist and Western psychology. Patients often gain freedom when they recognize that thoughts are not facts; they are just thoughts.

Yet traditional cognitive-behavioral techniques that focus upon the identification of certain depressogenic thoughts—followed by thought refutation and thought substitution—have limited therapeutic effect for some patients. How often have we sat with someone who says, "I know that my thinking is crazy" or "I know why I think this and that it's distorted," yet gets little therapeutic mileage out of the insight? What Segal, Williams, et al. (2002) recognized in the power of mindfulness training was the potential for patients to fundamentally change their relationship to all thinking, not just negative thinking. They found that watching thoughts come and go without engaging them, and returning repeatedly to present experience, decreased the frequency of ruminative thinking.

When ruminations are a feature of the patient's depression, the following observations and questions are helpful:

- "You expressed that thought as if you believe it to be true."
- "Have you noticed that you think differently about this when your mood changes?"
- "You seem tired when you express that thought. Are you tired of it?"

Feelings Change

The fact that feelings change can bring great relief to a person who is depressed. As we bring more attention to experience moment by moment, it becomes readily apparent that everything is in flux. Our bodies, a growing child, and the natural world are all powerful and constant reminders of this truth. Patients struggling with depression often forget this. A patient says, "I can't bear this" or "I can't live with this." In exploring the experience, the patient sees that he or she is indeed managing to tolerate whatever pain is occurring at the moment. What is unbearable is the fear that the state will never change.

Mindfully attending to experience on a more subtle level enables a depressed person to realize an important insight: even while depressed, he or she is not always experiencing depression. No two moments are the same. Years ago, a friend who was dying of AIDS said in the last weeks of his life, "You know, the mind is amazing. Here I am in my last days; some moments I'm terrified, some moments I feel the angels coming, and in other moments, I still enjoy a juicy piece of gossip." If we think that some state has a uniform texture, we are not looking closely enough. As mentioned earlier, the tendency to overgeneralize experience is correlated with depression (Williams et al., 2000). MBCT teaches mindfulness skills to counter this tendency. In the course of mindfulness-informed psychotherapy, we can foster awareness of the changing nature of experience by offering the following suggestions:

- "Tell me about times in the last week, however fleeting, when you did *not* feel depressed."
- "What can you tell me about your experience right now? Notice any changes in your feeling, however subtle."

This is delicate work. When someone is in the throes of crisis or loss, it can be profoundly unempathic to say, "This will change." Timing is important. We are attempting to nurture awareness of the changing nature of all phenomena to assist someone in being able to stay with present experience, however painful. It is by staying with whatever is happening that the lack of solidity of a mood or state of mind is discovered.

Fertile Silences

The meaning and function of a patient's silence in a given moment is endlessly variable. In bringing mindfulness to moments of silence, our awareness is more finely attuned to what is being conveyed wordlessly. Some silences feel like walls erected for protection. We intuitively sense this and try to make the situation safer by inviting the patient to talk about not talking. Some silences are avoidant or defensive, bespeaking a refusal to be with difficult experience. We challenge these silences. Other silences are angry. We comment on the anger when we feel it.

Still other silences are fertile; there is a palpable sense that the silence is teeming with life and is best left undisturbed. We are sitting with someone who is conveying "being"—in his or her silence. We join with this activity of being, and our silent participation is experienced as active support for the person's freedom to be quiet. These moments of wordless communion can be transformative, and nothing need ever be said. The experience stands alone.

Like word-filled times, wordless times within the therapy hour can change. When we sit with someone, co-enveloped within the silence, there is a sense akin to watching a changing sky. A silence that felt free and rich starts to feel arid or tense. A silence that seemed to move lightly and meander suddenly feels full of feeling. Mindfulness attunes us to these varied textures of silence and assists us in discerning how to be with our patients in these moments. Sometimes it is hard to sense the quality of the silence, and we wonder whether to say something, and if so, what? This is particularly relevant with depression. Is the person feeling alone and abandoned in the silence or free to move about and inhabit it? Is our silence experienced as permissive or disinterested? A comment such as "I'm wondering if the silence is fertile or if it is impeding you in some way" shares the question. It also nicely models that we are finding our way together. Asking "Do you need company?" or commenting that the quality of the silence seemed to change, can be invitations for more contact and exploration.

Finding the Heart of Depression

Treatment requires getting to the heart of the depression and bringing loving attention to this terrain of the patient's experience. Mindfulness is a tool of sufficient power and subtlety for the task. Theories are helpful in providing us with a general map of human experience. It helps to know where to direct our attention, but theories fall short. By definition, they are at best excellent pointers: They are not the landscape.

We can only go the last distance by surrendering to the moment-to-moment, co-created experience. We participate in something of which we are dimly aware—trying to shine the light of understanding at the same time. What mindfulness brings to this endeavor is our added capacity to be present with the density of the experience, the depth of pain, the ways in which our patient felt left alone, and then left him- or herself. We lend the draft of our presence, we tolerate the hours and hours, when it cannot yet be experienced. We attempt to sit with someone, free of our own need for something to happen.

When a person arrives at his or her experience in this bare way, it is painful. We respect why there had been a turning-away. We do not just understand the hopelessness or despair; we can experience it with the patient. The person feels *raw*. It is a form of open-heart surgery.

A middle-aged man who had struggled with suicidal feelings for most of his adult life had begun to experience the depth and pervasiveness of his self-hate. In one session, he was facing himself in this stark way. He had been looking down at the rug. As he looked up, he said, "I can't look at you." In the resounding silent minutes that followed, there was a palpable shared sense of his anguish. We were both being tested. Could we each face his inability to face me in this moment? Could we face his hate? In the wordless, mutual staying with his experience, new ground was forged.

Mindfulness sustains us in the pain of uncertainty. A trust develops that the ground is just what we have right here. The life is in the blood. Healing is in the flow. These are the moments that most deeply test our capacity to breathe fully with whatever comes. Precisely because there is such sensitivity in this deep terrain, the person with whom we sit senses the degree to which we can do this. In the atmosphere of our presence, viability is experienced.

MINDFULNESS OF TREATMENT CHALLENGES

The helplessness and hopelessness that so characterize depressive experience get mirrored in our experience sitting with depressed patients. As discussed in Chapter 3, as we grow in our capacity to be fully present with whatever occurs in our own experience, we are increasingly able to open to whatever the patient brings.

Engaged Equanimity

In mindful presence, our relationship to experience is one of *engaged equanimity*. To be engaged means to be present, available, and not to turn away. It is a cornerstone of our capacity to empathize and deeply understand our patients' experience. When we are fully engaged, we open ourselves to the impact that our patients and their suffering has on us, just as we acknowledge our impact on them.

> A woman with a severe trauma history was recounting one of her father's beatings. She stopped speaking at one point, and I asked her about it. She said that she had noticed pain on my face and didn't want to upset me. This exchange was an opportunity for us to examine her assumption that my feeling for and with her would be a problem. Often the feelings of a parent were a problem, not in and of themselves, but because the parent couldn't hold them responsibly. She was able to then express what had been frightening to her about my expression. It was the fear that in my feeling, I would *leave* her rather than *be* with her.

Awareness of the moment-by-moment flow of experience develops *equanimity* (Salzberg, 1995), enabling us to remain fundamentally undisturbed by life's vicissitudes. Equanimity implies a nonjudgmental openness: a trust in the *ultimate workability of all experience*. Engagement and equanimity balance one another. When equanimity is coupled with engagement, we are able to connect intimately with someone in the depths of his or her experience, without being inducted. We are moved, yet we do not leave our seat. It is the coexistence of these two threads that appears to be a central factor in healing.

Patients who are depressed present formidable challenges to engaged equanimity—particularly in the form of suicidality, boredom, and hostility. In working with each of these, the task is first and foremost not to be "killed off." By "killed off," I am not implicating the patient's aggression. We are killed off if we are not present in the moment. It is this capacity to *live with* in the truest sense, to discover the life or pulse right in this experience, that is transformative.

Suicidality

When a patient wants to commit suicide, we experience powerful emotions. Depending on the particular features of the case, we might feel frightened, angry, or self-critical. Suicidality can be experienced as an indictment of the treatment. In our formal training as therapists, these thoughts and feelings are loosely referred to as *countertransference*. If we are aware of them, we are less likely to be driven by them in our interactions with our patients. Mindfulness practice expands this awareness such that we notice more subtle levels of our reactivity, and are hence better able to remain present.

With mindfulness, we notice more readily when we have become less available. We may distance either by minimizing dangerousness or through overmanagement—asking too many questions, trying to bring certainty to a fundamentally precarious situation. The patient may sense this shift and consequently shut down. This can happen outside of both the patient's and our own awareness. Suddenly we are lost to our patient, and he or she is lost to us in a vital way. This movement, however subtle, has impact on the interpersonal field and will contribute to our patient's feeling even more alone. Suicide risk is increased.

If we are not distracted and distanced by our own fear, we can inquire further. Paradoxically, we might discover something new and vital in the patient's suicidality. What is the intent? Is it to relieve suffering? Is it revenge? Does it feel like an exercise of real choice in the context of abiding feelings of powerlessness? Often the life is found only in being where we do not want to be and hearing what we do not want to hear. Intimate connection is made when we demonstrate that we can tolerate hearing what is going on in this moment, and we can engage with the patient in the full horror of his or her experience. Andrew Solomon (2001), in *The Noonday Demon*, chronicles his own depression: "You cannot draw a depressed person out of his misery with love. . . . You can, sometimes, manage to join someone in the place where he resides" (p. 436).

Mindfulness fosters a quality of *active humility*. We cannot save a person's life, yet we may be the lifeline. We must neither take responsibility for something we cannot ultimately control, nor run away from the responsibility of being in direct relationship with the individual's experience. Our task is to identify the turnings away, the little moments of abandonment as they occur.

> I recall a woman struggling with an unremitting depression. One day, our conversation felt lifeless and she felt distant. I commented that I didn't feel her to be very much in the room. She looked at me directly and said, "You're a problem." She was silent for many minutes. She went on to say that she wanted to kill herself but didn't know what to do with me. She didn't want to hurt me; she knew that we mattered to one another. A dense reckoning between us followed. I told her that she didn't need to stay alive for me. I also said that my deepest sense was that her suicide would not be an expression of freedom, but a further extension of the cruelty toward herself with which we had begun to be intimate.

We have all had times like this, when the full encounter of two minds and hearts is access to a deeper truth. As presented in Chapter 5, the recognition can be deep, the connection vast, and in such moments, time and space are expanded in life's power and mystery. Something is found or created or remembered. We are trying to be present to this opportunity in more and more moments as we sit with someone. We are present to life asserting itself. The wellspring of possibility is touched in this collective place, turning toward aliveness.

Boredom

We have all experienced the sudden desire for caffeine or the furtive glance at the clock when sitting with certain patients. At times, we ask superfluous questions, trying to engage ourselves in the conversation. We are trying to "get something going." These attempts facilitate a pseudoencounter, absent of real contact with our patient. Often, either the therapist or the patient is running from some unacceptable thought or feeling that needs the therapist's attention. We might ask ourselves, "What is hard about staying in this moment?" At such times, mindfulness of the breath can bring us more into the room. In staying with our breath, or feeling our bodies seated in the chair, we make contact with at least one aspect of present experience. This mitigates our being distanced from the patient by our boredom.

Boredom also occurs when we are lost within the clinical hour. We are searching for "where to go" or "where to take our patient." We are occupied with self-doubts or doubts about the enterprise. If we are thinking and feeling this way, the patient may also be doing so. Again, addressing what appears true in the moment helps. A statement, such as "I'm not sure where we are right now," is an invitation to join us in the ambiguity. Things may be unclear, yet very alive, if we stay with what is occurring.

If we are bored because the patient is bored, we can simply say, "You seem bored. What might it be like to be with this boredom, to stay with it just as it is?" This quality of inquiry, which points to the experience of the present moment, is a challenge to someone who is depressed. Through this invitation to be with what is actually happening, we are challenging two habits of the depressed person: experiential avoidance and the tendency to engage with ruminative thoughts *about* experience instead of *having* experience.

> A man with a long history of depression spent the first few therapy sessions reporting worries about his wife's health, his financial security, and environmental destruction. Although we discussed these concerns, there seemed to be no easing of his worries. I commented on this. I asked him whether the worrying, although painful, had the effect of distancing him from his actual experience. He paused and said, "I don't want to go into what I'm actually feeling, because I'll feel a lot worse." He went on to say that he had had suicidal thoughts since his teen years. He didn't want to discuss this because he had no hope that he could ever feel any differently.

We had been participating in a pseudotherapy, talking about concerns that were actually a form of turning away from his deeper pain. He had many assumptions about his suicidal feelings, but he had not checked these assumptions in years. The boredom ceased. It was painful. As he increasingly turned toward his experience in this deeper way, he was able to touch a sense of aliveness.

Hostility

It is difficult to sit with the intense and pervasive hostility that depressed patients may have toward themselves and others. We also feel angry and hostile. It feels risky to bear witness to a patient whose self-criticism is relentlessly harsh. We lose patience. We join in ridiculous exchanges, in which we find ourselves trying to protect the patient from him- or herself by refuting self-critical statements.

When mindfulness makes us aware of such a dance, it is useful to note this with the patient and inquire about it.

> While working with a very bright man who bemoaned how incompetent he was, I found myself yet again countering with contradictory data. Upon noticing this, I remarked that I found myself disagreeing with him, and that this did not seem to help. He laughed and said, "I know what you mean; we've done this before." I suggested that we might be missing something in doing our patterned dance. He asked, "Like what?" I said I wasn't sure, just some sense that we were missing him in some direct way. His eyes welled up. He was silent for a moment. "I'm afraid there's nothing there." We stayed with his fear. There was life in the fear. Again, I had no sense of where we "needed to go," only the sense that we had moved away from his present experience in our debate. Simply noting what was occurring gave him more access to himself and increased our intimacy.

It is also difficult when hostility is directed at us. Again, speaking truthfully is important. Mindfulness helps us notice when we soft-pedal our remarks, reinforcing the patient's sense that something is too ugly or painful to be expressed more directly. It is hard to accept a patient's anger or hatred. Statements such as "Tell me about your hate" or "What does the hate feel like in your body?" invite formerly repudiated feeling onto center stage for understanding and connection.

MINDFULNESS OF THE THERAPY RELATIONSHIP

The treatment relationship is an ever-changing field. Rather than just a foundation or context for intervention, it is an intervention itself. While the therapy relationship was the central focus of Chapter 5, in this section I discuss how it is particularly relevant to depression. Relational therapists place the experience of connection or disconnection within self and between people at the heart of healing work (Jordan, Kaplan, Miller, Stiver, & Surrey, 1991). Similarly, this approach sees issues of relationship as central to working with depression, with mindfulness as a technology for investigating and experiencing the vicissitudes of connection and disconnection.

Disconnection from Self

Isolation is a central feature of depression. The patient is cut off in some way. The nature of this disconnection varies within and between patients, and a patient's experience of it is exquisitely personal. To enter into this territory with the patient, the territory first has to be found. Mindfulness informs a quality of deep listening that attunes us when we get near this territory.

Depression is most often an absence of real feeling. A patient who was severely depressed acknowledged, after many months, "There are rooms locked off within me. I have not let you into those rooms. There are rooms that even I haven't gone into." He was speaking of rooms of feeling—feeling that had been too difficult to bear. Ironically, treating depression always involves feeling more, not less. The adage that one needs to "feel worse before feeling better" might be rewritten for depression; one needs to *feel* before feeling better.

In depression, the cutoff always points to an experience of pain. Paul Russell described good treatment as "involvement in a psychological space where the patient has heretofore been alone and incompetent" (1996, p. 202). We convey that whatever the patient's experience is, it is possible to have it in the context of our relationship.

> A patient who had struggled with many bouts of depression talked of witnessing his father's nightly drunken rages at his mother and running outside to the beach to get away. I commented, "And no one followed you." He then said that it had never even occurred to him that someone might follow him. This revealed to him that he assumed his feelings were both unbearable to himself and also not acceptable within any relationship. He entered the room in a more real way from then on.

While mindfulness-informed treatment attempts to reconnect with lived experience within any moment of feeling, timing matters. In certain instances of trauma work and acute depression, when the patient is flooded with diffuse feeling, mindful attention is employed to label and bracket the feeling in the service of more organization. Ultimately, with more consolidation, the patient benefits from the practice of *having* a feeling rather than *being had* by a feeling.

Disconnection from the Therapist

Mindfulness enables us to ask our patients more genuinely about all dimensions of experience, including the therapy relationship. Often patients try to protect us from their experience, particularly when it is negative. This is fertile territory with depressed patients. Perhaps our company is felt. The therapy relationship encourages patients to enter into new, often raw, painful, or lonely inner experience. We invite them to have their whole experience, to breathe with whatever is going on.

Often there is a disconnection or perhaps the sense of our absence. Paradoxically, it is often in the moment when a patient can share that he or she does not trust us fully that trust is deepened.

> A patient was speaking about how defective she felt. She looked up and then looked away. I inquired. She said, "You're leaning forward, but I really don't feel you with me." She then associated to the ways in which she had always protected her mother from her early painful experiences of her mother's depression and profound absence. There was intimate connection in her expression and my reception of her feelings of disconnection. It is not simply that she could *be* with this feeling and that I could *be* with her feeling. Nor was it simply a sense that *we* could be with her experience. There was simply *being* and *living the moment*. Something loosened, giving way to increased life.

Yearning

The absence of interest or desire is a classic symptom of depression. A deepened therapy relationship is often the first context in which a person can safely experience some aspect of wanting or yearning. This is a harbinger of new life in the room, frequently subtle and easy to miss. Often we look for signs of life in all the wrong places.

> A depressed, middle-aged man came into treatment because his wife of 30 years had engaged in numerous affairs throughout their marriage. In our work together, it became clear that he and his wife experienced the world of desire very differently. She was driven by her desires; he was unaware of any desire. In one session, my patient made a passing reference to being attracted to someone. I inquired, but there was not much energy in his response. Was my timing wrong? Was he too ashamed to discuss it? As he was writing his check at the end of the same session, he looked at me squarely in the eye and said, "You know what I'd really like? I'd really like you to clean that window." His comment did not feel hostile. In this request was his freedom to want something. I commented that it was the first thing that he had ever asked of me. He responded, "No. Last year I asked you to pull down the shade once because of the sun." For him, these small requests were the first expressions of increased life and the freedom to have wants.

Uncertainty

We attempt to accompany our depressed patients into the territory of their emotional impasse. By definition, this territory is uncharted. The relational territory is also uncharted. Our patients hope and like to believe that we have the road map and know every landmark. We know that we do not. We only trust that the way can be found. Trust deepens with increased tolerance of uncertainty.

We often forget this fundamental reality. Sometimes we are swayed by the power of our patients' distress. Some relational moments are exquisitely hard to meet and we turn away, or respond superficially, or hide in trained responses. We may turn a question back on the patient, "What do *you* think?" to avoid feeling vulnerable ourselves.

A 30-year-old mother of three young children came into treatment very depressed, with a history of multiple early losses. After a number of weeks, she said, "I realize that I need to feel what I'm really feeling and catch up with myself in a deep way. But I also have three young ones who need me not to be a basket case! What do I do?" Of course, she knew that this was not a simple question, and I knew that a simple response would have been inadequate. Conditioned replies may help us through a difficult moment, but they squander opportunities for experiencing something more alive, such as uncertainty or awkwardness. A response such as, "What are your thoughts?" or "What would you say to yourself?" can help to some degree, but these responses fall short of the fullness of the moment. On the other hand, a straightforward "I don't know what you should do" might be defensive and foreclose the discussion. I responded that it was a dilemma and that we needed to be together in the "muddy middle of it all." The response was not eloquent, but it was born of awareness of all that we did not know in the moment.

MINDFULNESS OF THE PATIENT'S BEHAVIOR

Self-criticism is a cardinal feature of depression. It is useful when addressing patient behavior to distinguish between self-judgment and discernment. Judgmental thinking gets its bad name for good reason; it stops further exploration. The patient voices self-judgment about a behavior, and it becomes the end of the discussion. Discernment, on the other hand, is the wisdom that comes when we experience things as they truly are. Mindfulness makes a powerful contribution to our faculties of discernment by opening the field of awareness to unrecognized experience and consequences. For example, awareness can be focused on how smoking tobacco feels with each inhalation, what it is like to attend to the cigarette butts and ashes, and the likely health consequences. By inviting our patients to be discerning about themselves and their lives, we are not trying to get them to see or believe something preconceived. Instead, we are inviting our patients to be empiricists and to investigate their direct, *lived* experience.

Three considerations are useful as we explore behavior with the patient: (1) mindfulness of intention, (2) restraint from harm, and (3) kindness toward oneself. It is best to be flexible, curious, and respectful; and to relate the discussion to the patient's expressed desires at the outset of treatment.

Mindfulness of Intention

In the first therapy session, we typically inquire about precipitants, problems, and pain. Often we neglect to ask about deeper intentions, desires, and values:

- "What is your heart's desire?"
- "What is truly important to you?"
- "How do you most want to live?"

How closely is the patient's living aligned with his or her heart's desire? If a person can be more aware of what he or she truly wants, the relationship to behavior shifts away from "shoulds" and "should nots" to more spontaneous, proactive action.

One of the components of ACT involves helping patients clarify values and then develop a *willingness* to behave in ways that are more consistent with these values (Hayes, Strosahl, et al., 1999). The goal is for patients to live their deeper intentions. The difficulties that arise while patients are attempting to change behavior are to be welcomed as opportunities for mindful awareness.

Paradoxically, depressed patients are often waiting to "feel better" *before* doing things that are therapeutic. We can ask:

- "Need you wait to *feel* like doing something before you *choose* to do it?"
- "We've been noticing that your feelings change. Must they be your deepest bearings for deciding what to do?"

Restraint from Harm

We ask depressed patients whether they have any intention to harm themselves. Although clinicians who treat depression naturally focus on preventing suicide, it is useful to consider the full continuum of self-harm. Usually when a patient is speaking about this, there is a turning away: The voice drops off or the patient looks aside. We sense that we are hearing a programmed tape on the subject. We might mention that the vitality in the words seemed to drain out as the patient was speaking. We bring the patient to awareness of how it feels to discuss the matter. Eventually, we invite the patient to develop a lived, nonjudgmental awareness of the self-injurious behavior.

The ways in which a person can subtly harm him- or herself are as varied as the individual. We can ask each person to feel and listen for the subtler, self-inflicted hurts. One patient, a highly successful saleswoman, quietly harmed herself by overextending to others. She would endlessly commit her time and energy for projects that were depleting. As she attended to this, she found it increasingly painful to keep doing it to herself. She joked that there should be an "Overextenders Anonymous" group. She observed that she had to shut down to herself to continue this self-inflicted pain. With this patient, as with others, it was helpful to explore the notion of the *activity of restraint*. By practicing restraint from self-harming behavior, there is a reduction in the turning away from oneself that is a prominent feature in depression.

If we can join our patients in their difficulty and invite them not to abandon themselves in their particular hell, there is the chance that they can experience something directly in a new way. Perhaps they discover how dead they are when they do something. Perhaps they are able to sense the hurtfulness or cruelty in their behavior. Mindfulness brings light to this aspect of experience that has formerly been in shadows. The behavior is both an outcome of deadening and necessitates further deadening to be maintained.

For depressed patients, self-harming behaviors are well practiced. Their acute awareness of this contributes to a sense of hopelessness about developing new behaviors. Within the mindfulness-informed model, all these discouraging thoughts and feelings are merely mental events. They are what they are *and* one can choose a different trajectory in the next moment. The following clinical vignette illustrates this point:

> Ginny, an ardent Christian in her 60s, was in therapy because she was depressed and severely overweight. Ginny opened one of our sessions talking about the demands of caring for her elderly father and then quickly shifted to her eating habits that were "terrible and not even worth talking about." I asked Ginny if her eating habits entered her prayer life.
>
> She replied, "He doesn't want to hear it. I gotta do something about it. You can't, he can't, it's nobody's fault but my own. I'm dis-

gusted with myself." I asked Ginny if this disgust helped her. She snapped, "Of course not!" and then said, "May I change the subject for a moment?"

Ginny then told a story about a refugee family that needed money for relocation. Although Ginny had scant resources, she sent a relatively substantial donation to them. She went on to say, "God was speaking to me. I sat with it for 3 weeks and it still felt right, so I sent the money and it felt so good. I know it sounds really crazy, but I really checked it out, and it was just the right thing to do."

I said that it seemed as if she felt some real authority and trust about it.

Ginny nodded. I asked her if she considered letting God move in the same way with her struggles with her weight.

"What do you mean?"

I explained that she seemed to abandon her relationship with God when it concerned her weight, but she was intimately connected with him in these other areas of her life.

"Hmmm. I never thought about it like that. How do you mean, 'let him move'?"

"I mean bring him into every moment—much like you do in many ways—but also the moment when you reach for the potato chip or after, when you've had the chips and nail yourself. Let him be in there with you in these moments too."

Each moment is a new moment. In this new moment, we can restrain from harming ourselves, even if we have been harmful in this way thousands of times before.

Kindness toward Oneself

In addition to increasing awareness of behaviors that are self-harming, mindfulness can be brought to kindly actions. In psychotherapy, we shy away from the word *kindness*. The ubiquitous term *self-care* is more medical and less sentimental. Yet self-care may not capture the spirit or therapeutic attitude that kindness conveys. Recent contributions to the psychological literature are reviving the notions of kindness and compassion in psychotherapy (Ladner, 2004) and particularly in the treatment of depression (Gilbert, 2001).

When we ask patients about the ways in which they are kind to themselves, we are engaging them in a more intimate, experience-near way. We ask directly, "What is something that you do that feels like a kindness toward yourself?" This type of question reveals a great deal about the patient, developing awareness about ways of being that are consistent with his or her heart's deeper intentions. Perhaps the kindness is captured in a fleeting moment. A man with a history of severe childhood abuse said one day, "I had a moment of feeling dignity as I played the piano." This word, *his* word, *dignity* became an important bearing point in our work together. He learned to identify and value the feeling of dignity and to soften toward himself.

Cultivating a moment-by-moment awareness of being kind to oneself puts a patient in direct contact with possible obstacles doing so. Obstacles may include habitual thinking, resistance, internalization of the negative introject, negative conditioning, or repetition compulsion. Understanding why we are not kind to ourselves can be freeing. Yet simple, mindful observation can also help us gain freedom from our repetitive, anachronistic behaviors: We can choose kindness at any moment. Exploring this issue recently, a patient said, "I noticed how I'd positioned my radio in a way that it hurt my shoulder every time I reached to change the station or volume. I've done it this way, hurting myself, a thousand times. I finally moved the radio." Each moment is a new opportunity to notice and to practice kindness.

An Offering

There is so much to be found right here, in this present moment. In *The Noonday Demon*, Andrew Solomon (2001, p. 443) writes, "The opposite of depression is not happiness, but vitality." By being mindful within the therapy encounter, we cannot give someone happiness. We can, however, help our patients to feel more alive.

CHAPTER 8

Anxiety Disorders
Befriending Fear

CHRISTOPHER K. GERMER

The only thing we have to fear is fear itself—nameless,
unreasoning, unjustified terror which paralyzes needed
efforts to convert retreat into advance.
—FRANKLIN DELANO ROOSEVELT
(First inaugural address, March 4, 1933)

Anxiety disorders present a clear opportunity for the clinician
to observe mindfulness principles in action. An assumption
of the mindfulness paradigm is that we compound our suffering by trying to avoid it. The anxious person is particularly determined to avoid
the discomfort of fear. A feared stimulus can be *external*, such as snakes
(simple phobia), a mall (agoraphobia), or office parties (social phobia);
or it can be *internal*, such as a racing heart (panic disorder) or blasphe-
mous thinking (obsessive–compulsive disorder). Most anxious patients
recognize that their fear is irrational, but recognition is not sufficient to
alter avoidant or escape behavior during periods of heightened arousal.

Mindfulness is a technology for gradually turning the patient's attention toward the fear as it is happening, exploring it in detail with increasing degrees of friendly acceptance. A mindfulness-based approach
includes exposure, which is a key ingredient in effective treatment of
anxiety. The distinguishing characteristic of the mindfulness approach is

a gradual shift in the patient's *relationship* to anxiety from fearful avoidance to tolerance to friendship. We learn nonavoidance and nonentanglement until the fear subsides.

Efforts to treat anxiety probably date to the beginning of human history. Even the historical Buddha, psychologist that he was, reportedly spoke of anxiety and its treatment:

> Why do I dwell always expecting fear and dread? What if I subdue that fear and dread keeping the same posture that I am in when it comes upon me? While I walked, the fear and dread came upon me; I neither stood nor sat nor lay down until I had subdued that fear and dread. (Nanamoli & Bodhi, 1995a, p. 104)

The Buddha appears to have recognized exposure as a treatment. When questioned, he might have simply considered it as a healing aspect of mindfulness.

WHY A MINDFULNESS-BASED APPROACH TO ANXIETY TREATMENT?

The short answer is: Since anxiety is unavoidable, it is fruitless and often counterproductive to try to eliminate it. Anxiety probably developed through evolution to keep us alive. Whereas *fear* is a short-term response to imminent danger, *anxiety* is apprehension about events that might endanger us in the future. Anxiety becomes maladaptive when it is in response to perceived danger that is not real. Anxiety becomes a *disorder* when it interferes with a person's ability to function (American Psychiatric Association, 2000).

Anxiety disorders tend to have multiple causes. Some anxiety disorders, such as panic disorder and obsessive–compulsive disorder, have a genetic component (Gratacos, et al., 2001; Rauch, Cora-Locatelli, & Greenberg, 2002). Others, such as posttraumatic stress disorder (PTSD), may be more obviously environmental, although repeated stress can lead to structural and functional neurological changes (Bremner et al., 1995; Yehuda & Wong, 2002). What they all have in common is intolerance for the experience of anxiety. Effective treatments address, directly or indirectly, the patient's adversarial relationship to anxiety symptoms.

Mindful Awareness versus Negative Metacognitions

Thinking about mental events is known as "metacognition" (Flavell & Ross, 1981; Toneatto, 2002). We humans are continuously engaged in discursive or metacognitive thinking—describing our internal experience from the simplest sensation ("My heart is pounding") to the broadest beliefs ("I am defective"). Traditional cognitive-behavioral treatment (CBT) attempts to replace maladaptive metacognitions with beneficial metacognitions through examination of a patient's distorted thinking. Examples of distortions are catastrophic, overgeneralized, and dichotomous interpretations (Beck, Emery, & Greenberg, 1985), and irrational negative beliefs or schemas about oneself and the world (Wells, 1997; Young, Klosko, & Weishaar, 2003).

Anxiety disorders are sustained by negative metacognitions (Toneatto, 2002). An innocuous bodily response may be interpreted as dangerous ("Uh-oh!"), and corresponding efforts to ward it off make things worse. It is often counterproductive for therapists to join the patient in trying to remove a symptom if the patient's aversion to anxiety remains the same. An example is "relaxation-induced panic," the panic that erupts when a patient is trying to relax (Borkevec, 1987). The belief that anxiety is bad can cause panic whether the patient is either relaxing or under stress.

Mindful awareness is different from metacognition insofar as mindfulness involves participant observation without evaluation ("good" or "bad") or entanglement in the particular mental content. Mindful awareness simply says "yes" to experience.

It is *awareness of*, rather than *thinking about*, mental events. Some metacognitive beliefs may be beneficial, however. These are akin to what Buddhist psychology calls *insights*. Insights may be understood as quasi-metacognitions; *quasi* because they are both intuitive and rational, and *metacognitions* because they are indeed observations about mental events. Toneatto identifies a number of beneficial insights that may emerge in the patient's mind through mindfulness practice. Among them are the following: (1) Most of our thinking is conditioned through experience and is not necessarily objectively true; (2) pleasant and unpleasant thoughts will occur throughout our lifespan whether we like it or not; (3) all thoughts and feelings are temporary; and (4) although we may be gripped by a thought, thoughts are illusory—like flickers on a movie screen.

A mindfulness-based approach to treating anxiety involves becoming less identified with our thoughts: simply noticing the event, as it is occurring, with acceptance. For example, a traditional CBT approach to catastrophic thinking would be to identify it ("I will die of a heart attack") and challenge it ("Will you? What are the chances? What else could a heart palpitation mean?"). A mindfulness-based approach would instead encourage the patient to explore the feeling of a racing heart and related thoughts in great detail, as they arise ("Heart beating . . . thinking I will die . . . always seems to beat faster when I think that . . . thinking about heartbeat . . . could be the pizza I just ate"). It is like cutting up a scary film into individual frames and laying the frames on the kitchen table for examination. The film loses its horrifying impact upon scrutiny. The process of being aware, moment to moment, dismantles the fear by distinguishing the raw facts of experience from the frightening conclusions we draw shortly thereafter.

The Neurophysiological Basis of Anxiety

Researchers are making interesting progress in understanding the neurophysiological basis of anxiety and its treatment. Using positron emission tomography (PET), Schwartz, Stoessel, Baxter, Martin, and Phelps (1996) found that exposure and behavioral response prevention with patients with obsessive–compulsive disorder generated observable changes in the brain. Similarly, CBT produced brain changes akin to medication effects in social phobics (Furmark et al., 2002). Davidson (2003) is developing an integrated neurophysiological model of approach and avoidance tendencies, based on the functions of the prefrontal cortex and the amygdala. Mindfulness meditation has been shown to activate the left side of the prefrontal cortex in practitioners over an 8-week training period, with a corresponding increase in positive affect (Davidson et al., 2003).

Our knowledge of brain behavior can be creatively applied to psychotherapy. Patients find that understanding what is going on in their brains when they are anxious helps them step back and become less reactive. Jeffrey Schwartz (1996) turned PET scan observation into a mindfulness-based treatment strategy for obsessive–compulsive disorder. Schwartz helps patients disengage from obsessive thinking by reminding them it is merely a brain habit—brain lock—and shows patients pictures of brains to prove his point.

The biological pathways of anxiety are complex but increasingly understood (Bremner & Charney, 2002; Davis, 1992; LeDoux, 1995, 2000). Sensory input is evaluated for danger before conscious awareness by the amygdala (located just below the cerebral cortex), which sends a message to other brain structures, including the hypothalamus. The hippocampus is close to the amygdala and stores emotional memory, so traumatic memories can trigger alarm even before we are consciously aware of danger, or when we merely imagine danger. The hypothalamus, when activated, uses corticotropin-releasing hormone (CRH) to signal the pituitary gland to signal the adrenal glands to start producing adrenaline and noradrenaline. This sequence is known as the hypothalamic–pituitary–adrenal (HPA) axis. Other hormones secreted by the adrenals, known as glucocorticoids, also prepare the body for emergency action. Unfortunately, chronic activation of the HPA axis can result in a host of stress-related disorders. This subject is discussed further in Chapter 9.

Improving Treatment Compliance

Ross (2002) reports that about 19 million Americans have an anxiety disorder, making it among the most common psychiatric disorders. Of people who suffer from anxiety disorders, 60–90% can lead normal lives with CBT and/or medication. However, difficulties with compliance may occur in the application of cognitive-behavioral strategies in the field.

There are a number of challenges. Sometimes the lengthy homework assignments are discouraging to patients. Often therapists are insufficiently trained in CBT techniques (Goisman et al., 1993) or simply unwilling to help a timid patient face a feared situation. Patients may refuse exposure assignments. Particularly patients with PTSD can become emotionally overwhelmed during therapy and drop out of treatment (Schnurr et al., 2003). In one naturalistic study of panic disorder, only 18% of agoraphobics had recovered during the first 22 months following an episode, and among the recovered agoraphobics, 60% relapsed (Keller et al., 1994). Admittedly, many of those patients did not receive empirically validated treatments. However, transfer of technology from the laboratory to the field is often fraught with difficulties such as comorbid conditions; social, financial, or health concerns; multiple demands on a patient's time; substance abuse; or mixed motivation due to secondary gain. There are at least three reasons why the mindfulness-based approach in this chapter might improve treatment compliance.

First, the treatment protocol is *flexible*. This approach honors the treatment alliance, the patient's motivation, and the patient's unique life circumstances. Techniques are selected in collaboration with the patient based on patterns of avoidance of his or her unique problem areas. The therapeutic process (i.e., mindful acceptance), rather than technique, is kept at the forefront of the treatment.

Second, the treatment is *positive and accepting*. Many existing treatments are based on a deficit model: Something is wrong with the patient that must be fixed. In this mindfulness-based approach, change occurs by recognizing *what* is occurring in the present, and by allowing it to unfold in a relaxed, spacious way. To progress in treatment, patients must stop judging and fighting against themselves. The need for this shift is obvious to many patients, since unsuccessful efforts to change themselves are what brought them into therapy in the first place. From a mindfulness perspective, illness itself (or dis-ease) is merely a reflection of how we grasp or push away mental contents—not a personal defect.

A third rationale for this approach to treating anxiety is *therapeutic fit*. Many patients are now seeking therapists who themselves meditate or have a mindfulness frame of reference. The therapeutic alliance has consistently correlated with treatment outcome (see Chapter 3), and matching patients to treatments appears related to positive outcome (Devine & Fernald, 1973; Mattson, 1995). Mindfulness-based treatment is a particularly congenial treatment paradigm for some patients.

MINDFULNESS-BASED TREATMENT OF PANIC DISORDER WITH AGORAPHOBIA

I present here an example of mindfulness-based treatment of anxiety, using the example of panic disorder with agoraphobia. While panic is the most thoroughly researched anxiety disorder (Antony & Swinson, 2000), I am unaware of any published, mindfulness-based, treatment protocols for panic disorder at this time. There are general treatment guidelines for mindfulness-based treatment of anxiety, however (Barlow & Wilson, 2003; Brantley, 2003; Kabat-Zinn et al., 1992; Lopez, 2000; Miller, Fletcher, & Kabat-Zinn, 1995).

Since 1981, I have specialized in cognitive-behavioral treatment of panic disorder. The treatment presented below, a program I have been developing since 2001, uses some familiar cognitive-behavioral strategies, as well as more recent mindfulness-based exercises. It usually takes 10–15 individual outpatient sessions to complete in a relatively uncomplicated case.

The treatment structure was inspired by mindfulness-based cognitive therapy (MBCT). In the study by Teasdale et al. (2000), those patients with three or more episodes of depression who learned mindfulness skills had roughly half as many relapses as the no-treatment control. The gains applied only to chronic, *ruminative* patients rather than to less chronic patients, who were probably responding to environmental stressors. Since patients with panic tend to ruminate about threats to their tenuous emotional balance (anticipatory anxiety), it seemed that mindfulness might be similarly helpful in panic disorder.

Furthermore, the treatment of panic disorder with agoraphobia has moved over the years from exposure to feared *external* situations, such as malls and subways, to interoceptive exposure, or desensitizing the patient to *internal* cues for panic, such as dizziness or a pounding heart. This shift in treatment focus from outer to inner stimuli suggests a natural progression toward mindfulness practice, which attends especially closely to experience arising inside the mind and body.

Insight-Guided, Mindfulness-Based Psychotherapy

This treatment program is insight-guided. (The approach is distinguished from insight-*oriented* treatment, which is associated with psychodynamic psychotherapy and focuses on repressed thoughts and feelings.) Specific insights about panic serve as a heuristic for guiding the patient toward increased mindfulness. The following list of these insights is in no way exhaustive but represents common themes in the treatment of panic disorder that should be familiar to most clinicians. I hope that mindfulness-based psychotherapists understand these insights from personal experience, so that they can be discussed with the patient in a nuanced manner and applied in jointly created experiential exercises.

1. Anxiety is a fact of life. It protects us from danger. It is built into the nervous system and unavoidable.
2. We cannot control precisely when, where, and what we feel or think. Mental events occur in the brain, often before we are conscious of them.
3. Trying to control or avoid our experience is futile; often, it makes it worse.
4. The brain makes mistakes. When we panic, the brain perceives danger when there is none.
5. Problems occur when we *believe* in the reactions of the body to a false alarm by the brain. We suffer from a terrifying illusion.
6. Panic is never permanent. It has a beginning, a middle, and an end.
7. Treatment is the gradual process of redirecting attention toward the fear, exploring it in detail as it arises, and befriending it.
8. Our progress is measured, not by how seldom we panic, but by how much we accept our anxiety.
9. Cure entails becoming disillusioned with our fears. They become ordinary mental events occurring in the brain.

The reader may notice that brain function is emphasized in this treatment of panic disorder. Mindfulness treatment can proceed without that element, but, as mentioned earlier, an understanding of the role of brain functioning seems to afford patients more objectivity in relationship to their symptoms. It also reduces stigma: "It's not me, it's my *brain*!"

Experiential exercises are chosen mainly from the mindfulness-based techniques listed in Chapter 6. They are selected based on what experience the patient has difficulty seeing or accepting, or on the insight that we are trying to cultivate. More often than not, the *patient* will have his or her own ideas about how to approach and tolerate a body sensation or situation more fully. Borkevec (2002) suggests that when we pay careful attention to the present moment, we can trust that an adequate, adaptive response will appear.

Psychopharmacological intervention may be necessary in mindfulness-based treatment of panic disorder if the patient is unable to regulate attention sufficiently to function in life, or to begin psychotherapy. Otherwise, medication should be evaluated according to whether it supports experiential avoidance or exposure.

A Case Example

The composite case presented here illustrates how a therapist might work with experiential avoidance in anxiety disorders in general, and with panic disorder in particular, using an insight-guided, mindfulness-based approach. There are six segments to the treatment: (1) assessment, (2) awareness of the body, (3) awareness of the mind, (4) befriending fear, (5) befriending oneself, and (6) relapse prevention. The segments loosely follow in this order. Similarly, the key insights, questions, and practices associated with each segment may vary depending on the patient's circumstances.

Cara, a 45-year-old, Italian American, married mother of two children, had her first panic attack at the age of 15, when she used marijuana and spent an entire night shaking with fear, gasping for breath, and imagining death. This initial episode was followed by periods of intense anxiety and panic, lasting many months each, when Cara went away to college, and again at age 30, shortly after her first child was born. After the birth, Cara was put on a low dose of Klonopin and attended psychotherapy for 5 years with three different therapists. Her condition worsened and she stopped driving on highways and missed work a few days each month due to anxiety. Eventually, Cara stopped taking her medication because of concerns about side effects, quit psychotherapy, and became increasingly agoraphobic and panic-stricken.

Cara ventured into my office on the recommendation of a close friend who had benefited from mindfulness-based treatment. Cara could not travel outside her city limits or go shopping without her husband. She averaged two panic attacks per week. Cara's symptoms included a racing heart, shortness of breath, dizziness, chest pain, nausea, sweaty palms, blurry vision, depersonalization ("totally detached from my body") and derealization ("like on a movie set"). Cara also reported that she had been having nocturnal panic attacks once or twice each month. She tearfully confided that she was a "weak person" and probably a difficult therapy case. In the initial interview, Cara could not identify any events in her life that contributed to her seeking treatment at that particular time, 30 years after her first panic attack, but later in therapy, she realized that her daughter had just turned 15, Cara's age when she had her first panic attack.

Cara's physical health was compromised by obesity and gastro-esophageal reflux disease (including chest pain, burping, and throat soreness), for which she took medication. She never engaged in physical exercise, because an escalated heart rate reminded her of a panic attack. Prior to our initial interview, Cara saw a cardiologist, who ruled out a heart problem. She did not want to consider medication for panic due to her fear of side effects.

There were no other significant stressors in her life. Cara had good support from her family and friends, and did not abuse any substances. Her family was moderately secure financially, her two children were healthy, and she had a satisfying job.

Cara's family history was positive for depression and "nerves" on both sides of the family. In a family with three children, she was the only child who suffered from anxiety. Cara said that she always tried to look like a "strong person," but did not feel strong. Her father was actively alcoholic throughout her childhood and humiliated Cara when she cried, saying she was "stupid" and "too sensitive." Cara reports that that "started a war with my feelings—I became hypervigilant." Her mother told her never to cry in front of her father.

Session 1: Assessment and Introduction to Treatment

Key insights

1. Avoiding fear sensations causes panic.
2. You come by your panic naturally.
3. The wisdom of acceptance.

Questions

1. What internal cues trigger your panic?
2. Describe your panic.
3. Why is fear unacceptable in your life?

Practice

1. Complete a Mind Stream Inventory.

Cara presented most of the preceding information during an initial, 2-hour interview. My first goal was to establish rapport with Cara by understanding something about her struggle and her personality: Where does it hurt? What does she value?

It was clear that agoraphobia was unwelcome, because Cara wanted to be seen as a strong person. Her hypersensitivity to internal cues and her intolerance of changes in her body can probably be traced to her father's intolerance of her sensitivity. Cara gave me a detailed inventory of her body sensations, and we developed a hierarchy of internal triggers of panic, starting with (1) pounding heart, (2) chest pain, (3) choking, and (4) shortness of breath. The most catastrophic outcome was always death. Sometimes Cara feared the embarrassment of being seen as out of control. We discussed the futility of trying to control all bodily reactions, how fear of fear perpetuates the panic cycle, and how her health concerns had all been unsubstantiated by her physicians.

We began the psychoeducation process in the first session, emphasizing the naturalness of symptoms. The concept of acceptance was introduced using the inverse scales of anxiety and willingness (Hayes, Strosahl, & Wilson 1999, pp. 133–134); the greater one's willingness to feel, the less one's anxiety. She determined, tentatively, that acceptance is a better option than fearful control and frozen inactivity. She agreed to try to develop acceptance by understanding how her body functions under stress, how stress is intensified, and how to tolerate changes of all kinds in her body.

At the end of the first session, Cara was introduced to the Mind Stream Inventory (MSI), which I developed as part of this program. The MSI is a self-monitoring thought record. Cara was asked simply to write down, at least three times a day when anxious, or shortly thereafter, her succession of thoughts, feelings, body sensations, and actions. This exercise turns the patient *toward* the experience of anxiety with curiosity. Noting and labeling the stream of mental events introduces the patient to moment-to-moment awareness. The MSI is similar to the Mindful Monitoring Record (Roemer & Orsillo, 2002), but it captures a longer string of briefer mental events.

The stage was set for treatment in the first session by getting the patient's history, establishing rapport, introducing the rationale for treatment, providing psychoeducation to objectify the problem, and introducing a simple exercise to begin practicing mindful awareness.

Session 2: Awareness of the Body

Key insights

1. The brain raises false alarms about danger.
2. Panic is a temporary state.

Question

1. How does your body experience fear?

Practice

1. Three-Minute Breathing Space (Segal, Williams, & Teasdale, 2002, p. 184).
2. Present-moment awareness of sensation (eating, sounds).
3. Body Scan Meditation (Kabat-Zinn, 1990, pp. 92–93).

Cara had some difficulty exploring the evolution of panic in moment-to-moment detail on the MSI. (Patients usually improve at this during treatment.) Cara also reported that she did not have any panic attacks during the previous week, and she wondered aloud whether that was due to the homework assignment, even though it was hard to do. She seemed to be developing curiosity about her panic. Between our sessions, Cara recognized that she became more anxious before menstruating, that her fear escalated on the way to work, and that she often has a nervous stomach.

In our second 2-hour session, we discussed how the amygdala uses sense impressions to provide a rapid, preconscious screening for danger and often sends out a false alarm. We discussed how, with detailed, moment-to-moment awareness, we may be able to recognize this alarm early on; that is, we can catch the anxiety as a trickle before it becomes a torrent of panic.

We also explored each of Cara's symptoms from a biological point of view. Since Cara was afraid of a palpitating heart, we discussed the adaptive importance of increased blood pressure and heart rate in preparing for self-protective action. Her chest pain was either muscle tension in response to fear, or a symptom of acid reflux. Cara agreed to investigate her chest pain further at home through mindful attention. Shortness of breath alarmed Cara during panic episodes. We discussed the hyperventilation syndrome and how the brain makes an incorrect assessment that there is insufficient oxygen in the blood due to an oxygen–carbon dioxide imbalance.

Fortuitously, Cara developed a tight throat and fear of choking during the session. We did an exercise of eating a nut slowly and mindfully. Cara learned that by paying attention to the taste and feel of chewing and swallowing, rather than to the thought that she cannot swallow, she could swallow quite naturally. Feeling unable to swallow was a psychophysiological response to her fear (see Chapter 9). This led to a broader discussion about mindfulness in everyday life and the value of paying careful attention to whatever we are doing in the moment.

Cara agreed to do "mindful nut eating" a few times at home. We discussed the rationale of focusing on the present moment to disengage from her fearful, future-oriented thoughts. We experimented in session with mindful awareness of ambient sounds in the therapy room and outside. Two additional exercises were introduced: (1) Three-Minute Breathing Space (TMBS; Segal, Williams, et al., 2002, p. 184), to anchor her attention in the present moment, and (2) Body Scan Meditation (BSM; Kabat-Zinn, 2002a), to help Cara explore and befriend her unpredictable and anxiety-provoking body. I taught Cara the Breathing Space and gave her a written handout of the instructions. Cara was also given a compact disc of the BSM. Finally, she agreed to try completing the MSI a few more times.

We summarized the insights of the week: Panic has a beginning, a middle, and an end. It ends naturally and inevitably. Panic is more likely to end if we accept it. If we focus on present-moment sensations, such as the breath, we are not contributing to more panic by fighting it. Paying attention to sensations and fighting sensations are very different. Furthermore, there is nothing to fight against, because the fear is a false alarm by the amygdala anyway. We can safely observe the body and let the fear go.

Sessions 3–5: Awareness of the Mind

  Key Insights

  1. We cannot control what we think and feel.
  2. We believe false alarms and get hijacked by fear.

  Question

  1. What thoughts and feelings arise automatically when you panic?

  Practice

  1. Complete the Mind Stream Inventory.
  2. Mindfulness meditation (10 minutes/day).

Cara reported at the third session that her menstrual cycle had begun, and she had suffered two nocturnal panic attacks and one panic attack at work. She said, "I am afraid of my own body!" She noted that she had had a heartburn episode perhaps 1,000 times in her life and had thought it was a heart attack during 800 of them: "A tape keeps playing 'heart attack' in my mind!" During the week, Cara experimented with reminding herself that her doctor, who did a Holter monitor test, had specifically said that she had a healthy heart. That seemed to soothe Cara a little. She also identified specifically where her pain was located, how it seemed to radiate from her esophagus, and how it subsided when she was distracted by other events in her life. Cara's skill at mindfully attending to her symptoms was improving.

Cara tried the BSM, but said it was too hard to find time for it with two children at home. (Fear of her own body probably contributed to not finding time for the BSM.) Cara also tried the TMBS and said that she could not do it, because it reminded her of her tight throat and shortness of breath. However, she found listening attentively to sounds enjoyable. Eating mindfully worked for her and alleviated her fear of choking by perhaps 10% at home. These discoveries were encouraging.

We focused on automatic thoughts and feelings during Sessions 3–5. Cara diligently filled out the MSI at least twice daily when she was anxious. She started coming up with injunctions that she repeated to herself: (1) "Let go and let God," (2) "Surrender," and (3) "Breathe!" Cara found herself repeating rational statements to herself regarding her panic: "It's just my thinking and these thoughts are a bunch of junk!" and "I have to just accept my anxiety and stop searching for a heart problem!" Cara also started looking into a yoga class to help her "make the mind–body connection".

This phase of the treatment was particularly interesting. Cara recognized that her brain was simply repeating old habits. "Dr. Phil says thoughts are mental habits only," she reported. Cara also became intimately aware of how her attention was hijacked by a false alarm of the brain and that her expectation of dying from her chest pain was an illusion. But, she exclaimed, "It is tough to remember my fear is an illusion when it is so intense and distorted!" By carefully exploring her thoughts as they arose in the present, Cara gradually became disillusioned with her fears. For example, one MSI sequence she brought into therapy went as follows:

1. Heart beating.	10. I hate this.
2. Not NOW!	11. Let go and let God.
3. What if it is a heart attack?	12. You are OK, just shaking.
4. Uh oh.	13. Teeth chattering.
5. Am I feeling it in my shoulder?	14. It will end. Just shaking.
6. It's getting worse.	15. Watch the belly move.
7. I am panicking.	Breathing is good.
8. Panic is not dangerous.	16. Trembling.
9. I am such a mess.	17. Heart beating.
	18. Just panic. It will stop.

Cara was clearly improving in her ability to identify and name her sequence of thoughts, feelings, sensations, and behaviors. She was encouraged that she could recognize her experience as "panic" rather than a heart attack, before the panic worsened. She also discovered that careful observation of the moment-to-moment details of her experience made her feel better. This is an example of how mindful awareness of mental events "upstream," at an early stage of information processing, can interrupt the subsequent elaborations that lead to panic.

Cara agreed to try formal mindfulness meditation for 10 minutes each morning before her children woke up. She was given a compact disc by Jon Kabat-Zinn (2002b) to help her explore this practice. Cara also agreed to continue her work with the MSI, and she wanted to write down all the positive self-statements that she seemed to be discovering for herself.

Sessions 6–10: Befriending Fear

Key insights

1. Progress is measured by how much I *accept* anxiety, not by how seldom I panic.

Question

1. To feel safe in my body again, what physical sensations and external situations do I need to explore and accept?

Practice

1. Mindful exposure.
2. Practice mindfulness (meditation, MSI, etc.).

By this time, Cara's cue for a heart attack—pain in the shoulder—had been realistically reframed as acid reflux pain. She lost the fear of choking as a result of her repeated experience with mindful eating. Shortness of breath seemed to disappear on its own, without additional exercises, perhaps as a consequence of general mindfulness. Panic continued to arise spontaneously at least once a week, but with lesser intensity and shorter duration.

Cara continued to meditate daily for 10 minutes. She noticed, however, that meditation on the breath, even on the belly, made her shorten her breathing. This can happen if the patient is either anxious or zealous about breath meditation. Therefore, we switched the object of her attention to "stillness of the body." The object of meditation was the sensation of her hands resting quietly in her lap. Cara said that the practice made her feel calm. She learned that her feelings come and go, and that she has the ability to sit still through all her emotional changes. Cara lengthened the meditation to 20 minutes daily. The instruction was merely to "notice what took your mind away" when her attention strayed from her hands, and to gently return her awareness to the stillness of the body. This exercise is usually enough meditation for panic patients; it produces calmness and stabilizes attention.

The following key mindfulness-based insights were discussed in this phase of treatment:

1. Anxiety is not a setback; *fighting* anxiety is a setback.
2. How can you practice letting go of fear if you do not have the *experience* of fear?
3. The point is to grow in *acceptance* of your body and mind, not overcome panic.

4. Progress is measured by how much anxiety you can allow in your life, not by how seldom you panic.

Patients usually begin to expose themselves to fear-inducing stimuli by the sixth session. The logic of learning to tolerate fear sensations brings a natural wish to test oneself: "How long can I be in the meeting? What will I be going through?" Cara came up with a clever plan of assigning points to herself for doing certain challenging, acceptance-based tasks. She decided to "learn acceptance of fear, one event at a time." Cara contracted with me to earn a certain number of points each session. She challenged herself to experience a pounding heart by doing aerobic exercise. (Cara, after at least 15 years of not exercising, found that her athletic husband was fully supportive!) Cara collected points for using a NordicTrak. She also got points for crying, breathing through fear, and admitting her fear to others—all in the name of rewarding acceptance.

Cara came up with a plan to shop alone gradually, to drive her daughter to another town, and eventually to take an aerobics class. When anxiety arose, her strategy was to focus on what she was doing at the present moment. She also told herself, "Breathe! Physical symptoms are just anxiety," and "Don't fight it—that will make it worse."

Session 11+: Befriending Oneself

Key insights

1 I may feel I am defective, but I am also OK.
2. We continually construct our world from past experience.

Question

1. What core belief about yourself is hardest to admit?

Practice

1. Mindfulness meditation (daily).
2. Other mindfulness practice.

During this phase, Cara addressed her conviction that she was a "weak person," hoping to stop modeling fearfulness for her daughter. Cara read *The Highly Sensitive Person* (Aron, 1996) and took comfort that her presumed weakness might also be a strength. This was a new perspective after a childhood filled with her father's angry rebukes. Cara discovered how deeply she rejected any unease in her body, because most of her body sensations only got her into trouble as a child. She saw how trying to stay calm kept her away from interesting life experiences.

Feeling like a weak person was associated with sadness. Cara observed, "My daughter makes me remember what I was like at her age. I was afraid, hurt, and lonely. I remember the feelings even more than the circumstances." Feeling weak as a result of her father's criticism was frightening, sad, lonely, and painful, and any of these feelings could evoke Cara's core belief that she was a "weak person."

Core beliefs about ourselves, or schemas, are lucidly described by Young, Klosko, and Weishaar (2003) and have been blended into the mindfulness approach by Tara Bennet-Goleman (2001). Schemas are intertwined feelings, thoughts, and actions. Many of us have one or more core, maladaptive, largely unconscious schemas that shape how we relate to our world. Examples of schemas are abandonment, approval-seeking, vulnerability, failure, subjugation, entitlement, mistrust, enmeshment, and deprivation. Each patient may eventually find a word that best captures the shameful, hidden "truth" about him- or herself. In panic disorder, being "defective," "weak," or "crazy" are prime suspects. Treatment is not complete until the core belief about oneself is identified and mindfully observed. With mindful observation, the belief is seen for what it is—a false idea. Some understanding by the patient of his or her personal history is often necessary for this level of deep acceptance, which, in Cara's case, already occurred through previous treatments.

The other mindfulness skills that continued to interest Cara were a newly discovered yoga practice, meditation on "stillness of the body," self-statements (especially "Let go and let God"), and occasionally the MSI, when Cara became anxious.

Closure: Relapse Prevention

Key insights
1. I will always be more anxious than I would like to be.
2. Anxiety will come and go.

Questions
1. When am I most likely to be hijacked by fear?
2. How shall I cultivate mindfulness in everyday life?

Practice
1. Practice mindfulness every day.

In the final phase of treatment, it is important to recognize that panic is likely to reappear periodically. Anxiety is inevitable, and a person with a panic history may be genetically predisposed to have more anxiety than average. The assumption of the mindfulness-based approach is that panic is a result of conditioning—brain habits that will automatically reemerge in certain contexts. If a patient with panic believes that he or she has overcome panic, his or her intention to be mindful may lapse and the panic habit may return in force.

In the final, relapse prevention phase of treatment, the patient should try to remember which circumstances make him or her vulnerable to panic. For example, Cara recognized that she was more likely to panic when tired, before her menstrual period, when outside in the open air, and when she recalled her alcoholic father. These are times when mindfulness is likely to diminish and the patient returns to fighting fear. The patient should be encouraged to remember the most effective mindfulness skills that help him or her accept the fear.

Finally, the patient with panic should be encouraged to maintain the skill of mindfulness *throughout life*, so that anxiety is less likely to mushroom into panic disorder. Ideally, meditation should be practiced daily, usually for 20 minutes, but many patients do not have a taste for it or do not have sufficient social support. However, mindfulness skills for everyday living, such as breath awareness, journaling, contemplative walks, and other techniques (see Chapter 6) are more easily folded into the daily routine. In our case example, Cara reduced her frequency of meditation to once or twice a week after her panic attacks stopped. Cara's preferred mindfulness exercises at the end of treatment were to pay attention to what she was doing in the present moment and to practice mindful yoga daily. When I asked Cara for her permission to use our clinical material in this book, she remarked, "I have a lifelong habit of avoidance. This book may help people like me with the habit of acceptance."

OTHER ANXIETY DISORDERS

Let us briefly consider other anxiety disorders from the point of view of mindfulness-based treatment. The sustaining feature of all anxiety disorders is *avoidance* of internal and/or external cues for fear. The source of distress is critical in designing a treatment program (Craske & Hazlett-Stevens, 2002). Each anxiety disorder poses a unique challenge to the anxious individual and his or her therapist.

Generalized Anxiety Disorder

The treatment program for generalized anxiety disorder (GAD) by Lizabeth Roemer and Susan Orsillo (2002) brought mindfulness and acceptance-based treatment of anxiety squarely into the clinical arena. Their program triggered a healthy debate about the integration of mindfulness and acceptance techniques into CBT (Antony, 2002; Borkovec, 2002; Crits-Christoph, 2002; Craske & Hazlett-Stevens, 2002; Hayes, 2002; Mennin, Heimberg, Turk, & Fresco, 2002; Roemer & Orsillo, 2003; Wells, 2002). The treatment is based on *pervasive worry* in clients with GAD: worry that things could go wrong in the future, nonspecific worry, worry that involves a lot of mental chatter, and worry that expresses itself in restless sleep, overwork, meticulousness, and fatigue. Previously existing treatments helped less than half of patients with GAD (Borkevec, 2002). Roemer and Orsillo (2002) argued that a general attitude of awareness and acceptance, in the present, would be an antidote to the GAD pattern of attempting to control or reduce nonspecific anxiety. Pervasive worry demands a pervasive shift in attention and attitude.

Their treatment protocol employs psychoeducation, early cue detection, mindfulness techniques, monitoring, relaxation, and mindful action. Roemer and Orsillo's (2002) innovative treatment approach is currently being empirically tested.

Obsessive–Compulsive Disorder

The source of distress in obsessive–compulsive disorder (OCD) is ruminative thoughts (obsessions) that do not respond to reassurance, and behaviors (compulsions) that temporarily reduce distress. Patients with OCD are trying to make things safe. An example of obsessive worry is "Did I lock the door?"; a compulsion might involve checking the door three times before going to bed. OCD is the fourth most common psychiatric disorder, following the phobias, substance use disorders, and depression (Robins et al., 1984). The standard of treatment is pharmacotherapy with behavioral treatment (*in vivo* exposure and response prevention), although 25% of patients decline exposure therapy (Greist & Baer, 2002).

A mentioned earlier, Jeffrey Schwartz (1996) developed a treatment protocol for OCD based on mindful awareness and his neuroimaging research. The program is novel, easy to implement, and targets the patient's tendency to get locked into repetitive cycles of thinking or behaving. Schwartz first educates the patient about brain functioning and OCD, and then suggests four R's: *Relabel* ("It's not about an unlocked door, it is my OCD"), *Reattribute* ("My brain is doing this, not me"), *Refocus* ("Why not do something useful, like reading a bedtime story to my child"), and *Revalue* ("These repetitive thoughts are disturbing and a waste of time"). The patient is expected to practice new patterns of brain activity and extinguish old ones. Overall, the patient learns to decenter from the thoughts that hold him or her hostage, making room for new possibilities. I am unaware of controlled outcome studies of

Schwartz's approach, but my clinical experience indicates that patients both enjoy and benefit from it.

Social Phobia

People with social phobia are primarily distressed by the possibility of embarrassment or humiliation in social situations. Panic attacks may occur in social or performance settings, and the patient typically learns to cope by avoiding situations such as school, dating, or the workplace. Often people avoid the problem with "liquid courage": alcohol. Medication can be used to block social anxiety, but as-needed use of medications can also be a form of avoidant behavior. Effective treatments include cognitive restructuring (more realistic assessment of threat), exposure, and social skills training (Cottraux et al., 2000). Like most anxiety disorders, there is a genetic component to social anxiety (Mancini, van Ameringen, Szatmari, Fugere, & Boyle, 1996).

A mindfulness-based approach to social anxiety might attempt to cultivate a general skill of mindfulness, or nonreactive acceptance of what is occurring in the body in the present moment, and then apply mindfulness to situations in which the fears and body sensations are particularly intense. An ACT approach may be helpful here, by nurturing the life aspirations of the patient and encouraging him or her to allow the mind and body to react naturally as those goals are pursued. This approach showed some success compared to CBT in a study by Block and Wulfert (2000), by reducing behavioral avoidance.

Specific Phobias

Specific phobias include fear of flying, heights, blood, snakes, mice, and, potentially, any other stimulus. The origin of phobias may include classical conditioning, biological preparedness due to the inherent dangers of certain common phobias, genetic factors (Vythilingum & Stein, 2004), and unconscious conflicts. *In vivo* exposure is the treatment of choice, and medication is usually not necessary. A therapist rarely sees a patient only for treatment of a specific phobia, unless there is an impending confrontation, such as a blood test, an airplane flight, a move to an apartment building with elevators, and so forth.

Mindfulness-based treatment can facilitate exposure by having a patient first turn toward the fear as it arises in memory (imaginal desensitization), then explore it in great detail. The patient may be asked to describe each moment of bodily sensation as it arises, along with the stream of thoughts. The patient would invariably become mindful of the intention to flee, and might restrain the body for a few moments to further explore the avoidance reaction. When the patient can do all of this imaginally, he or she can begin the same precise, moment-to-moment exploration *in vivo*.

I sometimes explain to phobic patients that we want to pass the fear through a microscope: First we see the tissue, then the cell, then the molecules, then the electrons, then the vast space between electrons. The deeper we probe, the less fear we see. The fear can exist only as long as we look at the experience superficially.

Posttraumatic Stress Disorder

It is estimated that more than 50% of the U.S. population has been exposed to a traumatic event (Kessler, Sonnega, Bromlet, Hughes, & Nelson, 1995). Trauma becomes a disorder when the traumatic event is persistently reexperienced (flashbacks), when related situations are avoided, when the person feels emotionally numb, or when there are symptoms of persistent arousal. Trauma appears to affect parts of the subcortex, such as the amygdala, thalamus, hypothalamus, hippocampus, hypothalamus, and brain stem, that are less accessible to conscious or verbal thought (Hull, 2002). PTSD involves remaining in a state of biological readiness long after the threat has passed.

The best example we have of mindfulness and acceptance-based treatments with traumatized persons is dialectical behavior therapy (DBT; Linehan, 1993a; Robins, 2002). DBT is the standard of treatment for patients with borderline personality disorder, many of whom have a history of trauma. Two of the modules in Linehan's program are acceptance-based: Mindfulness Skills, in which the patient observes, describes, and participates in moment-to-moment experience; and Distress Tolerance, in which the patient is taught to endure distress without acting on the discomfort. Linehan quips, "You can feel like a mental patient, but that doesn't mean you have to act like one" (cited in Carey, 2004, p. D6).

Mindfulness must be skillfully applied when therapists work with trauma patients. When to shift attention *toward* or *away* from traumatic memories—attention regulation—is perhaps best described as a wisdom skill, based on the needs of the present moment. The rule of thumb is to assess the stability of attention: "Can the patient experience the pain without being overwhelmed?" (Please refer to Chapter 6 for more on trauma and mindfulness techniques.) Intellectual understanding alone is insufficient to heal trauma in the body–mind, but mindful awareness of bodily experience, without reactive avoidance, may be beneficial. Bessel van der Kolk (cited in Wylie, 2004, p. 36) says that trauma patients need the "therapist's attuned attention to the moods, physical sensations, and physical impulses within. The therapist must be the patient's servant, helping him or her to explore, befriend, and trust their inner felt experience."

WORKING MINDFULLY WITH ANXIOUS PATIENTS

I would like to briefly mention four considerations when working with anxious patients in mindfulness-based treatment.

First, it is important that the therapist have personal experience with mindfulness, ideally from a meditation practice. It is one thing to *suggest* to a patient that he or she accept feelings as they emerge and quite another to have the *personal experience* of sitting with intense emotional difficulties, with curiosity and an open heart, and watching them transform. The patient will have faith that his or her worst fears are indeed manageable if the therapist is also convinced from personal experience.

Second, the therapist must be able to communicate effectively about the paradox of goal-directed behavior and nonstriving. Mindful awareness is a means to symptom reduction, but to achieve this, we need to fully abandon the goal and allow ourselves to be absorbed in awareness of the present. A patient once wondered aloud, "How to *not* do it to just get better!" The therapist is required to have faith that the treatment goal will indeed be achieved if it is temporarily suspended. The therapist is a role model for nonattached commitment to the therapy process.

Third, the therapist needs to know the difference between passing through negative mind states, such as anger or sadness, and ego disintegration. Practicing mindfulness is in the service of emotional balance and alleviating suffering, not an end in itself. Mindfulness exercises can have adverse effects if not applied wisely. Our patients are avoiding their experience because it hurts. We want to create a positive experience of the formerly avoided fear. We are trying to artfully move the patient from freedom *from* fear to freedom *in* fear.

Finally, mindfulness itself cannot be captured in a technique. It is an elusive way of being. Our strategic exercises, such formal mindfulness meditation practice, or the MSI, are merely props. Waking up to our lives in each moment requires considerable intention and effort. It is a lifelong endeavor that we undertake for ourselves, and can share with our patients, using whatever means at our disposal.

CHAPTER 9

Psychophysiological Disorders

Embracing Pain

RONALD D. SIEGEL

Nobody likes pain. Throughout history, people have gone to great lengths to get rid of it. While some physical discomfort is inevitable, a remarkable variety of medical disorders are actually maintained by our attempts to feel better. Mindfulness practice can help to resolve these conditions and enrich our lives in the process.

One of the first systematic treatment programs explicitly to teach mindfulness to patients was designed for the management of chronic pain (Kabat-Zinn, 1982). While there have not yet been many large-scale, controlled studies using mindfulness-based programs to treat pain or illness, reviews of preliminary data have been quite encouraging (Baer, 2003; Grossman, Niemann, Schmidt, & Walach, 2004). Over the past two decades, medical applications of mindfulness have broadened, and the practice has been integrated into the treatment of a wide range of physical disorders with psychological components (Goldenberg et al., 1994; Kabat-Zinn et al., 1998; Kaplan, Goldenberg, & Galvin-Nadeau, 1993; Logsdon-Conradsen, 2002; Saxe et al., 2001; Shapiro, Bootzin, Figueredo, Lopez, & Schwartz., 2003; Tacon, McComb, Caldera, & Randolph, 2003).

The distinction between the mind and the body, so familiar in Western discourse, is misleading. Subjective mental states are influenced by physical factors, such as medication effects, exercise, and diet. Conversely, a host of physical disorders are influenced by psychological factors. The most common are *psychophysiological* disorders, in which persistent mental states, usually involving negative emotions, create changes in tissues, which in turn cause symptoms. Examples include headaches, gastrointestinal distress, dermatological disorders, and muscular–skeletal pain of all sorts. Because these disorders are often maintained by a mix of medical, psychological, and behavioral factors, clinicians have evolved flexible, integrative interventions in an attempt to address all of these elements. It turns out that psychophysiological disorders seem particularly well suited to treatments that incorporate mindfulness.

One such intervention is the Back Sense program—an approach that my colleagues and I developed to integrate cognitive, psychodynamic, behavioral, and systemic interventions, along with explicit teaching of mindfulness practice for the treatment of chronic back pain (Siegel, Urdang, & Johnson, 2001). The program goes beyond the early uses of mindfulness for pain management, drawing on recent innovations in rehabilitation medicine and psychology to resolve the disorder fully for many people. Patients can participate in the program by following a published self-treatment guide (*Back Sense: A Revolutionary Approach to Halting the Cycle of Chronic Back Pain*; Siegel et al., 2001) or through treatment with a mental health or rehabilitation professional.

In this chapter, I discuss the program as an illustration of how mindfulness practice can be fruitfully combined with other psychotherapeutic interventions to treat psychophysiological disorders. The chapter explores the benefits to patients of formal mindfulness practice, as well as how principles derived from mindfulness practice—such as relaxing control, tolerating discomfort, staying with negative emotions, and returning attention to the present—can inform other components of treatment. It also discusses how the approaches used to treat back pain can readily be adapted to treat a wide range of stress-related health problems.

AN EVOLUTIONARY ACCIDENT

While almost everyone experiences occasional back pain, for 5 million Americans at any given time, chronic back pain (lasting more than 3 months) is a nightmarish disability that interferes with every aspect of their lives (Agency for Health Care Policy and Research, 1994). Until recently, most orthopedists would tell you that the disorder is so prevalent because of an unintended consequence of evolution. This story, told to countless patients, explains that our spines became stressed when our ancestors learned to stand up and walk on two legs. The increased pressure on our disks (small cushions between the vertebrae) and other structures of the spine supposedly leads to damage over time that accounts for the epidemic of back trouble among modern humans.

To the surprise of doctors and patients alike, recent research is challenging this idea. The new evidence points to a cycle of psychological stress, muscle tension, and fear-based avoidance of activity as the true cause for the vast majority of sufferers (Siegel et al., 2001). It appears that a different evolutionary accident is the more likely culprit, and mindfulness can help us to respond to it effectively.

Fight or Flight

All mammals share an ancient, sophisticated emergency response, often called the "fight-or-flight" system. It functions remarkably well in times of danger and probably has had enormous adaptive benefits throughout evolutionary history. When a mammal is threatened, its sympathetic nervous system and hypothalamic–pituitary–adrenal (HPA) axes are activated, resulting in increased epinephrine (adrenaline) in the bloodstream, and many other physiological changes (Sapolsky, 1998). Respiration, heart rate, body temperature, and muscle tension all increase— the better to fight an enemy or flee from danger. Vision and hearing even become more acute. At the same time, long-term processes such as digestive activity and immune system response tend to shut down. Stress physiologists tell us that this is adaptive: There is no need to exhaust resources digesting your own lunch when you are about to become someone else's (Sapolsky, 1998).

Let us look at how this usually works. Imagine that a rabbit grazing in a field notices a fox. It freezes, hoping not to be noticed, while becoming more vigilant and physiologically aroused in preparation for running away (rabbits are not big fighters). If the fox wanders off without seeing the rabbit, soon the rabbit's parasympathetic nervous system becomes active, and its physiology returns to a resting level. This system works wonderfully for rabbits and undoubtedly has contributed to their survival.

Imagine now for a moment that the rabbit possessed a highly evolved cerebral cortex like ours, allowing for language and complex symbolic, anticipatory thought. Once the fox has left, the rabbit might begin to think: "Will he return? Will he find my family?" Even once the immediate danger has passed, the rabbit could find itself thinking about the fox—not to mention whether it can save up enough carrots for retirement and other concerns. All such thoughts would continue to activate its fight-or-flight system, which would remain stuck in the "on" position.

Though admittedly oversimplified, this is what happens to humans. Our capacity for symbolic, anticipatory thought, while extraordinarily adaptive in allowing us to construct complex civilizations, is ill suited to coexist with our mammalian fight-or-flight system. Rather than our transition to walking upright, it appears that *this* evolutionary accident is responsible for the epidemic of chronic back pain, as well as a host of other psychophysiological disorders. Virtually every physiological change brought about by the fight-or-flight system can cause or exacerbate a stress-related symptom if the system remains continuously active. As we will see, mindfulness practice can be very salutary, interrupting the overactivation of our fight-or-flight system to which we are predisposed by evolutionary accident.

The likelihood that we will develop chronic, stress-related symptoms is increased dramatically if we misinterpret these symptoms when they arise. Before we introduce mindfulness practice into treatment, it is therefore important that our patients be well grounded in the most accurate possible understanding of what causes their symptoms.

BAD BACK?

Let us return to the problem of chronic back pain. Most patients and, until recently, most health care professionals have naturally assumed that persistent back pain must be due to damage to the disks or other structures of the spine. After all, if we cut our finger, we see blood and feel pain. We automatically surmise that back pain functions similarly, even if the "injury" is not visible to us.

There has recently been an explosion of research findings that question this, however. They all point to a lack of correlation between the condition of the spine and the presence of pain. Education about these findings is a necessary part of effective treatment programs, for understanding the research helps to alleviate patients' concerns about being damaged or fragile. A few examples serve as illustrations:

- Approximately two-thirds of people who have never suffered from serious back pain have the same sorts of "abnormal" back structures that are often blamed for chronic back pain (Jensen et al., 1994).
- Many people continue to have pain after "successful" surgical repair. There is little correlation between the mechanical success of repairs and whether or not the patient is still in pain (Fraser, Sandhu, & Gogan, 1995; Tullberg, Grane, & Isacson, 1994).
- People in developing countries who do "back-breaking" labor,

and use ergonomically primitive furniture and tools, have the lowest incidence of chronic back pain—not what we would expect if damage to the spine were the culprit (Volinn, 1997).

Along with the data questioning the assumption that damage to the spine causes chronic back pain, we find many studies implicating psychological factors:

- Psychological stress, and particularly job dissatisfaction, predicts who will develop disabling back pain more reliably than do physical measures or the physical demands of one's job (Bigos et al., 1991).
- Back pain patients show significantly increased muscle tension in their backs when placed in an emotionally stressful situation, while other pain patients do not (Flor, Turk, & Birbaumer, 1985).
- Chronic back pain is unusually prevalent among people with trauma histories or those who live in stressful situations, such as war zones (Beckham et al., 1997; Linton, 1997; Pecukonis, 1996).

THE CHRONIC BACK PAIN CYCLE

Taken together, these sorts of studies suggest that psychological factors, rather than structural abnormalities, are often the cause of chronic back pain. This occurs through a cycle that has many parallels with the dynamics of anxiety disorders described in Chapter 8. Its core components are irrational fear, increased psychophysiological arousal, misinterpreted symptoms, and behavioral avoidance. Patients need to understand this cycle before they can effectively use mindfulness practice to help interrupt it. The following case is a typical example of how it unfolds:

Last winter, Robert's back started to hurt after he shoveled snow. He had experienced pain like this before, which usually resolved within a few days. This time, however, the pain was still there after two weeks. In fact, he was occasionally experiencing pain running down his leg to his foot.

Robert began to worry. He had been enjoying working out at the gym—both to stay in shape and to relieve stress. When he hurt his back, he stopped exercising, waiting for his back to heal. Alarmed that the pain was persisting, he made an appointment with his physician.

Robert's doctor heard his report of sciatic (leg) pain and became concerned, suspecting nerve impingement in his spine. Magnetic resonance imaging (MRI) indicated a bulging disk, and the doctor suggested that Robert take antiinflammatory medication and avoid activities that might further dislodge his disk.

Prior to his injury, Robert had been having a difficult time at work, because the company was not doing well, and his boss had been extremely tense. Robert had felt stressed before his back problem began, but was now becoming even more anxious and agitated. Every day he awoke to the same pain. Robert began to fear that he might never get better.

Robert was becoming caught in the *chronic back pain cycle* (Siegel et al., 2001), which can begin with an injury from an accident or overexertion, or can appear to begin out of the blue, without a clear physical precipitant (Hall, McIntosh, Wilson, & Melles, 1998).

Once pain has persisted longer than expected or reached high levels of intensity, fear becomes a factor. Because chronic back pain has become an epidemic, virtually everyone has had contact with someone who has suffered with it and was not helped by his or her doctor. The prevalence of MRIs, with their ability to reveal random variations in spinal structure in great detail, contributes to fear by presenting patients with images of a decaying spine.

Fear and worry about one's back has several negative effects. Like Robert, most people respond by abandoning physical activities that previously helped to reduce psychological stress and keep their muscles strong and flexible. Distressing thoughts, coupled with this inactivity, lead to anxiety, frustration, and anger, all of which add to the arousal of the fight-or-flight system. This arousal in turn contributes to muscle tightness, at the same time that the muscles are deprived of the natural movement that previously helped to keep them relaxed. A cycle of pain–worry–fear–tension–pain accompanied by disability becomes established.

Fear not only adds to pain by increasing muscle tension, but it also actually amplifies the pain sensations themselves. There is now considerable evidence that the experience of pain is not simply proportionate to the degree of disturbance to tissues (Melzack & Wall, 1965). People experience a given stimulus as far more painful when they are frightened than when they feel safe (Beecher, 1946; Robinson & Riley, 1999). Thus, concern about pain contributes to pain cycles not only by tensing muscles but also by amplifying the sensations of pain that the tight muscles produce. As we will see shortly, mindfulness practice, which can alter our attitude toward pain, can therefore both help to relax muscles and influence our experience of pain by changing our relationship to it.

Yet another component of the chronic back pain cycle involves mistaken attributions. Once a person becomes worried about back pain, he or she will struggle to figure out which movements or positions seem to make it better or worse. Once such a relationship is observed, every time the person engages in the activity presumed to be problematic, he or she becomes more anxious, and more tense. Increased pain usually follows, reinforcing the belief that a given action is hazardous. This conditioned reaction, termed *kinesiophobia* (fear of movement), has been shown to be a better predictor of back pain chronicity and disability than medical diagnosis (Crombez, Vlaeyen, Heuts, & Lysens, 1999; Waddell, Newton, Henderson, & Somerville, 1993).

The parallels between the chronic back pain cycle and the anxiety disorders described in the Chapter 8 are evident. They both result from overactivity of the fight-or-flight system. They also both involve future-oriented maladaptive fear responses, experiential avoidance, and false assumptions about the nature of the problem. Mindfulness—awareness of present experience with acceptance—can help to counteract these processes by increasing tolerance of discomfort and decreasing identification with worrisome thoughts.

THE RECOVERY CYCLE

Recovery from the syndrome requires interrupting the pain cycle. This involves three basic elements, all of which can be supported by mindfulness practice: (1) *cognitive restructuring*, (2) *resuming full physical activity*, and (3) *working with negative emotions*. Interventions may be individually tailored, placing more or less emphasis on each element depending upon which aspects of the pain cycle are most salient for a given patient.

Before beginning treatment, all patients should undergo a thorough physical examination to rule out rare but potentially serious medical causes for their pain. These disorders, which include tumors, infections, injuries, and unusual structural abnormalities, are the cause of only about 1 in 200 cases of chronic back pain (Agency for Health Care Policy and Research, 1994; Deyo, Rainville, & Kent, 1992). The physical examination is needed to avoid overlooking a treatable medical disorder, to facilitate cognitive restructuring, and to grant trustworthy permission to resume activity.

Mindfulness and Cognitive Restructuring

As long as patients believe that their pain is due to structural damage in the spine, they react to pain with fear and avoid activity associated with it, thus perpetuating the pain cycle. The process of changing a person's belief about this is challenging. Because the pain can be intense, it is often difficult at first for most patients (and many clinicians) to believe that muscle tension could actually be causing it.

Patients are presented with key research studies questioning the connection between back pain and structural damage, followed by an explanation of how the chronic back pain cycle functions. A vital part of this psychoeducational process involves helping patients to understand the nature of psychophysiological disorders. This is particularly necessary before patients will embrace a mental exercise such as mindfulness to treat a seemingly physical problem. Many patients are concerned that our addressing psychological factors means that we think their pain is imagined, or "all in my head." They may also fear being accused of malingering. As clinicians, it is very important for us to emphasize that the pain is caused by changes in the muscles, and is in every way real.

Once patients have learned about the chronic back pain cycle, it is suggested that mindfulness practice can help to interrupt it by increasing pain tolerance, reducing aversion reactions, disentangling from negative thoughts, and facilitating work with difficult emotions. Basic mindfulness meditation instructions (Chapter 1) are then introduced.

While the effect is gradual, mindfulness practice seems to increase the cognitive flexibility that is needed throughout treatment. By observing the arising and passing of thoughts without following or judging them, patients become less identified with the thoughts' content. Mindfulness practice also helps patients to see that thought is socially influenced: They notice that their minds are full of ideas picked up from doctors, friends, and others. Patients come to observe a key cognitive-behavioral and psychodynamic principal that has been discussed in other chapters in this volume: It is not events themselves, but our interpretation of events that determines our reactions to them. Direct experience of this helps patients with pain to entertain the idea that assumptions about structural damage, and even medical diagnoses, are changeable constructs—not objective conclusions about reality.

Observing the interplay among pain, fear, and behavior in one's own experience is also supported by mindfulness practice. Most of the time, patients are unaware of the role that cognitions and emotions play in their pain. With mindfulness practice, this awareness can be deepened.

Cathy had been suffering with back pain for years. Despite the fact that doctors had never found anything more than a mild disk bulge, she was convinced that she had a "bad back" and was in constant danger of reinjuring herself. She particularly avoided sitting for prolonged periods, as she was convinced that her body could not tolerate the pressure this put on her spine. As soon as she experienced a twinge of pain, she would get up and walk around.

Mindfulness practice was easy at first. She began while lying down. She was able to follow her breath and dealt well with the usual challenges of having a busy mind.

The practice became difficult when she was asked to try it in a chair. Cathy noticed that her attention was constantly moving toward her lower back, monitoring it for pain. She wanted to get up as soon as she experienced a twinge. Cathy also became aware that her urge to change position was motivated more by fear than by the intensity of pain itself. In her mind, Kathy would "budget" her chair time, thinking that if she already hurt after 5 minutes, she would never be able to sit for 20 minutes. When encouraged to keep practicing in the chair, she experienced fearful thought after fearful thought, accompanied by feelings of anxiety, increased back muscle tension, and more pain.

This use of mindfulness can dovetail well with cognitive-behavioral methods for observing thought patterns. For example, I sometimes ask patients to keep a pad with them and make a mark each time they notice themselves having an anxious thought about their backs. Most people abandon the exercise after a few hours, because they realize that they are constantly having such thoughts. Patients can also be asked to complete inventories, such as the Beliefs about Pain questionnaire (Siegel et al., 2001)[1] or the Tampa Scale of Kinesiophobia (Kori, Miller, & Todd, 1990), which help them to notice hitherto unacknowledged assumptions about their condition. Such interventions work well with mindfulness practice to increase awareness of negative emotions and cognitions, thereby making the idea of the chronic back pain cycle more plausible.

Using Mindfulness to Resume Activity

The second step of the recovery process, *resuming full physical activity*, serves many functions. It is an exposure and response prevention treatment for kinesiophobia and fears of disability, designed to change a patient's relationship to these experiences. Instead of avoiding activity in response to fear, he or she enters into activity and attempts to open to, or

---

[1]This and other *Back Sense* inventories may be obtained without charge from *www.backsense.org*.

befriend the fear that results (see Chapter 8). It is also a physical exercise for muscles that have become short and weak, and a means of reducing psychological stress.

Patients are asked to create a hierarchy of activities that they have abandoned, rating each activity as *pleasant, neutral,* or *unpleasant,* and *easy, moderate,* or *difficult* to resume, using the Lost Activities Inventory (Siegel et al., 2001). They are instructed to begin with those activities that they imagine would be most enjoyable and least difficult or frightening to pursue. This is designed to make the process self-reinforcing and to keep anxiety at a tolerable level.

When patients initially resume relinquished activities, their pain often increases, both because tight, weak muscles are painful to use at first, and because of the increase in anxiety that results from challenging a phobia. Mindfulness practice can be an effective tool to move patients through this difficult step.

Pain Does Not Equal Suffering

There is a famous talk attributed to the Buddha, in which he describes our typical response to pain:

> When touched with a feeling of pain, the uninstructed run-of-the-mill person sorrows, grieves, and laments, beats his breast, becomes distraught. So he feels two pains, physical and mental. Just as if they were to shoot a man with an arrow and, right afterward, were to shoot him with another one, so that he would feel the pains of two arrows. (Bhikku, 2004b, p. 1)

This ancient realization that the experience of pain is followed immediately by a response of aversion and suffering is readily observed in mindfulness practice. One of my patients expressed it in a succinct mathematical formula: *pain × resistance = suffering.* This insight, verified in patients' own experience, can allow them to move forward in resuming activity.

> Beth had been disabled several times by excruciating sciatic pain. She had spent thousands of dollars on ergonomic automobile seats, workstation chairs, and top of the line orthopedic mattresses. Whenever the pain returned, she would become despondent, desperately trying to identify its source. She hoped that she could keep it at bay, if she were sufficiently careful.
>
> Beth's brother was going to be married soon, and she very much wanted to be at the wedding. Unfortunately, she was terrified by the prospect of the plane trip, sure that several hours trapped in

an unmodified airline seat would cripple her. We decided to use mindfulness practice to help her prepare.

Beth began by sitting in an ordinary chair, following her breath. After about 10 minutes, she was invited to bring her attention to the sensations in her leg. She was asked to observe the sensations as precisely as she could, to notice whether she felt burning, aching, throbbing, or stabbing. Whenever she had a fearful or distracting thought, she was asked to return her attention to the actual sensations in her leg at the present moment.

At first, the sensations increased in intensity, and Beth was frightened. Over the course of 30 minutes, however, she noticed that the sensations actually became variable. They changed in quality, as well as intensity. Thoughts of "I can't stand this," or "I hope this isn't going to set me back" arose, and passed.

Beth was asked to see whether she could notice how her pain was actually made up of a series of separate momentary sensations, like frames in a movie strung together so quickly as to give the illusion of continuity. She was asked to continue noticing the detail, as she might when watching a sunset or listening to a symphony. Often this was difficult, because the sensations were quite unpleasant. Nonetheless, Beth was surprised to find that she could stay with the experience and, by the end, actually felt no more uncomfortable than she had at the beginning.

Several impediments to resuming activity are addressed during this sort of mindfulness practice. First, it becomes possible to see that pain sensations themselves are distinct from our aversion responses—our negative thoughts and feelings about the pain. These aversion responses constitute the experience of suffering (the second arrow in the Buddha's talk). This observation can be enormously freeing, because it allows a person to tolerate pain rather than feel compelled to avoid or alleviate it. If pain can be accepted, then a wider range of human activity becomes possible.

Second, by bringing attention to the present moment, anticipatory anxiety is reduced. It has often been observed that even in terrible situations, our fear is of the future. For example, when people become conscious following a serious automobile crash, their minds often race forward: "Will I be OK? Will my loved ones survive?" This concern about the future occurs even if they are in pain or bleeding. By bringing attention to the present, the anticipatory anxiety that feeds pain cycles is reduced. This lowers muscle tension and reduces the perceived intensity of pain.

Third, mindfulness practice helps people to feel "held." When a person is in pain and has no clear options for relief, he or she often becomes quite distraught. Mindfulness practice gives patients a structured activity that does not feed into the spiral of aversion responses, increased pain, and more aversion. The present moment can become a place of refuge rather than a threat to be avoided.

Once patients are less terrified of their pain, they are better able to move forward behaviorally by resuming abandoned activities.

Patients may need frequent reminding that uninhibited movement is not dangerous, and they may require repeated invitations to approach pain mindfully. In order to help extinguish conditioned associations between activity and pain, patients are encouraged to engage in their chosen activity several times weekly for a few weeks before moving on to the next challenge. They are usually able to observe fluctuations in pain level during this period, despite consistency in activity. This helps them to realize that the activity itself is not the problem.

Working with Intentions

Many patients are far more concerned about disability than about pain per se. Mindfulness practice can help them to realize that they need not be disabled by their pain sensations—that sensations need not dictate behavior.

> Michelle was a police officer who loved her work. Her back pain, which had lasted for over 2 years, began following an automobile accident that totaled her cruiser. Even though her medical findings were unremarkable, she was unable to sit in a chair for more than a few minutes. She had been given an administrative position, but now her post was about to be eliminated, and she had to either return to regular police work or lose her job. Michelle was afraid that she would not be able to sit all day in a cruiser and would soon be an unemployed single mother. To a competent, can-do woman, this thought was intolerable.
>
> Michelle was willing to accept that her pain was due to muscle tension, but this did little to lessen her misery. She was introduced to simple, breath-focused mindfulness practice, and took to it readily at first. She was able to observe her pain sensations and notice their changing quality. As time went on, however, the pain increased, and she began squirming in her chair. "I have to get up," she announced. "The pain is too intense." She was asked to try to stay with the sensations in her back for a few more minutes. When her squirming continued to intensify, she was directed to now bring her attention to the sense of urgency to get out of the chair—to focus her mind on the intention to get up itself. She was invited to locate this feeling of urgent intention in her body.
>
> After a few moments, Michelle reported that she felt the urge to rise as a tightness or pressure in her chest and neck. She was then

asked try to focus her attention on this area. Soon the sensations associated with the intention to get up—which were independent of her back pain—began to change and move around in her body. Her squirming stopped, and she was able to remain sitting and return her attention to the breath.

This experience had a profound effect. Until then, Michelle had not noticed any gap between her sensations of increased pain and her moving to relieve the discomfort. Observing that the *intention* to rise occurs in between, and can be worked with like any other sensation, significantly increased her sense of freedom. This gave her confidence that by practicing mindfulness, she could learn to sit for extended periods, which would allow her eventually to resume regular police work.

Strength, Flexibility, and Endurance Training

One way to accelerate both the extinction of fear responses to normal activity and the return of muscular strength and flexibility is through structured exercise training. Graded weight lifting, stretching, and aerobic exercises can help move patients beyond their fears that they are structurally compromised (Siegel et al., 2001). Once a person can deadlift 25 pounds, he or she is less likely to fear bending to pick up a child's toy or grocery bag. Systematic exercise treats both the kinesiophobia and the shortening and weakening of muscles caused by caution and inactivity. There is mounting evidence that vigorous exercise, even if it initially exacerbates pain, facilitates recovery (Guzman et al., 2001; Mayer et al., 1987; Rainville, Sobel, Hartigan, Monlux, & Bean, 1997; Schonstein, Kenny, Keating, & Koes, 2003).

When patients begin to exercise previously neglected muscles, they often experience increased pain. Rehabilitation programs often fail at this point. As with the resumption of other activities, mindfulness practice can be fruitfully applied to working with the fear and pain that arise when patients embark on a structured exercise program. After developing some capacity for concentration by following the breath, patients are instructed to bring accepting attention to the pain sensations associated with lifting weights, stretching, or participating in aerobic activity. This builds pain tolerance and reduces the likelihood that increased pain will cause counterproductive muscle tension.

Using Mindfulness to Work with Negative Emotions

For many patients, learning that their pain is not due to structural damage, seeing for themselves how the chronic back pain cycle operates, and resuming full activity is sufficient to free them from the disorder. For others, however, a return to normal activity is not enough. In our experience, these are generally people for whom emotional difficulties—beyond concerns about back pain—are contributing to persistent muscle tension. Often some combination of psychodynamic exploration and social skills training is helpful. Here again, mindfulness practice can support the recovery process.

There is evidence that people who have difficulty acknowledging affect suffer disproportionately from psychophysiological disorders (Schwartz, 1990), and that learning to identify and safely express emotion can reduce the frequency of symptoms (Pennebaker, Keicolt-Glaser, & Glaser, 1988). When we are unable to acknowledge or tolerate a thought or feeling, our fight-or-flight system reacts to its threatened emergence much as it reacts to external threats. Since life experiences continuously trigger disavowed cognitions and affects, our fight-or-flight system is frequently on overdrive. It is thus no surprise that increasing affect awareness can help to free some people from chronic back pain.

> By everyone's account, Eddie was a very "nice guy." He had not always been this way. As a boy, he was known for being provocative, and he often got into fights. He had a strict father who did not tolerate his transgressions.
>
> In adolescence, Eddie turned over a new leaf and became an exemplary citizen. As an adult, he rarely argued and was always well mannered. He reported that he often felt sad, lonely, or anxious, but never angry.
>
> Not surprisingly, Eddie was very compliant in following his treatment program. He recognized how frightened he had been about his pain and was systematically able to resume activity. He clearly wanted to please his therapist.
>
> Eddie was frustrated, though, that his pain persisted. As it became clear that he was unusually inhibited in recognizing and expressing anger, he was encouraged to discuss situations in which anger might arise.
>
> While he was able to identify some previously disavowed anger in this way, it was during mindfulness practice that his aggression became most apparent to him. He would notice that when angry thoughts arose, he would quickly talk himself into forgiving the other person.
>
> Eventually, Eddie recalled that he used to be angry a lot but had made a conscious decision to stop, since it only seemed to cause trouble. As his therapy and mindfulness practice continued, Eddie was increasingly able to notice and acknowledge a full range of feeling. His anxiety lessened, and he experienced less pain.

Mindfulness practice supports such psychodynamic exploration both by bringing previously unnoticed emotions into awareness and by helping patients to tolerate them. During mindfulness practice, thoughts, feelings, and memories are free to enter the mind, just as they are during free association. The processes differ, in that mindfulness practice does not encourage following each mental event to find its meaning. Nonetheless, both practices are likely to bring into consciousness affects and cognitions that we might otherwise not notice. Just as mindfulness supports the development of pain tolerance by helping us to see that sensations are impermanent and ever-changing, it also facilitates the tolerance of difficult emotions. Patients see that emotions arise, are experienced, and eventually pass. This is an important way that mindfulness practice functions in dialectical behavior therapy (DBT), which is designed for people who are readily overwhelmed by affect (Linehan, 1993a).

Not Relaxation Training

The uses of mindfulness that I have been discussing differ significantly from the more conventional application of relaxation training in the treatment of psychophysiological disorders. Such training can take many forms, such as *progressive relaxation* (Jacobson, 1938), *autogenic training* (Schultz & Luthe, 1959), the *relaxation response* (Benson & Klipper, 2000), or a host of guided imagery exercises. What these all share is the intention of gaining control over physiological arousal through some combination of manipulating muscle groups, developing concentration, or entering into pleasant, unthreatening fantasy.

Mindfulness practice differs from these approaches in that it attends to whatever is actually happening at the present moment, with acceptance. This investigative quality enables mindfulness to go beyond attempting symptom relief through reducing physiological arousal. As we have seen, it can facilitate cognitive change, increase tolerance of pain, uncover emotions, and increase our capacity to choose whether to act on our urges.

In the process, however, mindfulness practice may initially increase the intensity of symptoms by reducing distraction. As mentioned in Chapter 6, it can also increase autonomic arousal as upsetting thoughts, feelings, and memories enter awareness. Nonetheless, in the long run, mindfulness practice seems to allow our nervous system to settle down more consistently as we gain insight into the workings of our minds and feel less resistant to and threatened by the vicissitudes of our experience.

CONTROL

Many lessons that one learns through mindfulness practice are essential to working successfully with psychophysiological disorders. One of these involves finding an optimal balance between goal-oriented effort and letting go.

Mindfulness practice is full of paradoxes. It is often described as a "goalless" activity, since it involves paying attention to whatever is happening in the moment, including the experience of being distracted from paying attention to what is happening in the moment. This is sometimes confusing to beginners, who have difficulty deciding how hard to try to concentrate on an object of attention. They frequently imagine that their mind should be "blank," and feel that they are failing each time their minds wander. It can take some time before people are comfortable having some moments in which the mind is scattered, and others in which it is more focused. Eventually, they learn to put effort toward paying attention, while simultaneously letting go of the goal of remaining focused. Paradoxically, the mind naturally focuses when we no longer insist that it be focused.

Shunryu Suzuki, an influential Zen teacher, writes about this principle metaphorically: "To give your sheep or cow a large, spacious meadow is the way to control him" (Suzuki, 1973, p. 31). We see this paradox at work in psychophysiological disorders. It arises in all situations in which the overactivation of our fight-or-flight system creates an unwanted effect. This is because the very act of *trying* involves some struggle and, hence, some activation of the system. A person struggling with insomnia finds him- or herself more aroused and awakened the harder he or she tries to sleep; the man who fights against erectile dysfunction by trying to control his body finds that the strategy fails; *trying* to relax often backfires. Attachment to symptom reduction perpetuates symptoms.

This insight, called *creative hopelessness* in acceptance and commitment therapy (ACT), is particularly valuable for resolving psychophysiological disorders. To communicate the concept, ACT offers the metaphor of "Chinese handcuffs," the woven straw tubes into which you insert your index fingers, only to find that the more you try to pull them out, the more tightly the tube grips them (Hayes, 2002). To practice mindfulness effectively, or to work effectively with most psychophysiological disorders, patients must learn to differentiate between those areas over which they can exert control and those in which it is counterproductive to try. Generally, we can effectively control our behavior, but not our experience. A student of mindfulness can commit to practicing daily for a prescribed period of time but cannot control whether he or she will feel relaxed or tense, focused or scattered. Similarly, a patient with back pain can commit to systematically increasing his or her range of activity and to a program of stretching and exercise, but cannot control when pain will arise.

The idea that it is counterproductive to try to avoid pain is particularly difficult to grasp in modern Western culture. The torrent of messages we receive from advertisements leads most people to feel that if only they purchase the right remedy, they would never experience pain. Conventional treatments for pain reinforce this notion by focusing on pain relief. It can therefore be difficult to accept that relinquishing the goal of alleviating pain is essential for recovery.

Mindfulness practice can help. By observing that suffering comes from our reaction to pain, and learning to watch the coming and going of pleasant and unpleasant experiences, patients are able to cultivate the accepting attitude that ultimately can free them from a chronic pain cycle. They gradually learn to treat the pain as though it is completely out of their control, like the weather. The realization that psychological health involves a skillful balance between goal-oriented effort and acceptance forms a central component of most mindfulness-based treatments, including DBT, ACT, mindfulness-based stress reduction (MBSR), and mindfulness-based cognitive therapy (MBCT).

IMPERMANENCE AND MORTALITY

The experience of chronic back pain forces many people to confront existential realities. While few patients worry that their condition is fatal, it can make one lose faith in the health of the body. This often brings up anxiety relating to concerns far beyond the back pain, as thoughts of the body's fragility and impermanence enter awareness. Not surprisingly, such anxiety contributes to tension that can feed into the chronic back pain cycle.

All of the world's religious traditions have grappled with the fundamental existential reality of mortality. Patients who believe in God and an afterlife often turn to their religious tradition to find relief from this universal concern. For others, such beliefs hold little power, and the experience of chronic pain ushers in an existential crisis.

Mindfulness practice, stemming from a nontheistic, empirical tradition, can offer these patients a way to work with the challenge. Through practicing mindfulness, people often begin to see how all of life exists in the present moment, and that memories and thoughts of the future are psychological constructions. As has been discussed earlier, it also helps us to identify with a world larger than ourselves, and hence be less preoccupied with the state of our own bodies.

With therapeutic guidance, patients begin to sense that they can take refuge in the present moment and cultivate the capacity to face the reality of the body's fragility and eventual decay. There is an irony in this: Integrative treatment of chronic back pain incorporating mindfulness helps people to realize that their back is not actually damaged physically, and they can live normal lives. At the same time, it can help them to see that all life is impermanent, which helps to prepare them for the reality that the body eventually decays and fails.

TAILORING MINDFULNESS

Many variables go into deciding which mindfulness exercises are most suited to which patients. If patients find a particular exercise too challenging, they will not stick with it. Furthermore, some exercises are can actually be harmful to vulnerable individuals.

Trauma Survivors

I discussed earlier how mindfulness practice can support enhanced awareness and tolerance of affects, thus helping to reduce the chronic tension associated with the effort to keep such contents out of awareness. For individuals who habitually repress painful memories or emotions, however, this can become overwhelming. Since trauma survivors are significantly overrepresented among people with chronic back pain and other psychophysiological disorders, this is frequently an issue in treatment (Beckham et al., 1997; Pecukonis, 1996; Yaari, Eisenberg, Adler, & Birkhan, 1999). Such patients often become extremely anxious after a few minutes of following their breath, particularly if they are keeping their eyes closed. In these cases, the ratio between the "holding" effects of the practice and its power to uncover disavowed experience is tilted too far toward uncovering.

As discussed in Chapter 6, one solution to this is to use mindfulness exercises that turn the attention toward the outer, rather than the inner, world. Walking meditation, in which attention is brought to the feeling of the foot touching the ground, often works well and is compatible with the goal of increasing physical activity. Yoga exercises, which can be practiced mindfully, are another good alternative, because they combine flexibility training with mindfulness in motion.

Addiction to Control

Mindfulness practice may be difficult for people whose sense of well-being is tied to continuous involvement in goal-oriented activities. Frequently, such patients report that they do not enjoy vacations or other unstructured activities. These are the same individuals who trap themselves in psychophysiological disorders by scientifically studying every aspect of their symptoms, constantly trying to identify those variables that make them better or worse.

While mindfulness practice is potentially very beneficial to these people, they can find it quite threatening. Often, they will quickly complain of boredom and question the utility of the practice. Such patients require considerable psychoeducation about the role that their need for control plays in the disorder, and how mindfulness practice can help them to tolerate relinquishing control. Active techniques, such as walking meditation or mindful yoga exercises, are initially easier for these patients.

MINDFULNESS AND OTHER
PSYCHOPHYSIOLOGICAL DISORDERS

A remarkable number of other psychophysiological disorders are maintained by processes similar to chronic back pain. Together, these account for a large percentage of all physician visits. Both mindfulness practice, and its associated insights, can be effective in resolving these.

Other Pain and Muscle Tension Disorders

The same factors that cause and perpetuate chronic back pain are often at work in a wide array of other muscle and joint disorders. These include symptoms diagnosed as tendonitis, bursitis, bone spurs, plantar fasciitis, temporomandibular joint syndrome, repetitive strain injury, chronic headaches, and fibromyalgia. While many of these disorders can be caused by structural damage, injury, or disease processes, they are very often muscle tension disorders. My medical colleagues and I find that patients who are able to free themselves from their chronic back pain cycle often develop one of these other disorders if they continue to be psychologically stressed.

The process by which these take root parallels the chronic back pain cycle. It may begin with physical or psychological stress. Once the patient becomes concerned, he or she begins to focus on the painful area, often protecting it and abandoning normal activity. Worry and frustration set in, and a pain cycle becomes established.

Treatment for all of these disorders is similar. First, a competent medical workup is needed to rule out other causes of the pain. This is followed by psychoeducation, which can be challenging, because most of these pain syndromes, like chronic back pain, are often assumed by patients' health care providers to be caused by structural damage or disease. Next, patients are asked to list their abandoned activities. These are then reintroduced systematically, beginning with those that are pleasurable and minimally frightening. Mindfulness practice is used to develop tolerance for the associated pain sensations. Mindfulness exercises may also be used to increase awareness of disavowed affects and to facilitate relinquishing the attempt to control symptoms.

Gastrointestinal and Dermatological Disorders

Like muscle tension disorders, these conditions are widely assumed to have a physical disease process at their root. While some may be caused by infections, allergies, and other physiological processes, numerous cases of gastritis, irritable bowel syndrome, eczema, psoriasis, and related disorders are either caused or exacerbated by psychological stress (Blanchard, 1993; Friedman, Hatch, & Paradis, 1993). A wide variety of mind–body interventions have shown promise. Mindfulness meditation itself has been experimentally shown to speed healing of psoriasis (Kabat-Zinn et al., 1998)

All of these disorders frequently follow a pattern similar to that of chronic back pain. The initial symptom may be caused by a physical event, such as an infection, but once patients become preoccupied with their symptoms, their worry causes activation of the fight-or-flight system, which in turn exacerbates or perpetuates the problem. The more diligently a patient pursues medical treatment, the more preoccupied he or she becomes with the symptom, hence becoming trapped in a vicious cycle. Often medical interventions fail to alleviate the problem, and the same sorts of psychological interventions that have been discussed above are useful. Effective strategies include psychoeducation, self-monitoring of psychological reaction to symptoms, return to normal behavior, and guidance in working with negative, stress-causing emotions.

As with the other disorders, mindfulness practice can be quite useful to develop an accepting, tolerant attitude toward the symptoms, as well as to increase emotional awareness and to relax counterproductive attempts at control.

> Ed, a 45-year-old, successful businessman, came into treatment complaining of a number of gastrointestinal symptoms. One week, he would suffer from abdominal bloating and nausea; the next, he would be plagued by constipation alternating with diarrhea. He had been through numerous medical workups, none of which could identify a disease or structural cause for his suffering. He had taken

a wide variety of medications and had tried several restrictive diets. Each new intervention would appear to show promise and then fail.

Ed carefully monitored his eating, searching for correlations between what he ate and how he felt. He was always fearful that his symptoms would come at an inopportune moment, interrupting his work or causing embarrassment. Finding a cure for his condition had become the focus of his life.

We started with an explanation of how preoccupation with alleviating symptoms can contribute to psychological stress, which itself can cause symptoms. This was followed by an introduction to mindfulness practice for the purpose of observing anxious thoughts about his condition, as well as cultivating a nonrejecting attitude toward his symptoms. Ed's catastrophic fears were examined, and he was encouraged to take an emotional inventory—observing which emotions were most difficult for him. He practiced using mindfulness to "be with" his symptoms, emotions, and thoughts, without trying to fix them.

Since Ed was generally very action-oriented, this approach was difficult at first. Nonetheless, with continued support, he was able to see how fruitless his search for a cure had been, and how the search itself had kept him anxiously preoccupied with his gastrointestinal system. Over time, he began to eat normally again, letting the symptoms come and go as they would. His discomfort began to abate, and he started to realize that in many areas of his life, excessive zeal for control was the cause of his suffering.

Sexual Dysfunctions and Insomnia

These conditions usually also involve counterproductive attempts to control psychophysiological arousal. While the disorders can be caused by a physical disease process or physiological condition, patients and health care providers more readily identify these as having a psychological component and, consequently, need less persuasion to try psychological interventions. A number of empirically validated psychological treatments have been developed (Heiman & Meston, 1997; Smith & Neubauer, 2003).

Sexual Dysfunction

Sexual dysfunction treatment began with psychoanalytic interventions designed to identify neurotic conflicts rooted in early psychosexual development. The field was advanced dramatically, however, by the work of Masters and Johnson (1966; Masters, 1970) and their followers, who have focused on performance anxiety as a major cause (Singer-Kaplan, 1974). The most effective interventions prior to the advent of Viagra and similar medications have involved helping patients to stop fighting their symptoms and settle into creative hopelessness.

Consider, for example, the treatment of erectile dysfunction. After ruling out possible physical causes, therapists typically help men to understand that it is their very effort to control their erection that is creating the anxiety that interferes with a normal physical response. They then assign couples to engage in foreplay, but with instructions not to proceed to intercourse. "If an erection develops, so be it. If it doesn't, that's OK, too." The goal is to attend to the sensations of foreplay in the present moment and relinquish concerns about getting or keeping an erection.

Mindfulness practice is well suited to support such protocols. By learning to watch mental and physical experiences come and go, with acceptance, in the present moment, patients learn the art of not controlling their experience. If this is first practiced in formal mindfulness practice, it can generalize nicely to sex therapy exercises.

Insomnia

Insomnia has received a great deal of attention from the medical community, mostly in the form of an ever-expanding offering of pharmaceuticals. Most nonpharmacological treatments involve some combination of stimulus control therapy, sleep hygiene education, relaxation training, and sleep restriction therapy (Smith & Neubauer, 2003). Stimulus control therapy, the central intervention of the sleep disorders field (Chesson et al., 1999), involves having the patient reserve the bed for only sleep or sex. This means that if the patient is still awake after 15–20 minutes, he or she is instructed to get out of bed and do something else until sufficiently sleepy to try again.

Interestingly, most patients report that insomnia follows a pattern similar to sexual dysfunction. Anxiety about not sleeping leads to arousal, which prevents sleep. While some treatment regimens recognize this and even employ paradoxical suggestions to "stay awake" (Shoham-Salomon & Rosenthal, 1987), most interventions focus on the goal of getting to sleep.

There is an alternative, mindfulness-based approach that some patients find useful. First, medical and other psychiatric disorders are ruled out. Next, the dynamics of this insomnia are reviewed and the wisdom of giving up the fight against symptoms is explained. Patients are then taught mindfulness practice and invited to try it *instead* of sleeping.

People who engage in intensive mindfulness practice in retreat settings notice an interesting phenomenon: They need less sleep. Mindfulness practice apparently produces many of the restorative benefits of sleep and can substitute for it, up to a point. This is explained to patients, and mindfulness practice is offered as an alternative to lessen concerns about falling asleep.

Patients who are willing to practice mindfulness meditation during the day are asked to practice in bed. Worried thoughts about being tired the next day are allowed to come and go. If the practice brings relaxation that leads to sleep, the patient gets a good night's sleep. If not, the practice can nonetheless provide a rejuvenating experience, with the patient feeling far more rested in the morning than if he or she had spent the night trying to sleep. In either case, the struggle with insomnia is relinquished, which generally leads to a more normal sleep pattern.

It is interesting that this approach violates the cardinal rule of stimulus control therapy—reserving the bed only for sleep and sex. Nonetheless, by eliminating the central dynamic of the disorder, mindfulness practice can free many patients from chronic insomnia.

Parallels

There are many parallels among these various psychophysiological disorders. All can begin either with a physical stressor or a physical symptom caused by chronic arousal of the fight-or-flight system. Once begun, the symptom causes emotional distress, which increases the body's stress response, hence exacerbating the symptom. A vicious cycle is then established.

This cycle may be interrupted at several points. For most people, a combination of cognitive restructuring and exposure treatment through behavioral change is needed. For many, it is also important to explore other issues that may be contributing to their anxiety. All of these processes can be facilitated by mindfulness practice, and by applying insights derived from mindfulness practice to treatment.

SILVER LININGS

While few people ever say that they are glad to have had a psychophysiological disorder, it is not unusual for patients to appreciate the lessons they have learned through their recovery. In retrospect, many people come to understand their symptoms as wake-up calls, signals that their approach to life was in some way out of balance. A surprising number of people become drawn to regular mindfulness practice and to the philosophic principles with which it has historically been associated.

As the disorder resolves, patients begin to notice that their suffering stems from trying to control things that are out of their control, and that they can gradually learn to let go. The reality of the impermanence of all things becomes clearer. They may develop an appreciation for experience in the present moment, realizing that this is where life is actually lived. They also gain confidence that they can learn to bear both emotional and physical pain, and no longer need to rush to resolve it. A subgroup of patients is so taken by their recovery experience that they begin to investigate Buddhist or related teachings in depth. Their medical condition becomes a gateway to opening a spiritual dimension in their lives. When adversity becomes an opportunity for learning and growth, life is enriched.

CHAPTER 10

Working with Children
Beginner's Mind

Trudy A. Goodman

Try to be mindful, and let things take their natural course.
Then your mind will become still in any surroundings, like
a clear forest pool. All kinds of wonderful, rare animals will
come to drink at the pool, and you will clearly see the
nature of all things. You will see many strange and
wonderful things come and go, but you will be still.
—ACHAAN CHAH (in Chah, Kornfield, & Breiter, 1985, p. vi)

"Beginner's mind" is a familiar expression in the Zen tradition for qualities of mindfulness: openness, receptiveness, and readiness to learn. Mindfulness practice cultivates the states of openness and relaxed spontaneity into which beginners in life—children—are born. Children live in a different country. Therapists have to bridge a natural, cultural divide to connect with them. At times, therapy can be more challenging when relating to children than when working with adults. Beginner's mind can help the therapist enter into the world of the child.

In this chapter, I will explore how mindfulness can help clinicians connect with children and their families, as well as help parents do their job more effectively. This is an area that has to date received very little attention in either the professional or research literature, though mindful parenting has attracted popular interest. I also discuss programs and techniques for helping children and their families to cultivate mindfulness in a variety of settings.

RELATING MINDFULLY TO CHILDREN

What is unique about mindfulness-oriented child therapy? It is the intention and enhanced ability to return to the present moment again and again, with openhearted, nonjudgmental attention, to both the experience of the child and to one's own experience.

The Challenge of Working with Kids

Children do not communicate the way adults do. Many of their thoughts and feelings are expressed nonverbally, through play and body gestures. Mindfulness practice by the psychotherapist facilitates communicating with children, because mindfulness enhances nonverbal awareness. Moments of mindfulness are instantaneous, preverbal, preconceptual moments of clear seeing. The practice teaches us how to be aware of what is happening in the moment rather than engaging in discursive thinking or talking *about* experience.

Our operational definition of mindfulness—awareness of present experience with acceptance—provides a useful standpoint for relating to children. Children are more likely than adults to live in the present moment—in fact, they are notoriously confused by adult conceptions of time and sequence. I was reminded of this when treating a family with a 13-year-old daughter. When her mother told her a story about herself as a girl, the daughter responded, "Mom, I don't see how you can live in the past like that! Everything I think and do is now!" Mindfulness increases our capacity to relate empathically to a child's present-moment consciousness by helping us to experience life *ourselves* as a continuous series of present moments. It helps us to take concepts of time less seriously, much as children naturally do.

Acceptance is also critical to joining with children. Because of the intensity of their attachments, and because adults are working continuously to socialize them, children are very sensitive to acceptance or disapproval by others. The aspect of mindfulness that is nonjudgmental, accepting of what is—that understands without evaluating—creates a necessary atmosphere of emotional safety and trustworthiness in the therapy room.

Mindfulness can also help the therapist accept a frequently annoying aspect of child treatment: repetition. Kids are uniquely willing to return again and again to their chosen activities. The repetition of play that can be transformational and pleasurable for a child can be unnervingly tedious for the therapist. Mindfulness can help the therapist to sustain interest and emotional connection with children during these subtly changing, repetitive play sequences.

Mindfulness gives us the opportunity to know deeply, often in a nonverbal moment of realization, what is going on in the child. The child's world is different from our own; we can enter it with mindfulness by staying very present with what is happening in the moment. We can often rely on our child patients to give us feedback when we become *un*mindful, perhaps through their misbehavior or withdrawal. The children, with their beginner's minds, are our teachers.

Psychotherapeutic Presence

Psychotherapeutic presence refers to more than being in the physical company of another person. It refers to a felt sense of being with another, of *mindfulness-in-connection*. The opposite of therapeutic presence is absentmindedness or preoccupation. Children are especially sensitive to whether or not adults are emotionally engaged with them. The experience of being alone in the physical company of another can feel more abandoning to a child than actually being left alone.

> Cari, an 18-year-old patient, was upset after watching a home movie of her mother holding her when she was about 6 months old. In the movie, Cari was on her mother's lap, being bounced on her mother's knee. Both Cari and her mother were facing her aunt, who held the movie camera. Her mother periodically bent over baby Cari and nuzzled, poked, and tickled her, then quickly returned to talking to her sister. Cari was strangely troubled by this seemingly benign scene. She felt that her mother had been oblivious to her as a baby as her mother talked and jiggled her in a mechanical way. Her mother's interactions felt intrusive, motivated by her mother's need to make contact and reassure herself.

Although Cari was physically present with her mother, she felt that her mother was emotionally absent. Cari also practiced mindfulness meditation, and she drew a parallel between the feeling of being emotionally intruded upon by her mother and the patterns she observed in her meditation. Anxious thoughts would swoop into her consciousness when she was in a calm mental state, grab her attention, and pull her out of a state of peaceful presence, just as her mother did in the home movie.

Cari's experience illustrates two points. First, it shows how the quality of the adult's attention shapes the way a child attends to his or her own experience. Second, we see how mindfulness practice may enhance social cognition in general (Siegel, 1999). Cari believed that her own mindfulness practice enabled her to perceive the legacy of her mother's mental states more accurately.

This enhanced sensitive awareness applies to the therapist doing psychotherapy. Awareness of the movements of his or her own mind during treatment can help the therapist learn a lot about a child's inner experience: of warding off and being close, of being present or being absent; abandoned or abandoning.

Presence in Chaos

When Carlos, age 9, arrived in my office, he asked, "Is this a place for kids who hate themselves?" He quickly confided that he, indeed, hated himself. Carlos was not able to wait to get to know me before becoming absorbed in dramatic play. The themes emerging were violent and explicitly sexual. Both his disregard for being in a room with an unfamiliar person and the uninhibited explicitness of his play were disconcerting.

At one point in the first session, we each had a puppet on one raised hand and were advancing across the floor on our bellies, slithering slowly along in Carlos's game. He suddenly looked over at me and asked incredulously, "Is this your job?" His sense of humor notwithstanding, I saw that, for Carlos, the line between real and pretend was unclear. His ability to move in and out of fantasy was dizzying, and I was beginning to feel flooded by all the emotional material surfacing in his play. Being with Carlos, I felt inner chaos and a swirl of overwhelming thoughts and feelings.

Mindfulness helped to bring steadiness of attention in the midst of the whirling impressions of the session. With three breaths in and out, I steadied my own mind and recognized that my own chaotic mind state was a reflection of Carlos's. I felt his intense need to make sense of his world. This eventually became our clinical agenda.

I decided to introduce a mindfulness exercise to help us both. I suspected that Carlos might benefit from the same technique I used to disentangle from his emotional chaos. We developed a game called "three breaths" in which we would stop whatever we were doing, whenever he wanted, to explore how he was feeling. Carlos liked the control this gave to our interaction and to his own experience in the moment. He also learned increasingly to use words for vulnerable and difficult feelings. In this way, Carlos began to benefit from mindful awareness of his tumultuous inner life, and I was able to remain more connected to him.

This quality of mind, which we might call authentic presence, mindfulness-in-connection, or therapeutic presence, involves being aware of the fluctuations of our own attention while we are emotionally engaged with a patient. Thomson (2000) suggests that "authentic presence . . . must sit somewhere between therapist and client" (p. 546). This means that we may be open and receptive to the patient's experience but simultaneously remain aware that the drama is a play of consciousness. Mindfulness enables the therapist to be engaged yet disentangled from the patient's experience. We can pop in and out of our own reactions and learn from what our mind is doing, without losing connection with our patient. The process is subtler with children than with adults, because interactions with children are less verbal and structured; we must remain alert to visceral, preconceptual experience. It requires greater refinement of our attention.

Presence in Disconnection

We have seen how sustained mindful awareness facilitates connecting with children. Sustained awareness comes naturally as long as we are enjoying our experience and it remains interesting. However, unpleasant experiences also occur in therapy, and the therapist's attention often begins to wander off in response. Sustained mindfulness requires the intention to stay in the present with the child, accepting of all that the moment brings. The intention to cultivate mindfulness helps to discern the patterns of connection and disconnection that occur in the office.

> Maria, a fifth grader, was referred for therapy by her school due to social withdrawal and emotional passivity. While sweet and compliant, Maria was as emotionally disengaged in therapy as she was emotionally absent in the classroom. She was disinterested in most things, including her physical appearance, which is ordinarily a compelling concern at Maria's age. Her hair was unwashed, and she seemed generally neglected.

It was difficult to remain present in the room with Maria due to her emotional blandness and inability to engage in conversation. Despite my intention to be present with Maria in therapy, the temptation to space-out, to plan or daydream, was almost irresistible. I sometimes found myself dreading our sessions. All my efforts to return again and again to presence and connection did not seem to enliven our connection. I often felt exhausted after our sessions.

After 6 long, lackluster therapy hours spent mindful of—and willing to explore—the perplexing sense of something missing in the relationship with Maria, I shared my puzzlement with Maria's parents. A few weeks later, I received a call from Maria's father very early in the morning. He told me that he had been sexually involved with his daughter. He described the emotional numbness and longing that led him to seek that kind of comfort from her. He rationalized that his behavior might compensate for Maria's mother's neglect of the little girl, but Maria's father had no apparent awareness of his own role in that neglect. I acknowledged his courage in telling me about what had happened.

Maria had checked out of being present to herself and to others. She was living in a dreamy, dissociated semblance of being a normal schoolgirl, going through the motions, without even knowing what was really wrong. My reactions—wanting to leave, to check out of being with her—reflected Maria's feelings with painful precision. I discovered later that Maria's mother was herself a victim of abuse, and my sense of disconnection reflected her mother's pervasive emotional disengagement as well. Mindfulness of connection and disconnection can sometimes be uncannily revealing if we are willing to linger with it and allow it to reveal its truths.

Our intention to return to the present moment with curiosity and acceptance, despite how it may feel, is an essential skill when working with patients who are bearing suffering without words. Children, especially, bring their struggles to therapy nonverbally. What is confusing or opaque to the therapist will eventually become very interesting if we have the intention to return to it again and again. Mindful awareness can go anywhere, exploring all corners, independent of our theoretical frame of reference. The question is, "What is happening here, now, in my experience and in my patient's experience?"

Beginner's Mind

In the beginner's mind there are many possibilities; in the expert's mind there are few.
                                                    —SHUNRYU SUZUKI (1973, p. 21)

Teachers in most fields are eager to work with new students and often express particular interest in beginners. A beginner is eager to learn, asks excellent questions, is curious, and is generally receptive to information and experience. What a delight!

Our child patients are seeking the same receptiveness in their therapists. Can the therapist understand me, know me, be patient enough to feel my struggle and recognize my achievements? Does the therapist like being with me? To fulfill this tall order, the therapist must meet the child with few preconceived notions. In spite of the child's diagnosis or family history, he or she must remain aware of what it feels like to be with the child and what the child is feeling.

> Leni, a 3-year-old girl with rosy cheeks and a ponytail, was referred to me by a well-known pediatrician, who raised the question of whether Leni had autism. Her frightened parents wanted a second opinion. When I first met Leni, her averted gaze, her silence, and her willingness to leave her mother without a backward glance all seemed to confirm the diagnosis. Leni was not ready to acknowledge me or respond to my words; in fact, she appeared to be ignoring me. When Leni came with me into the playroom and sat down, she painted a picture of a little girl sitting in the back of a big gray car, all alone, being driven down a street surrounded by falling snow.
>
> In other ways as well, Leni communicated what it was like to live in her world. Her play was repetitive, she perseverated verbally, and her behaviors were neither welcoming nor rejecting. Still, as I brought my attention fully into the moment and became mindful of all the sense impressions that were occurring in the field of my awareness, there was a felt sense of this little girl's presence and a slight connection. I sensed her presence in the form of her diligence, her energy, her anxiety, and her stubbornness. Leni evoked those same qualities inside of me. Her mother confirmed that those were some aspects of little Leni's personality.

It became evident over time that Leni indeed suffered from Asperger syndrome. While the diagnosis was crucial for getting proper care and services during her school years, the focus of therapy was for Leni's parents and me to develop an understanding of the little girl, buried behind her atypical neurology. Leni's needs could be flexibly addressed by this understanding.

As we search for the person behind the diagnosis, the willingness to *not know* is a precondition for discovery (see the discussion of this in Chapter 3). The minds of beginners do not know. We often foreclose our minds due to anxious feelings, or by trying to fit a preconceived diagnosis. As therapists, we need to restrain this tendency and learn to rest in the midst of uncertainty, with balance and equanimity. I tried to hold my diagnostic understanding in suspension, so that it did not interfere with the task of making an authentic connection with Leni's individuality and experience. Mindfulness practice can be helpful in this regard; it trains the practitioner to suspend "cognitive construing" (Delmonte, 1987).

Child therapists in training often need to know that it is OK simply to be receptive, to sit with a child, relaxed in what is yet to be revealed.

Holding our concepts and theories lightly allows us to make a journey of codiscovery with the child. It is a collaboration in which our thoughts about treatment are deemphasized in favor of the "felt sense" (Gendlin, 1996) of the connection. The felt sense changes moment to moment, much like a child him- or herself. When the novice clinician asks for guidelines on how to think during the session, the answer is, "Not too much." If we feel the moment with the child, something will naturally occur to us when we need it.

Our beginner's mind is a gift to children. They are then free to come forward and inhabit our relaxed space of receptivity. Our peaceful state of being invites children to "come as they are," no part left out. All the scary, unacceptable, "strange and wonderful" creatures that live in the child's psyche are drawn to the "still forest pool" of our receptivity (Chah et al., 1985, p. vi).

Preverbal Awareness

Difficult experiences occur for all children, before they have the ability to speak. They are buried in the body and feelings of the child. Even for adults, the results of traumatic experiences are largely preverbal. Through mindful awareness, clinicians can help to integrate preverbal experiences that have been exiled from awareness. Mindfulness, especially with the component of acceptance, may make it safe for difficult experience to come forth, like animals emerging silently and warily from the forest. With familiarity in the preverbal realm of experience, and comfort therein, the therapist can remain quietly connected with the suffering child.

> Jason, a tousled 5-year-old with big brown eyes, had already been kicked out of every preschool program in which he was enrolled. He was entering a therapeutic school program when I met him. When limits to his behavior were set in the new school, Jason would start to scream, wail, flail his arms, and eventually collapse. Jason had apparently often witnessed his mother being beaten by her live-in boyfriend and naturally was unable to protect her. His mother compounded the problem by reacting to Jason's rages alternately with passive guilt and by verbally threatening to "tear [him] limb from limb." Both Jason and his mother felt helpless and out of control.

In his fantasy play in therapy, Jason could be a hero who saved people, a superman who could subdue any angry bad guy. Nonetheless, his small size and the vulnerability of a 5-year-old boy were keenly felt. The feeling of disempowerment caused by the limit setting at his new school led to eruptions of fear and rage. I chose a new approach with Jason. What would it be like to hold him with steadiness and calm in response to his storms, without anger or reactivity? This had a profound effect. His anger exhausted itself and he sobbed softly, allowing himself to be rocked and comforted as felt his unbearable sorrow.

As Jason learned to put his terror into words, he revealed that he was afraid his arms and legs would fall off. This fear echoed his mother's threats to tear him limb from limb. In the "country" where children live, words are swallowed literally. Jason was afraid I was going to pull off his arms and legs in retaliation for his anger. Little by little, Jason learned to tell the difference between his fears and reality. He learned that his arms and legs were securely attached to his body and that when his therapist stopped his rages, she would not hurt him. Jason's rages subsided.

The bulk of Jason's treatment was nonverbal. Children are especially attuned to the felt sense of others. Jason was positively affected by my efforts to remain aware of his struggle, nonjudgmentally, and connected throughout the course of his painful outbursts. Mindfulness seems to be even more contagious with children than adults. Surprisingly, Jason later recognized himself in other little boys when *they* had temper tantrums and he looked for opportunities to be kind and soothing.

Mindfulness in the presence of strong emotions takes practice—not years and years, but some period of regular practice and the intention to be mindful. My own intention to be mindful has been held for 20 years in a quote on the wall of my therapy office:

> By being in alert attention, by observing oneself, with the intention to understand rather than to judge, in full acceptance of whatever may emerge, simply because it is there, we allow the deep to come to the surface and enrich our life and consciousness. . . . This is the great work of awareness. (Maharaj, 1997, p. 112)

Most of our experience is indeed deep, a field of preconceptual and preverbal awareness. We learn to abide calmly in that domain during mindfulness practice.

Kids do not yet fully inhabit the verbal world, and adults sometimes cling to it too tightly. Adults have a tendency to foreclose a child's experience by offering verbal explanations or solutions. With mindfulness practice, this perceptual domain can become a safe resting place for the psychotherapist.

The Present Moment

As has been discussed in previous chapters, therapeutic work in the here-and-now is where our actual work with patients happens.

Daniel Stern's (2003) reflections on the "now moment" in psychotherapy, discussed in Chapter 5, sound like a description of mindfulness practice.

> There is no remove in time. [The moment] is direct—not transmitted and reformulated by words. . . . Moments of meeting provide some of the most nodal experiences for change in psychotherapy. They are often the moments most remembered . . . that changed the course of therapy. (Stern, 2003, p. 57)

Although Stern suggests that we lack a theory of such moments, Buddhist psychology has elaborated in great detail the many nuances of the present moment and how to attend to them in a sustained manner.

One problem with the present moment is that it is exceptionally fleeting. When we conceptualize an experience of the moment, it is already gone. With mindfulness, we move closer and closer to the simple arising and passing of preverbal experience—closer to the present moment.

Clinical researchers have videotaped infant–parent interactions and have observed microcommunications flashing back and forth between the two individuals as quickly as 10 times a second (Beebe & Lachmann, 1998; Tronick, 1989). The baby glances, the mother responds; her response is echoed by the baby, who shapes the mother's next response, and so on. Mutual, reciprocal call and response happens so quickly that it cannot be followed by the conscious mind of an observer. Awareness of the present moment brings us closer to seeing this subtle, nonverbal process, and thereby makes it easier to enter and participate in the world of the child.

How does a therapist enter into a relationship of such subtlety? A therapist who is attuned emotionally to the child patient probably participates in these microcommunications with intuitive, mindful awareness rather than objective, intellectual awareness. A sense of connection and understanding may be a result of a stream of reciprocal perceptions that are too fleeting to track. When this attunement is strong, the therapist is fully attentive to the patient and absorbed in the "flow." Through emotional attunement and authentic presence, effective therapists are fully engaged in elusive, successive, fleeting present moments.

With some children, explicitly calling attention to the present moment facilitates treatment:

> Nine-year-old Maggie challenged me. She had previously seen two experienced clinicians without success. She was emotionally disconnected, frequently teased at school, and very sensitive to criticism.

Maggie was frequently battling with her parents about her refusal to do homework. It did not help that her younger brother was an excellent student and very popular in school. The school counselor confided that the kids called Maggie "Poisonhead." Her parents did not know how to help Maggie feel less victimized, angry, and lonesome.

A therapy veteran before the age of 9, Maggie was hyperalert to anything that smacked of psychology. Disdainful and distant, she would deflect every arrow in my therapeutic quiver by throwing a fit, followed by sullen silence.

Late one winter afternoon, Maggie and I sat facing each other on the floor of my office in a pool of lamplight. I wanted to connect but was frustrated in a way that was so familiar to Maggie herself. The silence was tense and uneasy. My thoughts wandered out the window. It was twilight, one of those hushed moments when the whole world turns deep blue. I felt the deep peace of meditation. I spontaneously turned to Maggie and said softly, "Look, it's all blue out there." She looked. I asked her if she had ever noticed this blue twilight world. She was curious, attentive in a new way. It was a moment of meeting, of presence and peace. For one brief "now" moment, we entered each other's world. As Stern (2003, p. 54) writes, "As soon as a now moment arrives, all else is dropped and each partner stands with both feet in the present. Presentness fills the time and space."

A year later, I taught Maggie to practice mindfulness, sitting tall on an imaginary throne, focusing on the ebb and flow of the breath moving gently through the body. She learned to sit calmly, confident and absorbed, for 10 whole minutes, noticing her feelings and all the stories they tell, coming and going, appearing and disappearing, while she remained steadily there. She understood that she did not always have to believe her thoughts; she could choose to let them be, to let them go. She practiced in her room, sitting cross-legged on her bed, and found a haven in the present moment. To paraphrase Achaan Chah (Chah et al., 1985) again, Maggie found the still forest pool, where all her wild things, scary things, unacceptable things, could come out and drink their fill. Children can learn that all their "strange and wonderful creatures" can coexist peacefully in the same young heart.

Play

Play therapy grew out of psychoanalytic psychology. Young children are encouraged to represent symbolically and express what they are thinking and feeling in their own language—the language of play. By cultivating mindfulness, therapists may become more skilled in attention and develop other qualities that are integral to successful play therapy (Landreth, 2002).

The space of play is intimate and immediate. Children explore, recreate, redo. During play, children can transform difficult events in their lives and unbearable emotions into experiences they can assimilate. For therapists to enter the arena of play, they must be willing to temporarily abandon their logical, linear, and verbal modes of thought and expression. Clinicians develop comfort with the child-like emotional intimacy of play through intimate awareness of their own subjective experience.

The child patient usually has a greater capacity than the clinician to be absorbed in play. A relaxed frame of mind can bring the therapist closer to young patients, so that he or she can join the flow of play. While playing, kids can be big and powerful, they can control their world, and they can design the game so they always win and never get left out or lose. Children can create healing distance from disturbing or traumatic events by having them happen to others, and by effectively controlling their outcome.

> Six-year-old Hilary was hospitalized for an operation to correct a congenital heart defect. Well after recovering, Hilary had nightmares and was wetting her bed. She organized a game of "hospital" in which a fleet of doctors roared up on motorcycles (Hilary was afraid of motorcycles) to stick needles in their little patients. "There, there, don't cry," Hilary comforted the patients. Hilary also made sure that all the patients fully recovered from the sticking and probing, just as she did.

In the safety and protection of play therapy, Hilary took charge of a situation in which she had formerly felt victimized and frightened. She regained her sense of competence and the bedwetting ceased.

Play is essential for all people. Adults differentiate between work and play, ordinarily calling work the activity that we do for an extrinsic goal (such as money) and play activity for its own sake. Work is *doing*, with an eye to the future, and play is *being*—spontaneous, wholehearted activity in the present moment. Absorption in play, like in meditation, generally increases energy: Attention is unified and concentrated. (This may be one reason that children have so much energy!) When work, including clinical practice, becomes play, we find we have much more energy at the end of the day.

Resting in the forgotten world of childhood—fresh, immediate, spontaneous, wide awake, immersed in the reality of here-and-now—is a kind of mindfulness training for our adult minds. We can feel refreshed and renewed by working with, playing with, and being with our young patients. Children can become our best teachers in the development of mindful presence.

Family Therapy

Several of the therapeutic skills discussed here are relevant not only to individual work with children but also to family therapy. One goal of most family therapy is to enhance mutual understanding between children and their parents. Increasing the therapist's ability to relate to and understand children through mindfulness practice can support this work.

A great challenge of family therapy is remaining equidistant among family members, while remaining empathically attuned to each of them. This can be particularly difficult during moments of intense emotion or conflict. The ability to tolerate powerful affect, to remain with the process of the present moment, to be present in the midst of chaos, and to notice in detail nonverbal communication, all help the family therapist to navigate these tumultuous waters.

Beginner's mind is also very useful in family treatment. It is virtually impossible to plan family sessions effectively. Being in a room with several people, each with his or her own history and agenda, introduces so many variables that our only hope lies in trusting that we will be able to respond creatively and intelligently to whatever occurs. The comfort in being with new, changing, moment-to-moment phenomena that mindfulness practice brings is a real help to therapists in these circumstances.

As I discuss below, for family members that are open to it, actually practicing mindfulness together can also provide support to their growth and development.

Parent Guidance

Mindfulness practice can help a therapist to understand and relate effectively with children and their families in many ways. Even more important to the child's growth and development, however, is having a healthy relationship with his or her parents. Teaching mindfulness practice to parents has something essential to offer here as well.

Although at the time of this writing there seem to be no controlled studies on the effects of mindfulness practice on parenting skills, parents who have taken up mindfulness practice have been singing its praises in the popular media. Several books have been written on the topic (Kabat-Zinn & Kabat-Zinn, 1998; Kramer, 2003; Napthali, 2003), and there is at least one website sharing anecdotal reports of how mindfulness practice enhances parenting (*www.themindfulparent.org*).

Sometimes parents are angry with or alienated from their children, making it difficult to relate to them empathically. Other times, parents are hesitant to set necessary limits, out of reluctance to tolerate the disconnection or tension that usually follows. Most parental guidance interventions focus on one of these difficulties, either increasing parents' ability to relate empathically to their children (e.g., Faber & Mazlish, 1999; Green, 2001) or enhancing their ability to establish clear, consistent consequences for behavior (e.g., Barkley & Benton, 1998; Patterson, 1977). Developmental psychologists generally agree that effective parenting involves finding an optimal balance between these strategies (i.e., skillfully providing both love and limits).

Parents who practice mindfulness often report that it helps them to be better at both of these core dimensions of parenting. For the reasons discussed earlier in the context of child therapy, mindfulness allows for greater presence, awareness of connection and disconnection, openness to a child's nonverbal communication, and ability to join a child in play, all of which help children to experience their parents' love and understanding more fully.

Equally important are the perspective and the patience that mindfulness brings. Many parents report that they have great difficulty responding to their children's misbehavior in ways they think are best, rather than just reacting instinctively. The parent who is thwarted by a 2-year-old in the supermarket, or who is defeated in an argument with a teenager, may react with anger—even though he or she knows that this will be counterproductive. Even parents who would never come to the attention of the child protection system frequently commit these small "parenting crimes." Mindfulness practice can help parents to deal with conflict and set appropriate limits more skillfully.

When parents are attentive to the daily changes in their children, they develop a keenly felt sense of impermanence, in childhood and in life itself. Observing impermanence with mindful awareness can enable parents to tolerate the loss of connection they face when setting a difficult limit. The losses experienced in observing impermanence can give more ballast to parents, more courage to be with challenging experience.

Mindfulness practice appears to hold promise for those parenting infants as well. Infant-led psychotherapy, which entails attending carefully to an infant's behavior in the present moment, has been shown to increase secure attachment, cognitive development, and emotion regulation. The Watch, Wait, and Wonder (WWW) program, while not explicitly incorporating mindfulness, has achieved these positive outcomes by teaching parents to slow down and follow their child's lead in interactions (Cohen et al., 1999; Cohen, Lojkasek, Muir, Muir, & Parker, 2002).

Building on this, at least one explicit "mindful parenting" program has been developed and is currently under investigation. It is designed to enhance parents' capacities for attending empathically to infants (Reynolds, 2003). The program consists of weekly group meetings in which parents engage in a formal period of quiet observation, lasting from 20 to 30 minutes, and are encouraged to notice the details of their infant's behavior, as well as the quality of infant–adult interactions. "Parents are encouraged to slow down inside to the pace of infant life, so they may notice the tiniest details of their baby's experience—and tease apart their own as well as their baby's emotional responses" (p. 364). Initial anecdotal reports suggest that the program increases parents' awareness and understanding of their baby's behavior.

By helping people to see that all of their experience is a series of changing moments, and that their thought, and even their sense of self is constructed, mindfulness practice helps people to take things less personally. This is absolutely essential for good parenting, because it allows parents to recognize the needs of their child rather than instinctually respond out of personal injury or pride. Also, by increasing their capacity to bear emotion, parents can flexibly provide what their child needs developmentally—including setting difficult limits—even if, in the short run, this results in the parents being rejected or subjected to a tantrum.

Explaining alternative ways that parents might respond to their children is relatively easy for psychotherapists, but it is frequently more difficult for parents to actually implement. Habitual, automatic, emotionally charged, parenting reactions tend to be quite tenacious and resistant to change. By bringing awareness to the present moment, mindfulness can help parents pause to see the steps that lead up to their responses. Parents can observe their feelings in response to their children's behavior and also observe the intention to react automatically, before they actually respond. This pause provides a vitally important moment in which to consider alternatives.

Mindfulness therefore has a valuable role to play in parent guidance, both by helping parents to be more compassionate and loving with their children, and by helping them to set limits more skillfully. Parental mindfulness practice can take the simple form of asking parents to notice how emotions manifest in their bodies when they are with their children. When they find themselves becoming agitated in response to their child, parents can be shown how to follow their breath, or pay attention to their physical surroundings. For those receptive to the idea, more intensive family mindfulness practice of the sort described in the next section can be of even greater benefit.

MINDFULNESS-BASED PROGRAMS
FOR CHILDREN AND FAMILIES

Following are examples of programs for children with which I have had personal experience. They are not specifically psychotherapy programs, but they have implications for positive behavior change and family well-being. These examples are included to inspire the interested reader to develop new ways of incorporating mindfulness into the treatment of children.

Family Programs

Mindfulness Community Gathering

I direct and teach a family program that incorporates mindfulness in Los Angeles, California; it is called Growing Spirit.[1] At Growing Spirit, children do pleasurable activities that promote mindfulness and are taught meditations designed specifically for their age group. (See below for meditations that can be used with children in a variety of settings.) Parents are also supported in their mindfulness practice, and are taught both meditation and informal mindfulness exercises. The participating families share the intention to foster mindfulness, compassion, and wisdom in the crucible of their family lives. The program occurs monthly on Sunday mornings, and the mutual support of community appears to be a key factor in the program's continuity and apparent success. There is considerable shared experience between children, between parents, and between children and parents.

Meditation with children is ordinarily done in groups. Parents meditate for 30 minutes, followed by a 45-minute parenting discussion led by an experienced meditation teacher. Parents learn to apply principles of mindfulness to the work of raising children, and they share with one another their experience of doing this.

Kids and parents are together for discussion and a meditation circle at the beginning and at the end of the program. Children are often initially shy about participating in the circle (sharing their heartfelt needs and desires for themselves and others), but they generally leave feeling recognized and appreciated by the community.

Anecdotal reports by the parents suggest that the program helps their children to develop self-awareness, attentiveness, and the willingness to slow down and take a deep breath when feeling distressed.

---

[1]Detailed information may be found at *www.growingspirit.org.*

Children also seem to like the program: "I didn't know it would be so much fun. I want to go every time" (Max, age 4). "I like the eating meditation. It's relaxing" (Sara, age 8).

Family Retreat

My colleagues and I have been developing another family model, a 6-day, summer, residential family retreat, at the Insight Meditation Society[2] in Barre, Massachusetts. A similar program exists at Spirit Rock Meditation Center[3] in Woodacre, California.

The children's program of games and activities includes group skills and mindfulness training. Mindfulness training includes daily living skills found in Chapter 6, storytelling on subjects that encourage the children to increase awareness about their immediate lives and actions, as well as some meditation. We have found that children as young as age 5 and 6 are visibly affected by the atmosphere of stillness and reverence in the meditation hall. They love to sit and practice their meditation for about 10 minutes, and then jump up, batteries recharged by the quiet time, and go to their groups.

The groups are divided according to age, and activities vary accordingly. The dyad meditation from Chapter 5 is simplified for use between children, who observe each other's rhythm of breathing, attuned to their partner and themselves. Periodically during mealtimes, a mindfulness bell is rung. Everyone freezes, midsentence or midbite, and is silent for 20 seconds. Habitual patterns can be interrupted and observed. Children also learn and practice lovingkindness meditation and know that this is a tool they can use at home and at school when they are having a difficult time. Parents have time to practice meditation, listen to talks, and have lively discussions. Each day includes family time for swimming, playing, and sharing experiences.

Schools

A model for how mindfulness can be adopted in schools can be found in India, in the Universal Education School in Sarnath, India, founded by Valentino Giacomin and his partner, Luigina de Biasi. Both are retired schoolteachers from Italy, where they spent 10 years refining their curriculum for incorporating mindfulness in education.

More than 220 mixed-caste children from five poor villages in the

---

[2]Details at *www.dharma.org/ims/programs.*

[3]Details at *www.spiritrock.org.*

area attend either a full-day classroom education or a 3-hour evening program. The evening classes are for working children and illiterate adults. Many of the children have no clothes other than their school uniforms and come from homes where there is abuse, neglect, and other social problems. I visited this school in 2001 to see how mindfulness was being taught to children from an illiterate, desperately poor population in a simple and helpful way. In 1997, 42% of Universal Education children tested above average on achievement tests compared to 15% at comparable village schools.

Valentino's curriculum is adapted to the local Hindu culture and is designed to provide children with experiences and insights that might help them make wise choices later in life. One such insight is that our personal experience is individually constructed—that things themselves have no fixed qualities. I discovered during my visit that even a 4-year-old child is capable of understanding this. A girl who thought that her lunch tasted good, but whose friend did not like it, was able to say that her lunch itself was actually neither good nor bad: It depends on each child's taste! To witness small children capable of this level of abstraction was a surprise.

As I was talking to a 12-year-old boy in an art class, he suddenly froze, stared stonily at me, and refused to answer. This seemed very odd until I noticed that no one else was moving or talking. I did not realize the school had a ritual in which a gong is rung several times a day, inviting the children to stop what they are doing or saying for a minute of mindfulness. This exercise is taught as an active exploration of the nature of mind and perception. When the bell rang again, children waved their hands joyfully, ready to report and reflect on their experiences. The kids shared with the class what they noticed going on in the stillness. Even the little children could report their nonjudgmental awareness of sensations, sounds, and mental states, their thoughts and emotions.

I witnessed children ages 4–16 sitting together in silent meditation for periods up to 15 minutes. The Universal Education School would provide a wonderful opportunity for the systematic study of the effects of mindfulness training on the lives of its students, and the capacity for training mindfulness skills of different age groups.

Incarcerated Youth

A juvenile detention center houses a tragically desperate population of young people. This is one of the few settings in which there are published data on the use of mindfulness training with children. In a study of an intensive, 7-day meditation program for 101 adolescent male delinquents in Thailand, researchers found that the participants all felt the practice to be beneficial, with significant self-reported improvements in contentment and calm, concentration, and impulsivity (Witoonchart & Bartlet, 2002).

In 2002–2003, I taught mindfulness meditation to three groups of young adults at a prison in Los Angeles: one class of African American and Latino young men (ages 14–18), a second class for young women, and a third class in a special care facility for girls who attempted suicide or hurt others while incarcerated.

We began most classes in a circle, with introductions and check-ins to determine who was facing a trip to court, sentencing, removal to another facility, or had difficult news from friends or family. Then, a member of the group would lead a brief lovingkindness meditation for anyone who was suffering intense fear, despair, or grief. After several brief meditations (with simpler language usually reserved for younger children, see below), I led a 20-minute guided mindfulness meditation and discussion.

Several times in the course of the year, we received permission to hold a half-day meditation retreat in the prison chapel. From 9:00 A.M. to 12:30 P.M., we practiced sitting and walking meditation and some yoga. I brought donuts that were shared with the guards, who also dutifully monitored our every move. I was continually surprised by the prisoners' willingness to participate in unfamiliar and potentially threatening activities, such as slow walking meditation outdoors (with hands behind their backs, in pairs), where they could be seen by other young men during recreation time. These kids had the gift of desperation: Many were looking at long prison terms, even life sentences—in terrifying adult facilities. They had little to lose by trying something new. Some longed for a second chance and were determined not to return to the life that had landed them in jail.

One inmate, Derek, used his mindfulness skills in the following way: One day Derek was handcuffed and shoved into a metal cage "like an animal" for a drive to court. Along the way, Derek remembered his meditation instructions: "Just sit here and breathe!" Crossing his legs, he straightened his back and sat with poise and balance during the ride to court. He had found a way to express his dignity in the midst of a humiliating situation. The meditation alleviated some of his rage and resentment. He was able to present himself favorably to the judge and later reported his success back to the group.

Most members of Derek's group reported positive results from their mindfulness meetings—less violence, more sense of control, a way to deal with difficult emotions, and a rare feeling of safety and kindness during the group itself. Many of the participants practiced meditation only once a week, as needed, as an emotional self-regulation skill during difficult times.

MINDFULNESS EXERCISES FOR CHILDREN

These exercises can be adapted for children from preschool to adolescence. They are designed to help children cultivate some stability and flexibility of attention. Relaxation comes first, to release excess tension in the body and mind. Then comes the cultivation of mindful awareness by focusing on one of our five physical senses. This heightens attention, bringing greater interest to the object of meditation. The exercises lessen distraction and absentmindedness, and enhance acuity of awareness.

Bell-in-Space Meditation

This exercise can be readily adapted to different age groups. Children sit quietly, kneeling or cross-legged on cushions on the floor. The leader does the exercise while teaching it, speaking from within the experience. The leader gives the following instructions:

"Imagine yourself sitting inside an invisible egg. There is an invisible eggshell, a big circle all around you, front, back, up, down, and sideways. Close your eyes and stay very still. Relax into the quiet, not moving."

Teenagers: "Just rest there in the peaceful stillness, imagining yourself completely at ease. Expand into this space, as far as your mind can go, including the whole universe."

Younger children: "Imagine your arms and legs, your hands and feet, your whole body and your skin, too, all over. Now imagine the egg is filled with space that stretches way out in all directions, as far as you can see. Imagine you are blowing a bubble, and you blow, and blow, and it gets bigger and bigger, until you become that bubble, stretching all the way out into outer space. Now take a few deep breaths, following the breath all the way into yourself and then all the way back out into distant space. Let your whole mind feel bigger and bigger and just rest in that great big space."

The leader then rings a bell. "Now, see if you can hear the sound of the bell all the way to the end." (*Pause until the sound stops.*) "Now, see if you can count the number of times you hear the bell." (*Ring the bell at intervals of 30–60 seconds, over a period of 3–7 minutes. The leader will have rung the bell 3–9 times per meditation session.*)

The bell-in-space meditation can last up to 10 minutes.

Afterwards, ask how many bell rings the children heard. All responses are considered correct, because answers are simply the number of times the bell was heard. To heighten awareness, ask, "When the sound of the bell disappears, where does it go?" Children often offer thoughtful and profound answers to this question.

Wake Up Your Senses Meditation

"Feel all your attention gently falling from the top of your head down to your neck, lightly falling like a snowflake or a leaf drifting silently down from a tree. Feel your attention move down through your shoulders, your arms and hands, your chest, belly, hips and thighs, your legs, knees and ankles, into your feet, all the way down to your toes. Let your mind rest in your body, noticing all the feelings inside—tingling, shivers, prickles, nothing, warmth, coolness, softness, hardness, relaxation, or tightness. Notice how the sensations and feelings change when you bring attention to them. See if you can just feel the stillness of your body as you sit, in the midst of changing sensations, not moving." If the children are age 7 or older, the guided meditation can continue for 10 minutes, touring the five senses.

Touch: "Feel all the places where the body touches the floor, where your clothes touch your body, where your lips touch each other, where your eyelids touch each other." Children can also hold an object, such as a smooth stone, to explore tactile awareness. "Feel the weight of the stone in your hand. Is it heavy? Light? Smooth? Round?"

Hearing: Children can attend to auditory experience, listening to sounds of nature, or the sounds in the classroom or therapy office. "Can you let your ears simply hear sounds? Can you hear the sound of the rain? The sound of the airplane? Listen to the airplane the whole way, until it disappears. Just listen to sound without wondering about what you hear, without trying to figure out what it is. Can you hear (*leader makes a sound, a sigh or any sound*)— without calling it 'sigh' or 'cough', but just hear—(*make the sound*)?"

Smell: Spraying a slight fragrance may highlight olfactory experience. "Notice what you smell, the fragrance or scent that may be in the air. Notice if it is pleasant or unpleasant to you. If it's pleasant, see how your nose wants to smell more. If you don't like it, notice how you want to hold your nose or turn away. See what happens if you don't notice it at all."

Sight and taste: See the eating meditation below to explore visual and gustatory perception.

If the children are younger than 7 years old, each sense meditation can be very brief. If the children are age 7 or older, they can explore the senses for over a minute each and experiment with attention to *emotions* or *thoughts*. Between meditations, discuss with the children what the meditation was like for them. "Does our wish to pay attention change our experience? Do we notice more?" Older children can also begin to distinguish between sensory perceptions, and how we automatically label and think about our perceptions. Bring warmth, gentleness, and precise detail into the instructions.

Apple Meditation

Every child is given an apple. First, the children reflect on the apple as part of the interconnected web of kinship with all life.

"Where did it come from? The store? How did it get to the store? Where was it before? Where did the apple tree come from? A blossom? A tree? A seed? What nourished its growth? Rain? Earth? Sunlight? How many people, what kinds of work, helped bring this apple from the tree into your hand?"

Then, the children are taught an eating meditation.

"Before eating the apple, take a close look at it. What colors, shape, size do you see? Smell it. What does it smell like? How does it feel in your hand? Don't bite it yet! Get to know the apple, and notice: Are you in a hurry to take a bite? Slowly, take a bite, but don't swallow it yet! Discover what your tongue does while you chew. Chew in slow motion and see if you can feel your tongue moving the apple around and pushing it toward your teeth. What else happens? Is there a burst of tastes? What does it taste like? Is it sweet? Does it make you want more? Do you want to quickly take another bite before you swallow this one? What happens if you do that?"

The children learn how to slow down and be mindful of their sense impressions and impulses. They see the connection between pleasurable sensation, wanting, and being in a hurry to get more.

Lovingkindness Meditation

"Find a comfortable, relaxed sitting posture and close your eyes. Remember something you did that makes you feel glad inside. Cross your hands on your heart and send a smile into your whole body. Relax and feel all warm and happy inside. Let the feeling of happiness, peace, kindness and love spread from your heart through your whole body. Next, send some lovingkindness, warmth, and happiness to someone in your family. Now send love to a pet, if you have one. Or to a friend. You can send lovingkindness to your class at school and to your whole neighborhood, to your country, and the world. Send peace to all creatures, two-legged, four-legged, and be sure to include the flying, swimming, slithering, crawling ones. We don't want to leave anything out!"

Small children will often call out, "What about tadpoles?" or "Even spiders?" We concentrate our minds and hearts, radiating friendliness and compassion in all directions, spreading our lovingkindness over the whole world.

Mindfulness practice and clinical work with children nourish each other. Our mindfulness practice helps us to enter into the world of children by teaching us to hold our ideas more lightly. It trains therapists and parents to disengage from emotional reactivity, granting us enough stillness to pay attention to the child's experience, and our own, in this precious, relational, transformational moment. Our adult attention is continually swept away into discursive reverie, but the intention of mindfulness is to restore our "beginner's mind." With this intention, therapists and parents may learn to meet the child with greater clarity and authenticity, and learn from the child about living in the present moment.

CHAPTER 11

Mindfulness Research

SARA W. LAZAR

This chapter provides an overview of scientific work related to mindfulness and meditation. It is divided into four parts: (1) an inside look at meditation and its putative mechanisms, (2) research exploring whether mindfulness works in psychotherapy, (3) research on the biology of meditation, and (4) future directions for research. This review is not comprehensive, but is intended to provide clinicians with a feeling for the challenges, methods, and findings involved in the empirical exploration of mindfulness.

INSIDE MINDFULNESS AND CONCENTRATION

What is actually going on when we practice meditation? It may be helpful to review earlier concepts. Attention is focused awareness. *Concentration* refers to focused attention on a single object, such as the breath or a mantra, whereas *mindfulness* generally refers to exploration of the *distractions* to concentration, such as sensations, thoughts and feelings. The technique of mindfulness meditation (MM) combines concentration with mindfulness, especially in the early stages of the practice, when we need to stabilize attention more often. Concentration meditation (CM) does not include any mindfulness of distractions, except for noticing that the mind was "somewhere else."

Most mindfulness-based treatment research explores the mindfulness-based stress reduction (MBSR) program, which places a heavy emphasis on mindfulness skills in daily living (i.e., not only formal meditation practice). There are nonspecific elements in this and other mindfulness-based treatment programs, such as group support, psychoeducation, and cognitive-behavioral skills, that probably contribute to outcome. CM is the predominant ingredient in transcendental meditation (TM) (Alexander, Langer, Newman, Chandler, & Davies, 1989) and Benson's Relaxation Response (RR) program (Benson, Beary & Carol, 1974). Neither of these programs emphasizes mindfulness during daily living. Although CM will naturally produce some mindfulness, that is not its aim.

We need models to make sense of what we observe studying meditative practices. One model might be *cognitive*. For example, Delmonte (1987) considers CM and MM to have a common element—both lead to a decrease in *cognitive construing*. Cognitive construing refers to discursive or elaborative thinking. Delmonte suggests that discursive thinking is *obstructed* during CM and it is *suspended* in MM. In practice, both CM and MM train a patient to break his or her train of thought by returning focus to the breath, mantra, or other object of attention.

Another model might be *physiological*. Focus on the breath or repetition of a word will readily elicit the relaxation response, which is a decrease in measures of physical arousal, such as skin conductance, heart rate, and breathing rate (Delmonte, 1984; Wallace, Benson, & Wilson, 1971). Improvements in psychological and medical status may in part be due to reduced physical arousal and stress. This model pertains well to the CM data, since mental distractions are irrelevant. However, stress reduction is also a core aspect of the mindfulness program of Kabat-Zinn (1990). Although Kabat-Zinn's program and CM-based programs such as TM and RR are demonstrably effective as medical interventions, the biological and cognitive–neurological mechanisms through which they each work will likely be quite different. It is also possible that some patients may benefit more from one approach over the other, but, as of this writing, there have not been systematic studies to address this issue.

DOES MINDFULNESS WORK?

When we evaluate the effectiveness of mindfulness training for psychological or physical problems, we are investigating whether people benefit from intentionally *being with* the discomfort in their lives rather than employing the usual strategies of avoiding, denying, or trying to remove the problem. For excellent critical reviews of the clinical outcome literature on mindfulness and meditation, see Baer (2003), Bishop (2002),

Bonadonna (2003), and Grossman, Niemann, Schmidt, and Walach (2004).

The sheer volume of encouraging data suggests that MM has some salubrious effects on a variety of physical and emotional illnesses. Relatively speaking, there are not as many well-designed scientific experiments assessing the effectiveness of mindfulness programs. Many of the studies on mindfulness lack adequate controls. This is due, in part, to difficulty in creating a control intervention that adequately matches the core elements of the mindfulness practice. For example, to make a controlled study of MBSR, we would require an 8-week group format, with 40 minutes of daily homework that is compelling enough to get the participants to comply, but has no therapeutic value.

Baer (2003) reviewed 22 studies that used either the MBSR program or the mindfulness-based cognitive therapy (MBCT) protocol, which is itself modeled after MBSR. Other effective treatment programs with mindfulness components, such as dialectical behavior therapy (DBT) and acceptance and commitment therapy (ACT), were not included in Baer's review, because they were considered less specifically mindfulness-based. Conditions treated in Baer's studies included anxiety, depression, binge eating, chronic pain, fibromyalgia, psoriasis, stress related to cancer, and medical and psychological functioning among nonclinical populations. The majority of the studies used repeated measures, pre–post, or follow-up designs. Baer concludes that MBSR is "probably efficacious" (according to the standards of the American Psychological Association Division 12 Task Force on Promotion and Dissemination of Psychological Procedures; see Chambless et al., 1998) based on the limited number of controlled studies. MBCT for treating depression will likely reach that designation with more studies by independent investigators using comparison treatment groups. Baer (2003) adds:

> In spite of the methodological flaws, the current literature suggests that mindfulness-based interventions may help to alleviate a variety of mental health problems and improve psychological functioning. These studies also suggest that many patients who enroll in mindfulness-based programs will complete them, in spite of high demands for homework practice, and that a substantial subset will continue to practice mindfulness skills long after the treatment program has ended. (p. 139)

A similar conclusion about effectiveness, with a strong recommendation for more research, was drawn in the review by Bishop (2002). For those wanting more details, Table 11.1 includes a number of conditions that have been clinically tested with MBSR and MBCT, and the methodology and outcome of each study. In the rapidly expanding

TABLE 11.1. Mindfulness-Based Treatment Research: Outcomes and Issues

Condition	Intervention	Findings	Issues	Reference
Anxiety	Uncontrolled study of MBSR for GAD and panic disorder. Pre–post with 3-month follow-up. $n = 24$.	Significant decrease in Beck and Hamilton scores for depression and anxiety from pre- to poststudy, and maintenance of these changes at 3-month follow-up. Half as many patients reported panic attacks in the last week of the course compared to the week prior to the start of the course. Also, significant decreases in Fear Survey Schedule and Mobility Inventory for agoraphobia. At 3 months, 84% were still practicing formal mindfulness at least 3 times per week.	No control group. Half of the 24 patients were taking anxiolytics during the intervention.	Kabat-Zinn et al. (1992)
	3-year follow-up to previous study. $n = 18$.	The changes observed in initial study were maintained at the 3-year time point. Of the 18 subjects available at the 3-year time period, 16 practiced the informal technique of breath awareness in daily life and reported that the program had had a lasting value on their lives. 38% ($n = 7$) still engaged in formal practice at least three times per week.	Half of subjects underwent additional psychotherapy for anxiety during the intervening period. Suggests MBSR is not sufficient as a stand-alone therapy for anxiety. However, given the time demand of formal practice, the high continued practice suggests that this intervention has had a strong positive effect on the patients' lives.	Miller et al. (1995)
Major depression	Random assignment to TAU or TAU plus MBCT for depression. $n = 149$	No change in mood scores. At 1-year follow-up, patients in the MBCT group had a significantly reduced rate of recurrence or relapse compared to TAU. Although 90% of the 8-week intervention, there was significant dropout. Results were best for subjects who completed at least 4 weeks of the MBCT course.	Only patients with at least three previous depressive episodes showed improvement relative to TAU. Control group received only TAU; could be nonspecific effects due to attention, peer support, etc.	Teasdale et al. (2000)

(continued)

223

TABLE 11.1. (continued)

Condition	Intervention	Findings	Issues	Reference
	Random assignment to TAU or TAU plus MBCT. $n = 45$.	Significant increases in the proportion of specific memories recalled pre- and postintervention compared to control group.	Control group received only TAU; could be nonspecific effects due to attention, peer support, etc.	Williams et al. (2000)
	Random assignment to TAU or TAU plus MBCT. $n = 75$.	MBCT group had half the rate of relapse or recurrence compared to TAU. Better patient retention than in Teasdale el al (2000).	Patients with only two previous depressive episodes were less likely to complete the course.	Ma and Teasedale (2004)
Pain	Uncontrolled study of MBSR for chronic pain. $n = 51$.	50% of subjects had greater than 50% reductions in PRI; 65% had a reduction of at least 33%.	Uncontrolled.	Kabat-Zinn (1982)
	Uncontrolled study of MBSR for chronic pain (though a nontreatment comparison group was used). $n = 90$.	A 58% reduction in PRI and 30% decreases in BPPA and Table of Levels of Interferences scales were reported in a majority of subjects. Decreases of 35–50% in mean MSCL, TMD, and GSI scores were also found. No change in these measures were reported in the comparison group.	Uncontrolled. Comparison group was not well matched to the intervention group on pain (PRI) and emotional distress (TMD) scales.	Kabat-Zinn et al. (1985)

Disorder	Study description	Results	Comments	Reference
	Observational follow-up study of MBSR for chronic pain. n = 225.	Patients were contacted from 2.5 months to 4 years postintervention. Although PRI scores returned to preintervention levels within 6 months of intervention, all other scores (POMS, SCL-90-R, MSCL, and BPPA) remained at postintervention levels for up to 4 years. At 1 year, approximately half of subjects were still practicing formal meditation regularly (≥ three times per week); at 4 years, 30% were practicing regularly.	Uncontrolled. Used regression analysis, which was not statistically appropriate.	Kabat-Zinn et al. (1987)
Fibromyalgia	Uncontrolled study of MBSR modified for fibromyalgia. n = 59.	Half of patients had ≥ 25% improvement on at least 50% of outcome measures (VAS for pain and sleep, SCL-90-R, CSQ, MSCL, FIQ, and FAI). 19% of patients had ≥ 50% improvement on at least 50% of outcome measures.	Uncontrolled. Half of patients were classified as "nonresponders" (≥ 25% improvement on at least half of scales). Originally 77 patients were enrolled but 18 patients dropped out within first 2 weeks and were not included in analysis.	Kaplan et al. (1993)
	Controlled study of MBSR modified for fibromyalgia. n = 121 (79 participants, 42 wait-list or no-treatment controls).	67% of participants reported improved symptoms compared to 40% of controls. Furthermore, the change in fibromyalgia symptoms was 16% greater in participants than controls, and the decrease in the global severity index of SCL-90-R was 32% greater in participants than controls.	Wait-list control, could be nonspecific effects due to attention, peer support, etc. Intervention included education on pain, stress, and communication, which probably also contributed to change scores.	Goldenberg et al. (1994)
Binge eating disorder	Uncontrolled study of MBSR modified for binge eating. n = 18.	Significant decrease in number and severity of binges. Decreases were related to increases in eating control, satiety, and sense of mindfulness. Significant decreases in Beck anxiety and depression scales.	No control group.	Kristeller and Hallett (1999)

(continued)

TABLE 11.1. (*continued*)

Condition	Intervention	Findings	Issues	Reference
Mixed population	Observational study and 1-year follow-up of MBSR for a heterogeneous medical population (17% anxiety/ panic, 16% depression, 27% pain). $n = 136$.	Found 44% decrease in anxiety subscale of SCL-90-R and 34% decrease on depression subscale. Also found significant increases in health-related quality of life scores (SF-36) and a 28% decreases in physical symptoms on MSCL (8% decrease in pain). Most improvements were maintained at 1-year follow-up, including anxiety and depression ($n = 41$). At 1-year time point, 70% ($n = 31$) still practiced formal meditation more than three times per week.	No control group. Only 30% of participants responded at 1-year time point, it may be that these patients are not representative of the larger group (patients with significant improvements may have been more likely to respond to the survey).	Reibel et al. (2001)
Community volunteers	Randomized wait-list control study of MBSR on healthy subjects. $n = 28$.	Intervention group experienced significantly larger decreases in SCL-90-R scores, including 59% decrease for depression and 60% for anxiety (vs. 7% and 10% for controls, respectively). Also found significant positive changes in self-control and acceptance scales, and a small but significant increase in spirituality.	Subjects were college students enrolled in a behavioral medicine course; all but one were female.	Astin (1997)
	Randomized wait-list control study of MBSR on healthy students. $n = 78$.	Found significant decreases in state and trait anxiety (STAI), depression (SCL-90), and increases in spirituality and empathy (INSPIRIT and ECRS). Results were replicated in the wait-list group.	Notable that the postintervention time point occurred during exam period, a high stress period.	Shapiro, Schwartz, and Bonner (1998)

| Cancer | MBSR breast and prostate cancer patients. $n = 58$. | Found increases in patients quality of life and sleep quality while decreasing symptoms of anxiety and depression as measured with SOSI. Also found decreases in systolic blood pressure that persisted for up to 1 year postintervention and significant decreases in several immune parameters, including interferon gamma and interleukin (IL) 10 (both associated with depression in cancer patients). Also found a threefold increase in IL-4, which slows the growth of breast cancer cells *in vitro*. | Although no correlation between the changes in immune and psychological measures, the finding of significant changes in biochemical markers thought to be playing a role in disease progression gives hope to the theory that meditation might have a direct effect on medical outcome and not just on the patients mood. | Carlson et al. (2003, 2004) |
| | Randomized active control group or MBSR for stage II breast cancer. $n = 63$. | Study focused specifically on sleep disturbances. Found improving sleep quality, particularly in patients whose sleep complaints are stress related. Although there was no correlation between the amount of formal meditation practice and sleep improvement, there was a positive interaction between feelings of being refreshed after sleep and the amount of "informal" practice the patient reported performing throughout the week between classes | Groups differed significantly at baseline, possibly due to randomization before baseline measures were collected. | Shapiro et al. (2003) |

(*continued*)

TABLE 11.1. (*continued*)

Condition	Intervention	Findings	Issues	Reference
Psoriasis	Randomized trial of formal mindfulness practice during UV treatments (no classes or homework) versus UV treatment without mindfulness. $n = 37$.	Found significant differences between groups in number of days until skin clearing. Importantly, unlike the other outcome studies reported above, patients in this study did not receive any of the social support, psychosocial education, or cognitive therapy elements of a typical MBSR intervention. Furthermore, they practiced only mindful attention to the breath, no yoga or body scan, and only during treatment (not daily practice). Furthermore, the outcome was a purely medical one—time to skin clearing—which, like the cancer studies described above, suggest that MBSR can produce profound physiological effects that can directly influence health outcome, not just psychological outcome.		Kabat-Zinn et al. (1998)

Note. MBSR, mindfulness-based stress reduction; MBCT, mindfulness-based cognitive therapy; GAD, generalized anxiety disorder; TAU, treatment as usual; MSCI, medical symptom checklist; TMD, total mood disturbance; POMS, Profile of Mood States; STAI, State–Trait Anxiety Inventory; SCL-90-R, Symptom Checklist-90 Revised; GSI, General Severity Index; PRI, Pain Rating Inventory; BPPA, Body Parts Problems Assessment; FIQ, Fibromyalgia Impact Questionnaire; FAI, Fibromyalgia Attitude Index; CSQ, Coping Strategies Questionnaire; SF-36, Short Form 36; BDI, Beck Depression Inventory; VAS, visual analogue scale; SOSI, Symptoms of Stress Inventory; INSPIRIT, Index of Core Spiritual Experiences; ECRS, Empathy Construct Ratings Scale; UV, ultraviolet.

field of mindfulness-based therapy, new studies are coming out all the time. The reader is referred to the websites of mindfulness-based treatment programs, some of which are listed in Appendix A, for the most recent findings.

As mentioned in Chapter 6, DBT and ACT both include mindfulness theory and practice. (For a discussion of the mindfulness component in DBT, see Robins, 2002; for ACT, see Hayes, 2002; and for a mindfulness overview in both approaches, see Hayes, Follette, & Linehan, 2004.) Both of these multicomponent treatment programs are supported by a small but expanding number of randomized, controlled outcome studies (Hayes, Masuda, Bissett, Luoma, & Guerrero, 2004).

DBT and ACT have both been tested with difficult patient populations. The first controlled trial of DBT involved chronically suicidal patients with borderline personality disorder (BPD) (Linehan, Armstrong, Suarez, Allmon, & Heard, 1991). At 1-year follow-up, the DBT treatment group had significantly fewer parasuicidal acts, had fewer days in the hospital, and stayed in treatment longer than treatment-as-usual controls. DBT also has demonstrated success with BPD patients who abuse substances (Linehan et al., 1999, 2002). DBT is arguably the most thoroughly validated and widely used psychotherapeutic treatment for BPD (Bohus et al., 2000, 2004; Koerner & Linehan, 2000; Linehan, 2000), although longer term outcome studies still need to be done (Westen, 2000). The DBT approach has also been used successfully for treating eating disorders such as binge eating (Telch, Agras, & Linehan, 2001) and bulimia (Safer, Telch, & Agras, 2001).

Controlled outcome studies of ACT cover a broad range of conditions including depression (Zettle & Raines, 1989), workplace stress (Bond & Bunce, 2000), and math anxiety (Zettle, 2003). One remarkable study of ACT showed a 50% reduction in rehospitalization (after 4 months) of patients with positive psychotic symptoms after participating in only four sessions of ACT compared to treatment as usual (Bach & Hayes, 2002). See Hayes, Masuda, et al. (2004) for a review of ACT literature.

Interesting health-related findings on CM include increased longevity among elderly persons practicing TM in residential homes (Alexander, Langer, Newman, Chandler, & Davies, 1989) and decreased blood pressure among African American senior citizens (Schneider et al., 1995), both compared to control groups. Benson's RR program led to a decrease in the frequency and duration of epileptic seizures (Deepak, Manchanda, & Maheshwari, 1994) and significant decreases in severe premenstrual symptoms (Goodale, Domar, & Benson, 1990). The treatment outcome literature on concentration-based techniques, with the exception of those just mentioned, is fraught with similar methodological problems as the mindfulness literature.

THE BIOLOGY OF MEDITATION

Although there have been numerous studies of the basic physiological, neurological, and immune changes that accompany meditation practice, to date, there is no *direct* evidence of the actual mechanisms through which meditation exerts its effects. In this section, I review the available biological data on mindfulness meditation as of this writing. Importantly, most of these studies have used healthy subjects, not patients, so one must be careful when trying to generalize these findings to clinical populations. For more extensive, earlier reviews of the meditation literature, see Austin (1998) and Murphy, Donovan, and Taylor (1997).

Some of the biological studies have had conflicting results. This is due, in part, to the use of subjects who practice different styles of meditation, large heterogeneity both within and between studies in the amount of meditation practice each subject has undertaken, and lack of criteria for evaluating the proficiency of subjects who meditate. Some studies have mixed subjects with 2 months' to 20 years' experience, with little regard as to how this might affect outcome.

A strength of the nonclinical studies is that they often employ control conditions (usually simple rest) and meditation-naive control subjects. It is quite possible that people who choose to meditate may be very different than the average population, so putative differences between experimental and control subjects could be due to inherent differences in these populations, not meditation effects. Longitudinal studies will be needed to address these concerns directly, though several studies have demonstrated subtle differences between long- and short-term practitioners, which may argue against this hypothesis.

Cognitive Changes

Experienced meditators claim that practice increases their ability to concentrate and to deal with stressful stimuli. Various researchers have documented differences in these traits between meditators and control subjects, suggesting that the claims of experienced meditators have some validity.

Stress Reactivity

Cultivation of equanimity increases the practitioner's ability to experience negative events with less reactivity. Goleman and Schwartz (1976) hypothesized that meditators should demonstrate less physiological reactivity to unpleasant stimuli compared to controls. To test this hypothesis, they measured skin conductance response (SCR) from meditators and controls while the subjects viewed reenacted woodshop accidents. SCR measures the amount of sweat produced as an indicator of autonomic arousal. Compared to controls, the meditation subjects experienced a slightly larger initial increase in SCR but then returned to baseline levels more quickly, indicating that the meditation subjects had heightened responses to the negative images, but were then able to quickly "let go" of the images and return to a state of mental calm and equilibrium. Presumably, these subjects are not engaging in ruminative thoughts that would prolong their autonomic arousal.

Attention

Valentine and Sweet (1999) conducted a study to compare directly the effects of mindfulness and concentration meditation on sustained attention in both novice and experienced subjects. Intriguingly, all subjects practiced Buddhist meditation, but were classified as either mindfulness or concentration style depending on self-report as to their mental focus during meditation. Although the sample sizes were quite small (9–10 subjects per group), mindfulness meditators were significantly better in their ability to detect unexpected stimuli (tones with different repetition frequencies) compared to the concentration group. Furthermore, all meditators were significantly better than controls in their ability to detect all stimuli, suggesting that both groups had developed heightened attention as a result of their practice. When the two meditation groups were subdivided based on total number of years they had practiced, there were striking and significant differences between novice and experienced subjects in their ability to detect the stimuli, with subjects having *more* than 2 years of practice able to detect approximately 5% more of the stimuli than the subjects with less than 2 years of practice, regardless of meditation style. This last finding strongly suggests that the differences between the meditators and controls were due to practice effects and not to personality differences between groups.

Habituation

An early study by Kasamatsu and Hirai (1973) with four highly experienced Zen masters demonstrated that their electroencephalogram (EEG) patterns failed to habituate to repeated clicking sounds, while the pattern of nonmeditating controls did habituate. Becker and Shapiro (1981) failed to replicate these findings 15 years later using three groups of meditators and two control groups—with one control group instructed to attend to the sound closely and the other to ignore it. However, the subjects in the different groups were not matched for age (Zen, 37.8

years old; yoga, 31.5 years old; TM, 28.7 years old; two control groups, 26.5 and 29.5 years old). Furthermore, the sound characteristics and method in which the clicks were presented in the two studies differed, which might account for the differences. In the Kasamatsu and Hirai (1973) study, the sounds were presented through stereo speakers, while in the Becker study, subjects wore headphones. The physical sensations associated with the headphones would likely draw more attention to the ears and make all subjects more attentive to the clicks. Also, neither study reported the magnitude of the tones, so it is possible that in the second study, the sounds were louder or more intrusive, overcoming the subtle effects observed in the first study.

Neurobiological Changes

Although numerous studies have documented the ability of meditation techniques to change peripheral autonomic measures such as heart rate and breathing rate (see next section), our inability to directly observe brain activity elicited by these practices has limited our understanding of the mind–body dynamic. Efforts are now under way to define meditative states neurologically. There is interest in distinguishing between different meditation and yoga practices, as well as to compare meditative states with more traditional states of consciousness, such as simple rest or sleep. Comparisons of different styles of meditation may shed light on the neural basis of consciousness.

The tricky problem for studies on the biology of meditation is determining what exactly is going on in the mind of the practitioner. For example, a person who practices MM for 1 year may be much closer to a CM practitioner from the point of view of actual practice and brain behavior than a person who has practiced MM for 30 years. There may be precious little exploration of mental contents in a beginning MM practitioner. The issue of *what* we are measuring becomes more important when we reduce the time frame of observation to a few minutes in the laboratory. In moment-to-moment brain imaging studies, what is the practitioner actually doing? Focusing on breath? Being distracted? Being mindful of having been distracted? Returning to the breath from distraction? Our experimental technology is not yet capable of discerning these events.

However, the use of neuroimaging techniques *has* provided several important contributions to the understanding of mind–body interventions. First, there has been some debate in the literature concerning whether meditation induces a discrete state distinct from simple rest or early stages of sleep. Studies with EEG, functional magnetic resonance imaging (fMRI), and positron emission tomography (PET) clearly indicate that the meditative state is different from rest or sleep (Hebert & Lehmann, 1977; Lazar et al., 2000; Lou et al., 1999). Intriguingly, these studies also indicate that there is not a single, unique "meditative state"; rather, different styles of meditation practice lead to different patterns of brain activity. This is in line with subjective reports of meditation practitioners, who describe qualitatively different mental states after engaging in these different styles of meditation.

Neuroimaging Studies

Two neuroimaging techniques developed over the last 10 or 15 years, fMRI and PET, allow scientists to identify activity inside the brain during a wide variety of tasks. A small handful of meditation studies using these tools has been published.

Although PET and fMRI can both be used to identify brain regions that are engaged during meditation practice, each method allows researchers to evaluate different aspects of neural activity. FMRI data can be acquired throughout the entire brain continuously over tens of minutes, which allows the investigator to follow the time course of neurological activity during the initiation and deepening of the meditative state. For instance, data indicate that while the fMRI signal in many brain regions involved in attention and physiological modulation increases during Kundalini meditation (a form of mantra meditation), there are also regions, such as the sensory cortex, in which activity gradually *decreases* during this style of meditation (Lazar et al., 2000), which is consistent with a withdrawal of attention from physical sensations.

Alternatively, PET imaging produces just one picture per experimental state, so the scientist can only look at average brain activity during this time period, not at how it changes and develops over time. However, this technique can also be used to image specific neurotransmitters, such as dopamine. These properties have been utilized by researchers studying Yoga Nidra meditation. This style of meditation promotes increased awareness of the senses, but also utilizes imagery and concentration techniques to reduce emotional reactivity. A PET study employing experienced subjects who practice Yoga Nidra meditation indicated that several brain regions were activated during meditation, including the primary sensory cortex (Lou et al., 1999). The authors also found *decreases* in regions involved in executive control, emotion processing, and motor planning, consistent with the hypothesis that these functions are dampened during Yoga Nidra meditation. In a follow-up study, these same researchers demonstrated that Yoga Nidra meditation results in the release of dopamine in the striatum, which the authors argue is consistent with decreased motor planning and increased physical relaxation (Kjaer et al., 2002).

In another study of concentration meditators, Newberg and colleagues (2001) found decreases in parietal lobe activity. This region is involved in sensory integration, and lesions to this area result in a loss of a patient's ability to maneuver in space. The authors argue that decreased activity in this region during meditation is consistent with the subjective reports of mystical experiences, including the loss of sense of body sometimes reported (Newberg et al., 2001). This same region was associated with an *increase* in activity in the Kundalini meditators, who do not report out-of-body experiences (Lazar et al., 2000).

Electroencephalographic Studies

Although fMRI can give information about brain activity over time, the temporal resolution of the signal is fairly poor: Each image is a composite of several seconds worth of brain activity. In contrast, EEG signals have millisecond resolution but poor spatial resolution. These images give the scientist only a general brain region in which the activity is occurring and cannot reliably detect activity from deep subcortical structures such as the amygdala or hippocampus. The use of EEG has allowed scientists to identify dynamic changes in brain activity during meditation in a way that reflects different *types* of activity that are occurring (i.e., alpha, gamma, or beta waves), not just the regions that are active. Furthermore, EEG has an advantage over PET and fMRI, in that it allows researchers to assess brain activity in quiet and relatively naturalistic settings.

Since the 1970s, numerous studies have been performed using EEG to identify changes in brain wave activity during meditation. Many of the early studies used subjects practicing TM, which was very popular at the time, though others used subjects from multiple traditions, without discrimination. I focus on recent studies that have focused directly on subjects practicing some form of MM.

In the most relevant study on mindfulness meditation, Davidson and colleagues (2003) measured resting EEG patterns in healthy subjects before and after an 8-week MBSR intervention. Davidson had previously shown that patients suffering from depression and anxiety have increased EEG power in the right half of the brain while resting quietly, while psychologically healthy subjects have greater activity on the left. Although the study was small, the results indicated that a leftward shift in resting EEG patterns could be detected after 8 weeks of practice and persisted for 3 months following the study completion. Importantly, the observed changes were correlated with improved immune function. This longitudinal study is an important step toward addressing the criticism that there are preexisting biological differences between people who meditate and those who do not, and it also lends credence to the hypotheses that meditation promotes brain plasticity and emotional development.

Lehmann and colleagues (2001) studied a highly advanced Buddhist lama while he practiced five distinct exercises. Although all the exercises were of the concentration type, the study clearly showed in a single subject that different meditation practices elicit different patterns of brain activity. Furthermore, the regions activated were consistent with what was known about the functions of those regions (i.e., use of mantra-activated language areas, imagery-activated visual areas), which helps verify that the subject's neural activity was consistent with his subjective report.

Taken together, the neurological data suggests that meditation is a distinct state different than simple rest. Furthermore, different types of meditation engage different brain regions. From a neurological point of view, it is as yet unknown why engaging these brain regions should result in the psychological and physiological changes that are observed during meditation, but these initial studies provide important clues as to how to design future experiments.

Autonomic Changes

Effects on Breathing

Because relaxation is not the primary goal of mindfulness meditation, the physiological changes experienced by a group of mindfulness meditators are more heterogeneous than those of subjects practicing concentration-style meditation. Mindfulness practice can paradoxically raise the breathing rate of newer students, perhaps due to the effort to stay focused or to the new awareness of stressful thoughts and sensations. In one study of experienced mindfulness practitioners, there was a correlation between the change in breathing rate and the number of years the person had practiced MM (Lazar, 2004). Subjects with just a few years' experience had a small but significant increase in breathing rate of 1–2 breaths per minute, while subjects with 6 or more years of practice displayed decreases of 2–8 breaths per minute, suggesting that as meditators slowly develop greater concentration and work through various psychological issues, they will be able to access deeper levels of relaxation.

Effects on Heart Rate Dynamics

A relatively new measure of autonomic nervous system functioning is provided by analysis of heart rate variability (Malik & Camm, 1995; Pieper & Hammill, 1995). Variability in the interval between heartbeats has been correlated with prognostic outcome in heart disease: Patients with low variability are at greater risk for sudden cardiac death (Ho et al., 1997; Ivanov et al., 1996; Malik & Camm, 1995). Subjects practicing Tai Chi, Kundalini, Zen, and MM have all shown increases in heart rate variability during meditation relative to rest (Lehrer, Sasaki, & Saito, 1999; Peng et al., 1999). These findings suggest a strong relationship between the meditative state and the neuroautonomic control of heart rate fluctuations, as well as cardiopulmonary interactions.

FUTURE DIRECTIONS

Mindfulness is currently generating vigorous discussion in the scientific community (see *Clinical Psychology: Science and Practice*, May 2003, Vol. 10) and spawning numerous doctoral dissertations. Although the mindfulness approach to therapy appears to be effective, the jury is still out as to why and how well mindfulness works (Baer, 2003). There are a host of interesting questions for future research.

General Effects of Mindfulness Practice

- What are the *short-term* biological and psychological effects of mindfulness during meditation or moments of mindfulness in everyday life? Are there particular brain processes associated with specific clinical conditions that mindfulness practice either augments or reduces, which can provide clues to clinical interventions?
- What *long-term* effects can we see, physically and psychologically? In what specific ways does mindfulness improve physical and psychological health?
- In what ways does mindfulness practice change a person's cognitive abilities or style, such as attention, emotional regulation, flexibility, or reactivity? Do conceptual shifts occur, such as insight into the nature of suffering and mind? Can we measure whether it fosters wisdom? Do personal values shift with practice? Does a practitioner feel more connected to the world in general?

- Does mindfulness change *behavior*? If so, what behavior and how?

Mindfulness-Based Psychotherapy

This treatment category contains techniques that are directly taught to the patient.

- Are mindfulness interventions more effective than other techniques? If so, which strategies work best for which patients and conditions? What are the contraindications for mindfulness-based treatments? What is the relative value of formal sitting meditation versus mindfulness in everyday life skills?
- Why might mindfulness-based interventions work? Is mindfulness an indivisible, therapeutic process, or can mindfulness be dismantled into components such as present awareness, acceptance, or exposure? Which elements are most effective, and for whom?
- What are the nonspecific ingredients of multicomponent treatments? Does mindfulness add anything to these nonspecific factors?
- How much training should therapists get to teach mindfulness? Does level of training effect outcome?

Mindfulness-Informed Psychotherapy

This category refers to therapists who practice mindfulness themselves and have a theoretical understanding of how to alleviate suffering through mindfulness, but they do not necessarily teach their patients to practice mindfulness.

- Does mindfulness practice by the therapist lead to better therapy outcome? If so, how? What level of therapist practice is required?
- Do mindfulness-informed therapists actually differ from other therapists? Is a particular kind of therapist uniquely drawn to meditation?
- Is a working *theory* of mindfulness enough? What is the relative impact on therapy of theory versus practice? Is there a positive effect when both the therapist and the patient share a common theory of mind, and/or when both practice mindfulness?
- What are the relational qualities in therapy that may shift if the therapist practices mindfulness, i.e., what changes can we witness in therapy between patient and therapist?

SUMMARY

We have compelling evidence that volitional control of attention through meditation affects neurophysiology. We are not certain how these mechanisms directly affect mental and physical health, although cognitive and physiological models are contributing to our understanding. Mindfulness meditation practices have begun to demonstrate their utility in benefiting the health of our patients. Clinicians should feel encouraged by the research evidence to explore these strategies with their patients in innovative new ways, guided by attention to the individual needs of the patient and good clinical judgment.

PART IV

Past and Promise

CHAPTER 12

The Roots of Mindfulness

Andrew Olendzki

E mpirical studies are beginning to demonstrate the usefulness of mindfulness for alleviating psychological and physical problems, so it may seem entirely unnecessary to link mindfulness to its historical and philosophical roots. Modern researchers are also attempting to separate the essential and nonessential ingredients of mindfulness, in order to set aside those elements that might be merely cultural elaborations. This is surely a fruitful agenda for clinical psychology. However, as discussed in earlier chapters, the goals of the mindfulness tradition go beyond those customarily identified in clinical practice. To more fully understand what lies outside the clinical domain, it may be helpful to look to the historical setting of mindfulness and the system of thought underlying what we now call Buddhist psychology.

The practice of attending carefully to the details of one's present experience is probably as old as humankind itself. Doing so in a deliberate and structured way, however, seems to have particularly strong roots in the religious traditions of ancient India. It was in the forests and plains along the banks of the Indus and Ganges rivers that people began to explore the nuances of perceptual experience using methods a modern scientist might recognize as empirical, experimental, and repeatable—despite being entirely introspective. Carried out over the last four millennia, this program of self-study has yielded a descriptive science of the mind and body that is of growing interest to the contemporary thinker.

Ancient insights into the workings of human experience are preserved in the Hindu and Buddhist traditions, each leaving a rich legacy of sophisticated psychological material. Buddhist theoretical psychology, in particular, articulates a remarkably postmodern model of human consciousness, based on a process view of noncentralized, interdependent systems for processing sense data and constructing identity. Its practical psychology is anchored in the practice of meditation, which can range from mindfulness, through various stages of concentration, to deeply transformative insights that can fundamentally restructure the organization of mind and body. The most basic and accessible form of the ancient Indian meditative arts, referred to in this volume as *mindfulness meditation*, is beginning to have a significant effect upon a wide range of contemporary scientific and therapeutic professions.

ANCIENT ORIGINS

A Unique View of the Human Condition

Each in its own unique way, the ancient Buddhist and Hindu schools of thought shared the view that human existence centers upon a node of conscious awareness, more or less identified as a soul, which is embedded in a sensory apparatus yielding both pleasant and painful experience. The nature of this existence is flawed by the fact that pain is inevitable, lasting pleasure is unobtainable, and humans have limited ability to see themselves or their world very clearly. Death provides no solution to this existential dilemma they called *dukkha* (loosely translated as "suffering"), for they believed that a person just flows on from one lifetime to another, without respite. Each time around, one will always encounter illness, injury, aging, and death. The religious agenda of ancient India was organized around liberating the soul from these rounds of rebirth and suffering, and, in the process, attaining a form of profound omniscience.

This is all very interesting to us today; because of the emphasis on awareness and direct experience, the problems posed by these ancient traditions, and the solutions offered to them, have a familiar psychological orientation. Unlike the dominant Western religions, which are grounded in a historical story line and come equipped with specific belief systems, Buddhism and its contemporaries were much more agnostic on matters of metaphysical revelation and focused instead upon the practitioner's inner experience.

There is no particular religious explanation for why beings find themselves embedded in an unsatisfactory existence characterized by suffering, and there is nobody to call upon to bail them out. But through careful examination of the situation, they can begin to understand how their suffering is caused, and can therefore learn how to work on undoing the conditions creating the discomfort. In these traditions, psychological and existential suffering are understood to have their origins in basic human drives and reflexes, which are for the most part unconscious and therefore apparently beyond one's control. But these can in fact be uncovered, behavioral responses can be modified, and it is possible to reprogram the mind and body substantially to avoid their instinctual shortcomings. What is required is a radical psychological transformation.

All the early schools shared the view that humans are actively participating in the endless turnings of this unsatisfying wheel of life through a combination of desire and ignorance. Desire is the deep compulsion to pursue pleasure and avoid pain, while ignorance points to the unconscious and unexamined nature of most of our attitudes and assumptions about the nature of things. Together, they condition how we construct our reality, lurching from one moment to another trying, usually with only limited success, to satisfy an array of selfish and short-term needs.

The Importance of Experience

The Western intellectual tradition embraces rationality to govern unruly human nature. This can be seen in elegant and elaborated systems of law, social philosophy, and psychology. In the ancient Asian traditions, the rational and conceptual tools we value so highly in the West are seen as often being employed simply to rationalize and justify what we are driven to do, rather than offering much help in accurately understanding our predicament. So reasoning was not seen to offer much help. The revelation of ancient truths, so highly valued by Western traditions, was also distrusted, because there was no assurance that the first in the file of blind men passing along the tradition had actually known or seen anything in his own direct experience. Another set of tools was needed to unravel the tangles of body and mind that held the soul in bondage to suffering, and this is where yoga, asceticism, and meditation became the crucial vehicles for self-exploration and self-transformation.

Yoga, in its original context, has to do with discipline, the yoking of body and mind, the binding of both to the will, and the fastening of human life to a higher purpose of discovery. It involves both asceticism and meditation, each of which works on loosening the bonds that tie the soul to suffering. Asceticism addresses desire by depriving the mind and body of what it desperately wants. In the practice of restraint, one can taste the flavor of desire, turn it over and examine its texture, and expose the hold it has upon the psychophysical organism. Meditation has more to do with learning to observe and to be keenly aware of what unfolds in the mind and body moment by moment. Honing an ever-sharpening experience of the present, the practice of meditation sheds light on processes that are otherwise invisible for their subtlety, or overlooked for their ubiquity. All these techniques of experiential exploration were developed and cultivated over many centuries, and the lore they generated about the functioning of mind and body grew proportionally.

As discussed in Chapter 2, meditation has much in common with the scientific enterprise of empirical observation. One is simply regarding as objectively as possible the data of passing phenomenological experience, using the apparatus of direct introspective awareness rather than the microscope or telescope. While, until recently, not amenable to outside measurement, meditation is by nature experimental, insofar as one is carefully noting the effect of various internal and external changes upon experience, and its techniques and findings are shown to be more or less replicated by whoever undertakes its rigors. This is why these practices are not so foreign and exotic to the modern psychological researcher, and why the ancient sciences of mind and body are being invited to contribute to the contemporary investigation of human consciousness and behavior.

THE CONSTRUCTION OF EXPERIENCE

The Emergence of Consciousness

The contemplative practices of ancient India gave rise to a very different way of viewing what we generally refer to as the self and the world. The sense of identity that every individual develops, and the notion each has of the world in which he or she is embedded, is regarded by the Buddhist tradition as an elaborate construction project. It is an edifice so complex and nuanced that it takes years of careful development and a tremendous amount of energy and attention to keep it in place. Ours is a universe of macroconstruction, in which the continually arising data of the senses and of miscellaneous internal processing are channeled into structures and organized into schemas that support an entirely synthetic sphere of meaning—a virtual reality.

The mind is a world-building organ that pieces together a cosmos from the chaos of data streaming though the senses at breakneck speed. Beginning at the earliest possible age, human beings have to learn how to do this, and most of childhood development has to do with marching, one hopes, in some reasonable order, through various stages of growing complexity and, presumably, adaptation, during which the child learns to perceive the world as populated with stable objects accurately known. It is a delicate process, and much can go wrong. While the gradual building of identity that takes place over a lifetime is a well-studied subject in developmental psychology, the Buddhist tradition has considerably more to say about how world building can also be seen as occurring constantly, taking place each and every moment.

The process by which consciousness is constructed involves a number of components, which are illustrated in Figure 12.1. According to classical Buddhist analysis, the most elemental discernable unit of experience is a moment of *contact* between a sense organ, a sense object, and the awareness of that object. The coming together of these three factors, each itself the product of an entire process, sparks a synthetic incident of human cognition, an episode of sensory discernment, an event of "knowing" that forms the core around which human conscious existence is layered. *Consciousness* is thus an emergent, conditioned phenomenon, manifesting in a series of momentary occurrences, which is simultaneously the agent, instrument, and activity of awareness (Bhikku Bodhi, 2000).

The mode of the arising of conscious experience will be codetermined by the nature of the organ and the object of its awareness, with which it is interdependent. We call it *seeing* when the eye is used to discern an object, *hearing* when the ear is involved in noticing a sound, and depending on the other sensory supports, consciousness may manifest as *smelling, tasting, touching,* or *thinking.* This last is actually far more diverse than the term *thinking* usually covers and includes any mental event that is not already included in one of the other five sense modali-

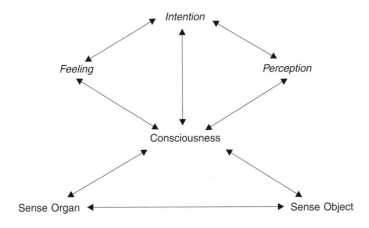

FIGURE 12.1. The construction of experience.

ties. According to Buddhist analysis, everything we are capable of experiencing will arise in one of these six ways, and our entire world of experience is woven from the strands of such simple units of awareness.

Of considerable interest to the philosopher, if not the psychologist, is that, in this view, none of the three elements of contact is ontologically primary, possessing a privileged and enduring role. The material world presumably underlying the objects of the senses is irrelevant to the analysis of the human situation in an instant of awareness: The organs are not in the service of an entity that is "having" the experience; and consciousness is not something that can exist other than in the instant of its being enacted. Mind cannot be reduced to matter in this model, and neither is materiality merely a projection of mind. Rather, each is an equally important facet of a single psychophysical organism, which itself does not *exist* as much as it *occurs*. Early Buddhist thought has little interest in conceptual speculations about such matters, choosing instead to cleave to a rigorous empirical phenomenology. What one can actually see unfolding under scrutiny of the moment is considered to be of far more interest and use than theorizing from abstractions.

Perception and Feeling

The moment of contact between organs, objects, and consciousness is the seed around which a more complex manifestation of mind crystallizes. Also co-arising with these three are perception, feeling, and intention. In Buddhist psychology, these terms have a unique and precise meaning.

Perception involves a host of associative functions that are learned gradually over time and are heavily conditioned by factors such as language and culture. It provides evaluative information about how the subject regards and construes the moment's experience; everything seen is *seen as* something; thus, every visual experience is automatically processed in light of previous understanding.

In this sense, perception is not the passive registration of the world received through the senses and represented accurately in awareness. In fact, it is a creative process of construction and categorization, drawing on past experience and the application of categories inherited from multiple sources. Consequently, it is not appropriate to say that we accurately perceive what is given; the act of perception often goes beyond the data present at the senses, potentially omitting details or filling in for missing information. Perception is also influenced by drive states; when we are hungry, we are more likely to notice restaurants than when we are not.

This process offers a degree of efficiency, although, as the Buddhists would say, at the cost of considerable distortion and projection. The creative aspect of perception occurs without our conscious awareness that we bring more to the sense experience than is given (Bruner, 1973). The same is true of all the other senses, including the perception of all nonsensory cognitive experience, such as dreaming, planning, and imagining. The reflexive construction of perception is as ubiquitous to all mental activity as it is to every moment of sense experience.

Feeling is a word used in technical Buddhist vocabulary to refer to the affect tone associated with every object of sense or cognition. To the raw knowing that underlies every moment of experience is also added a hedonic tone, so that everything seen is *seen as* pleasant, unpleasant, or neutral. This feeling tone is also a natural and automatic part of the processing of every object known in any of the six modes of knowing (seeing, hearing, smelling, tasting, touching or thinking) and becomes inextricably bound up with the way a moment is constructed.

In some cases, the clarity or strength of this charge is low, on which occasion the feeling tone is said to be neither pleasant nor unpleasant, but even when feelings are neutral, they play an important part in the texture of the moment. This process, too, ordinarily occurs outside of awareness, though it becomes an object of attention in meditation. Experience is so far seen to include five interdependent factors—an organ, an object, consciousness, perception, and feeling, all of which arise and fall together in the view of the attentive meditator.

The Role of Intention

One more psychologically important element, that of *intention*, is also added to this model of continuously arising factors. Intention has to do with the attitude taken towards what is happening in experience; it is the intentional stance one takes at any given moment. Whereas the other factors are primarily contributing to our *knowing* what is going on internally or in the environment, intention is more about what we are *doing* about it. While objects appear to the organs of perception and are barely noticed by consciousness, and while perception and feeling have somewhat more to do with shaping the subjective significance of the object, intention is a more active and creative function that has a great impact on how the moment's experience is organized and presented by the mind.

Intention can have an active manifestation, for example, in a moment of attachment or aversion to present experience, an intentional stance of embracing or resisting what is happening. Put differently, intention is the factor that responds to the pleasant or unpleasant qualities of the arising experience by trying to hold on and perpetuate the experience, or to reject or terminate it. This is the pleasure principle, described by Freud (1920/1961c), in microscopic action.

Intention manifests also as action when activities of body, speech, and mind are initiated—either consciously or unconsciously—by the choice or decision to act one way or another. A disposition to respond, mentally or behaviorally, to circumstances in a characteristic or patterned way is an expression of a subtle, passive influence of intention. In Western psychological terms, dispositions resemble traits. Dispositions are learned from experience. We might also call these learned behaviors, conditioned responses, or personality characteristics.

According to Buddhist psychology, a person is continually shaped by his or her previous actions and their resulting dispositions. The personality is composed of bundles of such dispositions, laid down and regularly modified over one's entire lifetime, and it is from the background of these accumulated patterns that intentions, perceptions, and feelings in the next moment are shaped.

Every action is thus conditioned by all former actions, and every action also has an effect on all subsequent actions. In ancient India, the word for this was *karma*. The great wheel of life, through which sentient beings "flow on" (as they conceived the mechanism of rebirth) from one lifetime to another, also functions on the microcosm: Beings flow on from one moment to another, continually being formed by previous selves and in turn continually forming and re-forming themselves and their world in each new moment. This is rebirth in psychological terms: Each moment is created anew from the conditions of previous events. Whether construed as occurring between lifetimes or between moments, the Buddhist notion of rebirth has to do with the perpetual re-forming of identity rather than the reemergence of a fixed entity suggested by the word *reincarnation*.

THE SELF

The Construction of Self

We can see from this basic overview of Buddhist psychology that a person is regarded as a process of continually unfolding dynamic systems, responding to a changing environment and perpetually reshaping itself as it constructs a meaningful order out of each moment's external and internal data. Mechanisms are in place to learn from experience and to retain information, and these structures stabilize over time such that each person acquires a unique set of characteristics. Some properties of this entire system change very rapidly, usually in response to some newly emerging stimuli, while other elements of character change very little or very gradually.

As this system becomes sufficiently complex, the word *self* begins to be applied, bringing a whole new dimension to the model. As long as the psychophysical organism can be seen as a complex but impersonal process, one is able to maintain some intellectual and emotional detachment. But when self arises in experience as an existential entity, when the subsystems *belong* to someone or are *owned* by a person, then the organism begins to respond in some very different ways.

According to classical Buddhist analysis, the application of the term *self* is a misunderstanding that causes considerable unnecessary difficulty. Much of this misunderstanding is rooted in the very way the mind has evolved to process information. It necessarily distorts reality in some important ways and on three different levels of scale: perception, thought, and "view."

To begin with, the mind takes information from an uninterrupted flow of phenomena presenting at the sense doors. Perception consists of fixed bundles of data extracted from this background perpetual flux, which amounts to constructing moments of apparent stability from an inherently unstable world. In Buddhist terminology, the mind is artificially creating virtual moments of "permanence" from an intrinsically impermanent universe. This is a distortion, and it is replicated at higher levels of processing. Thoughts, higher level operations built upon such bundles of perception, also consist of staccato images and concepts, and "views," or beliefs, are a further set of arbitrarily arrested attitudes and habits of mind.

The most important form of distortion fundamental to the way our minds operate has to do with creating the notion of self out of what is essentially an impersonal process. Selfhood is the expression of a particular kind of distortion of view, a situation that develops gradually from basic misperceptions, to the casting of whole sets of misinformed thoughts, and eventually to a deeply rooted belief system that becomes imposed upon all further perception and thought. Here again we see a cyclical pattern. Perceptions give rise to thoughts, which congeal into beliefs, and which then influence perception.

When the system operates optimally, it allows for growth, learning, and transformation. But when it is fundamentally misinformed, it can also give rise to a considerable amount of delusion. And this is what the Buddhists say is happening in the case of the ubiquitous belief in selfhood as a defining category of human psychology. They would not deny that stable patterns in this information-processing system provide a useful—perhaps even crucial—function in the organization of experience. But trouble arises when the constructed self becomes the main organizing principle, when it is unrealistically invested with qualities it does not innately possess, and, most importantly, when it becomes the node around which maladaptive behaviors coalesce. The self comes to be experienced as a central and dominant element of psychic life, mistaking what is a series of contingent patterns in constant flux for an enduring entity.

Self as a Cause of Suffering

Misunderstanding the nature of the self gives rise to suffering as it shapes our response to pleasurable and disagreeable experiences. While pleasure and pain are a natural part of every moment's experience, the reflexive *desire* for pleasure to continue or for pain to cease introduces a different element not originally present in the barest elements of the experience. Desire is essentially the expression of a tension between what is happening and the person's intent to maximize gratification of the pleasure principle. It is the movement of mind that seeks for the next moment to be different than the present.

If I am adapted to an environmental temperature of 70 degrees, for example, and the temperature falls to 50 degrees, a *feeling* of discomfort might arise. This is my body's way of expressing its present state of disequilibrium. Now a desire might also emerge from this situation, manifest in my very much *wanting* to be warmer, to restore the feeling of pleasure that comes with being in balance with the environment.

Here is where my level of understanding makes a big difference. If my understanding is sufficiently developed to realize how all this is just the natural unfolding of cause and effect in a depersonalized psychophysical system, the cold is merely cold; there is no expectation for it to be otherwise. Moreover, the presence of the cold is not a personal insult. Discomfort about the temperature may persist, but the desire for it to be different (i.e., the suffering) does not. This attentive but dispassionate quality is often described as *equanimity*, an attitude of mind capable of embracing both pleasure and pain, without being driven by them into the *action* of desire. Lacking equanimity and understanding, I might instead feel compelled to gratify my desire at any cost, an attitude the Buddhists refer to as *clinging* or grasping.

Much of our ordinary daily experience is colored by clinging. However, it is as dangerous as it is common, for a number of reasons. First there is the quality of compulsion, or being driven into action lacking in conscious choice. Without the mental ease to choose to act otherwise, we are in a cycle of conditioned responses, responding little differently than an animal or a machine might. We lose our humanity, our ability to act freely and with awareness.

Also, the pressing need to gratify the desire, whether it is in the pursuit of pleasure or the avoidance of pain, may lead us to overlook the needs and rights of others when they conflict with our own. Taking the former example to an extreme, we might hoard fuel and turn up the thermostat regardless of how much fuel is available for others, or we might even forcibly deprive a weaker person of clothing to keep ourselves warm.

Finally, clinging behavior reinforces the construct of selfhood. In the moment of grasping for something or pushing something away, the self as agent is created. This self experiences itself as the originator and beneficiary of this action. A sought-after object is labeled *mine* in the act of acquiring it, while a resisted or rejected object is defined in one's mind as *not mine*.

With this insight, the Buddhists are really offering a Copernican revolution to our understanding of selfhood and identity. It is not that a person *exists* (an assertion that so often goes unexamined) and then may identify with certain objects, ideas, and so on. Rather the person, conceived as an individual self with a particular identity, is *created* in a momentary act of identification. And with a *view* of selfhood underlying and shaping all experience, a person becomes motivated to create him- or herself moment after moment after moment. The solidity and coherence of the self is only apparent, emerging from innumerable instants of self-building, just as the apparent reality of a movie emerges from the illusion of continuity generated by numerous individual frames of film.

The self is born and dies, rises and passes away, moment after moment, whenever one grasps after or clings to the gratification of desires. Yet each time one desire is satisfied, another will emerge, suggesting that no meaningful sense of peace or fulfillment can ever occur. This is the etiology of suffering in Buddhist psychology. The Buddhist word *dukkha* is the term that denotes this suffering or unsatisfactoriness, a fundamental flaw in the mind–body operating system and thus in the human condition.

Identification with Self

Once we mistake the transient, constructed self for something enduring and central, we further reinforce it in our unexamined tendency to perceive that all experience is happening to "me." This is compounded by our use of the self as the yardstick of value; that is, an event is judged as good if I desire it and bad if I do not. Because of the way each moment carries a specific feeling tone, there is scarcely a moment that is not so judged. The world becomes divided into good *for me* and bad *for me*. So busy are we casting the world in light refracted through our desires, we miss the world as it is, intimate though impersonal.

The Buddhist analysis describes the self as a construct that arises with the requisite conditions and passes when those conditions are absent. It does not endure. However, once we come to mistake the self as somehow more real and enduring than it is, we have another problem on our hands. We spend much of our lives trying to fortify, defend, and aggrandize ourselves, fearing that failure to do so will result in our annihilation.

From this perspective the defenses, described so well in early psychoanalytic literature, are not enlisted so much against conscious knowledge of instinctual drives, but rather to buttress the illusion of self. Theorists as diverse as Alfred Adler (1927/2002), Ernest Becker (1973), and Erving Goffman (1971) have discussed how the drive to maintain self-esteem is a primary motive in psychological and social life. People often seek psychotherapy because of the elusive nature of achieving self-esteem. We calibrate our self-esteem by constant comparison with others, and we evaluate things and people based on whether they support or challenge our constructed identity. As a result, we can feel impoverished in the face of abundance. Others can become "part objects," judged by their value to our sense of self. When others become depersonalized in this manner, the way is paved for social cruelty.

Given the tremendous cultural value placed on the self in Western culture, it is no surprise that narcissistic disorders are so prevalent. From a Buddhist perspective, these disorders are mere exaggerations of a fundamental delusion about who we are.

MINDFULNESS AND THE HEALING OF SUFFERING

The Buddha characterized himself as a physician, whose primary work was identifying the malady afflicting humankind, uncovering its causes, using that knowledge to see how it can be cured, and laying out a program through which each person can find well-being. He demonstrated all of this first himself. According to tradition, the prince Siddhartha became the Buddha one night when he finally saw clearly how the mind and body create their own suffering and was able to so transform himself that suffering entirely ended for him. Having cured himself, he then went on to help others.

Even the earliest path of development articulated in the classical Buddhist tradition is quite rich and diverse. It was understood that different people have different strengths and weaknesses, different capabilities, and find themselves in a wide range of worldly circumstances. The Buddha understood, as any physician would, that the healing process involved far more than just medicine. The understanding and cooperation of the patient, the level of care and support available from others, and environmental factors, such as nutrition, rest, and time, all played important roles in determining the success of the protocol. Therefore, while the naming of the illness, the identification of its root causes, and the core elements of its cure are all quite standard elements of the tradition, the number of ways to go about effecting that cure are tremendously variable. Each generation seems to develop a regimen that is best suited to its own unique environment. This is what has allowed Buddhism to adapt to so many different cultures over two and a half millennia.

The starting point for the program of healing prescribed by the Buddha is mindfulness meditation. It will not effect the cure entirely on its own, but no real progress toward well-being can occur without it. Because suffering is constructed each moment in reflexive and unexamined ways, it is first necessary to be able to reveal something of the process. While, most of the time, a healthy human being is working hard at creating and maintaining the conceptual edifice of personal identity, mindfulness meditation invites us to attend simply to the field of phenomena, to *that which arises* at the level of absolute sensory and cognitive immediacy. Phenomena will appear or arise at any of the five sense "doors" of the eye, ear, nose, tongue, and body, or they will arise as objects of awareness in the "mind door" itself. The capacity to be aware of these data *as phenomena*, rather than as the objects of our conceptually constructed world, takes a great deal of training and practice.

Our reflexes and instincts are entirely directed to overlooking the details in incoming experience in order to reinforce ongoing projects at the macro-level of construction. In simpler terms, we are so invested in the larger picture of goals, strategies, and the validation of assumptions and belief systems that we are in the habit of relating to sensory and cognitive detail as *means toward an end*. Mindfulness meditation gradually teaches us to regard this ongoing stream of textured experience as an *end in itself*. The aim is not to undermine completely the conventional world we construct, but rather to put it into its proper perspective. By learning to view this otherwise overlooked level of raw appearances, we begin to reveal the *process* of identity building and world construction itself, instead of remaining entirely focused on the *product* of this process.

Mindfulness practice helps to reverse our tendency to lean ahead into the next moment, to rush forward to the level of macro-construction. By bringing deliberate and sustained attention to the field of phenomena itself, we train the mind to inhabit the more open, unformed space of freshly arising experience. The mind will naturally incline into its various construction projects (thoughts, memories, plans, fantasies, etc.), but as it does so, we are able to see more clearly *that* it is doing so, and *how* it is doing so. By observing the move from arising phenomena to thought creation, we begin to reveal the highly constructed nature of experience. From this starting point of heightened awareness of the mind's present-moment activity, a range of options for learning and growing becomes accessible. A detailed program of transformation was laid out in the early Buddhists literature (Nanamoli & Bodhi, 1995b), and has been continually elaborated by centuries of tradition.

CLASSICAL MINDFULNESS TRAINING

Mindfulness of Body

Classically, mindfulness is cultivated by being systematically applied to four general objects. The first is the body. Attending carefully to the physical sensations that arise in conjunction with breathing, for example, will yield an ever-present but continually changing set of phenomena to observe. The quality of attention brought to bear on these changing sensations can be gradually deepened as practice develops. The inbreath alone might at first seem to be accompanied by only a few discernable sensations at the nose, the abdomen, or as the clothing moves against the skin; but as skill increases, one will tend to notice more and more. Before long, a single inbreath might seem filled with a whole universe of nuanced physical phenomena, each, though exceedingly brief, with its own unique texture.

The same increasing acumen can be directed to the body as it assumes different positions: seated, standing, lying down, or walking. Each of these will provide its own universe of unique sensations, an endless landscape for phenomenological exploration. Also centering on the body, mindfulness might be developed by observing physical objects of touch as one moves through the range of normal behaviors such as eating, drinking, falling asleep, or waking up. Or one might augment one's capacity to discern the raw physical manifestations of resistance, movement, and temperature, which the Buddhists identify as the basic components of all physical sensation.

Another exercise is to "sweep" the body with one's mindful awareness, from the tip of the head to the soles of the feet, identifying the sensation in each of the different components of the body. The aim in all these cases is to become and remain aware only of the physical sensations arising through one of the sense doors, the "body door," without reverting to seeing, hearing, thinking, or any of the other modes of experience.

Mindfulness of Feeling

Mindfulness may also be applied to feeling tones. Here the practitioner will bring attention to the pleasant or unpleasant quality of every experi-

ence. It requires and develops the capacity to distinguish a bodily sensation, for example, from the feeling arising in conjunction with it. One
becomes able to discriminate physical sensations arising in one's knee,
for example, from the profound unpleasantness and even pain that is
arising with it. The *touch* of the bodily sensation is one phenomenon;
the *pain* of that touch is another. Classical mindfulness meditation seeks
to nurture this level of precision.

The same is true even of mental objects arising in the mind. Each
memory, thought, or imaginative image will be accompanied by a feeling
tone that is either pleasant, unpleasant, or neutral. Even when the feeling
tone does not easily resolve itself under scrutiny as being particularly
pleasant or unpleasant, as in the case of neutral feeling, it is still providing an ongoing, tangible sensation to all modes of experience that can be
discerned by the practiced meditator. The temperature in the meditation
room, for example, as experienced by the nerve receptors in the skin,
may not seem too hot or too cold but may nevertheless yield a constant
stream of feeling tones. Being able to unravel these two strands of
experience—an object known through a sense door and the feeling tone
accompanying that object—begins to reveal the restless movement of
mind and contributes to a deeper understanding of its constructed nature.

Mindfulness of Mind

As the mind itself becomes the object of mindfulness meditation, the observer is invited to notice whether or not this particular moment of consciousness is accompanied by one of the three root causes of suffering, or
afflictive intentional constructs—greed, hatred, or delusion. In any given
moment, the mind is either caught up by one or more of these or it is
not, and this is something of which one can learn to be aware. Greed
and hatred are the two polarities of desire, the intense *wanting* or *not
wanting* of an object, while delusion is a strong form of the basic misunderstanding that gives desire its power over us.

For example, when discomfort is detected in the body because one
remains unmoving in a seated position for some length of time, one can
notice the growing resistance to the sensory information being received
from the body. One can almost taste the building dissatisfaction, the
"wanting the unpleasant physical sensations to go away" or to change
into something else. At the next moment, one can experience the same
situation in another light, the "wanting pleasant physical sensations to
arise" in the body instead. It can be quite difficult to discern when the
not wanting, unpleasant sensations leave off and when the wanting,
pleasant sensations begin to arise and replace them. Exploring the tex-

ture of this ambiguity, even though it may manifest as confusion, is what mindfulness of mind is all about, and it contributes to a growing phenomenological intelligence.

In yet another subsequent moment, the meditator may well experience the realization that both wanting and not wanting are just turnings of the mind's habitual response mechanisms, following from contact with certain physical sensations in the context of certain attitudes. Such a minor but significant insight might be followed by a return to awareness of the physical sensations, but recontextualized in a way that enables greater equanimity or less personal investment. Such a shift in attitude might be accompanied by a physical or mental sigh, a further attentive relaxing of the body, and a fresh resolve to look carefully but patiently at experience in whatever mode it is actually arising. Through the eye of equanimity, the quality of wanting or not wanting is temporarily absent from the mind, and the texture of this state, too, can be examined.

In this brief example, one has become aware of how the mind is at first afflicted with aversion, desire and confusion, and then, following a moment of insight, how the mind manifests without these afflictions. By investigating the arising of these attitudes of mind in experience, mindfulness enters an evaluative stage that has the potential to transform. One might simply notice without judgment the variegated textures of physical sensations and even the alternating episodes of pleasure and pain; but as one sees a moment of aversive mind followed by a moment of nonaversive mind, or a moment of clear insight after innumerable moments of obscuration, one cannot help but notice the contrast.

It is not a matter of deciding conceptually that one is wholesome and the other unwholesome, for that is just the sort of *thinking about* experience that is counterproductive to the process. Rather, one develops an intuitive understanding, as a manifestation of insight or wisdom, about the relative effect of one mind state or another. We are still squarely in the realm of descriptive phenomenology rather than in higher level cognitive understanding.

Mindfulness of Mental Objects

A fourth foundation upon which mindfulness can become established, following on the body, feelings, and mind, is referred to as the mindfulness of mental objects or mental phenomena. Here one brings the same quality of nuanced awareness of that which arises to the actual content of mental experience. But since we are now at the culmination of the transformative path of mindfulness, it is not just a matter of being aware of whatever happens to arise and pass away in the mind. There is a detailed agenda, following the primary teachings of Buddhist psychology, of what to look for and how to work toward abandoning the factors that inhibit understanding, while cultivating the factors that augment it.

Five Hindrances

First, there are five *hindrances* or obstacles to clarity of mind that one can observe as present, absent, or arising in the mind when they had not been present. These are sense desire, aversion, indolence, restlessness, and doubt. One can also become aware of an attitude of nonattachment to such mental states that will cause them to pass away, and of an intentional stance toward such phenomena that will inhibit their re-arising in the future. Each of these five steps can be applied to each of the five hindrances. When one practices mindfulness in this particular way, these five qualities of mind will diminish and even cease, if only temporarily, and the mind will become considerably more clear as a result. Bringing focused awareness to the first hindrance of sense desire, for example, serves to uncover the innate reflex of the sensory apparatus to seek stimulation. Experientially, this presents as a subtle wanting that underlies all six of the human sense capabilities. Consciously working to set aside this stance of being primed for sensory stimulation, even temporarily, can bring an open-mindedness to the moment that allows for a greater range of response.

Five Aggregates

Next in the classical scheme comes bringing awareness to the five *aggregates* of experience themselves, namely, materiality, feeling, perception, consciousness, and formations (referred to earlier as intentions and dispositions). Here the exercise is to simply be aware of each of these strands of compounded experience, and to notice how each continually arises and passes away. This fivefold typology of experience is the Buddhist way of undermining the habitual tendency to reify personal identity. The tradition understands that people routinely assume the existence of a unified agent (the seer, feeler, thinker) underlying the flux of experience. Redirecting attention to each of these five categories gradually has the effect of emphasizing the flux of experience itself rather than the construction of a synthetic sense of unity. The phenomenological data merely reveal that seeing, feeling, and thinking occur; invoking the label of an agent noun (the "I" to whom it is happening) is unnecessary and unwarranted.

Six Sense Spheres

Following this, we have each of the six *sense spheres*, or sense doors, as an object of conscious awareness. In this case, the meditator observes, to take the first example, the eye or organ of perception and also the visual form or object of perception. These are referred to as the internal and the external manifestation of the sensory field. Moreover, the practitioner of mindfulness also notices phenomenologically how desire arises in conjunction with each of the sense spheres. Desire is not something general; in the momentary model of constructed experience, desire will always manifest for a specific mental or physical object.

Understanding the way any instance of desire is dependent upon and emergent from a particular sensory experience is an important insight yielded by these exercises in awareness. Having seen this, the practitioner is then in a position to notice, as with the hindrances, how abandoning one's attachment for this desire will facilitate its disappearance, and how attitudes can be expressed and repeated that will help effect its non-arising in the future.

Seven Factors of Awakening

Of great importance to the traditional form of mindfulness meditation is the awareness of seven positive factors in the growth toward wisdom. These are called the seven *factors of awakening*, and include mindfulness, the investigation of phenomena, energy, joy, tranquility, concentration, and equanimity (see Chapter 5 for a description of these qualities applied to psychotherapy). As before, one is guided simply to observe whether each of these is present or absent in any particular moment of consciousness, and when it is not present to see how it sometimes then arises. But unlike mindfulness of the hindrances, the object is not to abandon these mental factors, but to cultivate and develop them. Again, there can be an intuitive understanding of the beneficial effect that each of these mental states has upon one's mind and body in the moment, and one can learn what sort of intentional stance will develop these factors.

It is also the case that each of these particular states supports the others, so that guiding one's attention carefully through this list will gradually transform one's mind in the direction of greater wisdom and understanding. Again, mindfulness is the first step, and when the simple presence of mind upon currently arising phenomena matures, it will naturally lead to a deep interest in the coming and going of mental states. As each is investigated ever more closely, it will give rise to a natural energy and enthusiasm, which itself turns into a profound sense of joy that seems equally seated in the body and in the mind.

The joy is effervescent, apparently bubbling up from deep springs, but this will gradually be tempered by tranquility. One does not replace the other, but what then ensues is the paradoxical state of tranquil energy. Here the mind is both peaceful and alert; it is calm, relaxed, and at ease, but acutely aware, without effort, of the rising and passing of phenomena. The tranquility brings greater *concentration*, defined as a focus or one-pointedness of mind that will naturally take one object of awareness at a time, but with such skill that it can process innumerable bits of data very quickly. Finally, as each of these factors fulfills and completes one another, a profound equanimity of mind embracing all these qualities becomes established. In this state, say the Buddhists, one is capable of overcoming, if only for a time, the obscuring and distorting effects of desire and misunderstanding upon the moment-to-moment construction of experience.

A TOOL FOR OUR TIMES

Such is a brief overview of how mindfulness may be understood and developed in the traditional context of classical Buddhist practice. The end toward which the practice is devoted is nothing less than the complete and radical transformation of the human psychophysical organism. This transformation may be modest at first, involving occasional moments of insight into one's motivations, of freedom from the hold of some conditioning, or of refuge from the constant onslaught of selfishness and desire. But these moments are cumulative and gradually gain momentum as more and more of the underlying patterns of our psychological process become revealed.

Mindfulness leads to insight, and insight leads to wisdom. The kind of insight referred to in this context is not the conceptual insight into one's personal narrative, but a more visceral and intuitive glimpse of the conditioned, constructed, changeable, and impersonal nature of our mental and physical life. It is an insight that loosens the bonds of attachment and opens the heart to a wider context than the merely self-referential.

As unconscious patterns of behavior become exposed to the light of conscious awareness through the practice of mindfulness, they lose much of their power to deceive and compel us. The very way the data of the senses are organized each moment into the building of a personality and a view of the world begins to change. Eventually, recurring episodes of insight will contribute to more lasting alterations of the mind, a process the Buddhists refer to as the *deepening of wisdom*. This sort of insight changes us profoundly.

At its farthest point of culmination, the attainment of awakening (*nirvana*), greed, hatred, and delusion become entirely eliminated. A person is still constructing experience moment to moment by means of sense organs and perception, and experiences both pleasure and pain. The difference is that the pleasure will not give rise to the desire for more pleasure, and the pain will not be met with aversion or resistance. Action is therefore no longer motivated by grasping after satisfaction, and identity as a node around which self-interested behavior is organized no longer gets constructed. A person moves through the world responding appropriately to events as they emerge, and his or her life becomes an expression of the more altruistic intentions of generosity (nongreed), kindness (nonhatred) and understanding (nondelusion). We are left with a picture of a person who is content in any circumstance, free of involuntary conditioning, and in no way driven into action by compulsion. Such a person accepts the constant changeability of the world, no longer expects gratification beyond the meeting of certain contextual needs (such as eating or drinking when appropriate, but without attachment), exerts no claim of ownership over any object or element of experience, and, perhaps most importantly, does not suffer under the narcissistic delusion of inflated personal identity. Such a view of human potential suggests the transformation of the human psychophysical organism to a somewhat higher stage of evolution.

Is Mindfulness Universally Applicable?

Some forms of healing are based in truly universal human characteristics and qualities. For example, penicillin works independently of the culture of the patient, because our biology is one such universal characteristic. Systems of psychological healing, however, are more prone to being culturally specific, deriving their therapeutic power from their consonance with beliefs held within their host cultures. Healing methods indigenous to the Maori have little applicability in Toronto, and psychoanalysis as a treatment method has been a poor fit in non-Western societies. Our psychological lives are more influenced—if not determined—by culture.

It is nearly impossible to verify the universal nature of psychological constructs. The fact that Buddhism has successfully adapted to highly diverse cultures does not, by itself, distinguish it from other religious traditions that have also migrated. However, the focus of meditation on the deconstruction of conscious experience, the analysis of cause and effect, and the formulation of the nature of suffering, occurs at a level of mind that is so fundamental that it may be common to all humanity.

Culture creates a common language and unique forms for healing practices. Indeed, even Buddhist meditation practices vary enormously across cultures. What appears universal, however, is the fact that mental events continuously arise, and that we are prone to relate to them with desire or aversion. Perhaps this is why Buddhist psychology has been embraced cross-culturally. Suffering appears to be universal, as is our desire to be free of it.

The appearance of mindfulness theory and practice in Western psychotherapy is a modern instance of cultural adaptation of Buddhist psychology. The question remains whether psychotherapy, in its effort to make mindfulness useful in clinical practice, will neglect its potential for radical liberation, or whether Buddhist psychology and practice will invigorate psychotherapy with its broad conception of human potential.

CHAPTER 13

Positive Psychology

Awakening to the Fullness of Life

CHARLES W. STYRON

> The goal of warriorship is to express basic goodness in its
> most complete, fresh, and brilliant form. This is possible
> when you realize that you do not *possess* basic goodness but
> that you *are* the basic goodness itself.
> —CHOGYAM TRUNGPA (1984, p. 70)

MINDFULNESS AND STAGES
OF ADVANCED MENTAL HEALTH

Earlier chapters have touched upon the myriad applications of mindfulness practice to psychotherapy. Chapter 12 has reminded us, however, that the roots of mindfulness are in the Buddhist wisdom tradition. Mindfulness itself is remarkably simple: It is the application of mental faculties to the apprehension of "things as they are" (Trungpa, 1992, p. 192). It turns out, however, that apprehending things as they are is a very demanding project, because we each have proprietary versions of reality that we like to uphold. These projections of ours can be very difficult to see through and clear away, a fact to which any therapist sitting with a suffering patient over years can attest.

Mindfulness offers a rich possibility to psychotherapy that the field itself is only recently beginning to explore—the possibility of developing *positive* states of mind that go beyond symptom relief (Seligman, 2002b). In order to understand the potential contribution of mindfulness practice to positive psychology, it may be helpful to return again to its historical context and purpose.

The basic teachings of Buddhist psychology, the Four Noble Truths, boldly declare the possibility of complete and unobstructed "awakening" and delineate a path to travel in order to attain it. As discussed in Chapter 2, this awakening is commonly referred to as *enlightenment*, and it is a much larger project than overcoming depression, anxiety, or even trauma. Of course, the fact that mindfulness practice turns out to have application for all kinds of mental disorders that the clinician encounters in the psychotherapy office is wonderfully fortuitous. To conclude that such application is the primary purpose of mindfulness practice, however, would be very wide of the mark. It would be like using rocket fuel to kindle a campfire and subsequently concluding that such use was fundamental.

Expanding Perspectives: The Three Turnings

The Buddhist tradition has unfolded over many centuries, and during this lengthy period, the teachings have evolved considerably. Generally speaking, this body of instruction covers three overlapping and interrelated periods (referred to in the *Vajrayana* tradition as the Three Turnings of the Wheel of Dharma). These are three sequential, distinguishable phases in the development of Buddhist thinking, which I refer to here as the early, middle, and late periods. In the *early period*, the focus is primarily on individual suffering and how it is overcome. These teachings include the Four Noble Truths, first discussed in Chapter 2. Since this book has focused extensively on the use of mindfulness practice as a technology for understanding and overcoming suffering, it has drawn predominantly upon the teachings of the early period.

In the *middle period*, the Heart Sutra (Rabten & Batchelor, 1983) is one of the principal teachings. Its central message is that because everything continually changes, there is no place that one can ultimately hang one's hat, no place that one can psychologically call home once and for all. In Buddhist psychology, this realization of no ultimate reference point is called the *experience of no-self* (discussed briefly in Chapters 2 and 11). This realization prevents one from becoming overly identified with anything, particularly one's thoughts and concepts. A deep realization of no-self is also often referred to as the experience of *emptiness*, and it is accompanied, somewhat paradoxically, by the spontaneous arising of compassion.

The message of no-self, or emptiness, from the middle period can be rather unsettling, because we are very attached to our notions of who we think that we are. When these notions are convincingly challenged, it is like having the rug pulled out from under us quite suddenly, and a feeling of complete nothingness can set in. If this feeling becomes excessive, it can approach nihilism.

Fortunately, this tendency is tempered by the *late period* teachings, during which the concept of *buddhanature* is set forth. Buddhanature posits that each of us is fundamentally and unconditionally pure and whole. Obstacles and obscurations (e.g., a bad temper or an exaggerated sense of importance) are understood to be secondary and temporary, like clouds covering the sun. When they are cleared away, one's essentially compassionate nature shines through with vastness and equanimity. This final teaching is not a contradiction of the teaching of no-self: It is rather the statement that fullness and emptiness are complementary. The perfection and interconnectedness of phenomena (fullness) are apprehended when our projections and conceptualizations about them are cleared away (emptiness).

Fruition and Realization

Advanced stages of mental health are best framed in terms that recognize their excellence, without making them unattainable for the average practitioner. Although complete and unobstructed awakening is the ultimate goal of Buddhist psychology, it is probably more useful as a concept or an inspiration, rather than as a tangible reality. Whatever the case, it is by no means a prerequisite for entering the stages of health that are described below.

In *The Art of Happiness* (Dalai Lama & Cutler, 1998, p. 13), the Dalai Lama says, "I believe that the very purpose of life is to seek happiness. That is clear. Whether one believes in religion or not, whether one believes in this religion or that religion, we all are seeking something better in life. So I think the very motion of our life is towards happiness." From the outset, Buddhist psychology has inclined itself in this direction. Until recently, however, in Western annals, it has been associated predominantly with suffering. Buddhist psychology has long been an exceedingly ambitious happiness project, nevertheless, and its principal technology in this service has been mindfulness practice. To understand the possible value of Buddhist teachings for positive psychology, the following three subsections will look at some of the fruitions that result from diligent mindfulness practice.

As we look into these fruitions, a brief cautionary note may prove helpful. These fruitions do occur, but they tend to occur with more frequency and power when they are not overtly sought by the practitioner. It is a paradox. One must practice meditation with diligence in order to experience its beneficial effects, but at the same time, one must abstain from pursuing these effects as goals in themselves. Meditation practice is a lot like courtship in this regard; it benefits from a lighthearted approach, and it also benefits far more from what one gives to it than from what one seeks to obtain from it.

Early Period

Advanced students of the early period teachings are powerful emissaries for the efficacy of mindfulness practice. First of all, they are not beset with chronic struggles to overcome suffering in its myriad manifestations. They have tamed and trained their minds thoroughly, and they meet difficulties—yes, they do have them—with straightforward energy and skillfulness. They are grounded, rather fearless, and modest. They are also quite ordinary, but ordinary in a very positive sense. Everyday difficulties no longer stymie them, and they are zestfully present for their own experience, as well as for that of others. In their mindfulness practice, they learn to synthesize insight with cognitive reframes, as well as with overt behavioral changes. In other words, clear understanding is joined with clear thinking and adaptive behavior. Very little is left unexamined.

Middle Period

Advanced students of teachings in the middle period remain good early period students to the end, never feeling that they have outgrown the fundamentals. They begin to realize in their practice that positive mind states act as very powerful antidotes for negative ones. Additionally, they develop a deep-seated appreciation for the fact that nothing has turned out quite as they expected it would. They have experienced no-self intimately and have survived with a measure of cheerfulness. Concomitantly, the suffering of others has become extremely poignant and inescapable for them. It is ubiquitous. As a result, compassion has spontaneously taken residence in their being. Also, their own suffering has begun to pale in comparison to that of others, and they begin to put others first. They even begin to realize that working for the benefit of others makes them happier than working for themselves alone.

   This transition is traditionally referred to as stepping onto the path of awakened beings, the *bodhisattva* path (Sanskrit: *bodhi*, awake; *sattva*, being). This is the path of "peaceful warriorship," of indefatigable advocacy for gentleness and lovingkindness. In order to streamline this process and remove lingering egoistic obstacles, middle period students overtly practice the six virtues of generosity, discipline, patience, exertion, meditative action, and wisdom. Simply put, they pursue nothing less than completely ethical behavior. This is a tall order, of course, and is typically a lifelong process.

Late Period

Advanced students of the late period teachings remain good early and middle period students—again, never "graduating." At this level, however, negativity and obstacles of all kinds begin to be seen as transparent; they are nothing to fear. Respected, yes; feared, no. Obstacles, in fact, are perceived as being tremendous reservoirs of frozen energy waiting to be tapped. Diligent late period students have glimpsed their own unconditional basic goodness, and they are daring. They realize that delving into powerful negativity can often hold more ultimate potential for wisdom than steering clear. As a result, they will sometimes wade unhesitatingly into difficult situations, because they can see the possibility for transformation in them. They understand that conflicts and psychological pain are the fertile soil in which wisdom grows. When one meets an advanced late period mindfulness practitioner, the encounter inevitably reveals a person who is filled with radiance and bliss. There is not a whisker of pessimism or nihilism to be found. These practitioners exemplify the utter vastness of human potential.

POSITIVE PSYCHOLOGY:
THE SCIENCE OF ACTUALIZING POTENTIAL

Traditional psychology since World War II has focused on treating mental illnesses, with remarkable results. Until recently, however, the field has done very little to enhance mental well-being in the positive sense, and it has not carefully studied how to cultivate exceptional talent. Although this exclusion was not by design, there are good reasons why it happened. Funding for research was limited principally to the study of mental difficulties, as was reimbursement for clinical services. At present, for example, insurance companies reimburse for clinical services only when they are deemed to be medically necessary. Psychology has come to operate largely within the confines of the *medical model,* focusing on pathology.

Martin Seligman has a long history as a leading academic psychologist, and he spent the first 30 years of his career working primarily on problems of mental illness (Seligman, 2004a). More recently, he shifted his professional interests to the arena of positive human potential and growth, founding the positive psychology movement. As an experienced researcher, he has been passionately interested in ensuring that the findings of positive psychology be firmly evidenced-based. Seligman is not reluctant to entertain radical hypotheses. He believes, furthermore, that if positive psychology is to establish itself as more than just a temporary fad, it must demonstrate significant benefits from the outset. One of his initial undertakings in this regard involved studying happiness and ways to increase it, and his book *Authentic Happiness* (2002b) documents many of these findings.

As the preceding chapters illustrate, practitioners of traditional psychology are currently forging an alliance with mindfulness meditation practice. They are also beginning to draw quite extensively on the teachings of Buddhist psychology, particularly those embodied in the early period. Positive psychology, on the other hand, is in its infancy, and it is not quite ready for such an integration. It is not too soon, nevertheless, to begin drawing parallels between its findings and those of the middle and late periods of the mindfulness tradition.

The Benefits of Positive Emotion

Historically, the psychological literature has not made a significant theoretical distinction between positive and negative emotions, although negative emotions have received far more attention. Studies and articles on negative emotions, for example, were more prevalent in a sampling of *Psychological Abstracts* by a factor of 14 (Myers, 2000). As a result, the constructs that have proved useful for the study of negative emotions have been automatically applied to the study of positive ones. Recent findings in positive psychology demonstrate, however, that this practice has been misguided (Fredrickson, 2003). Positive emotions have their own substantial benefits. The mindfulness tradition would take no issue with this finding, of course, having reached the same conclusion centuries ago.

Longevity

The Nun Study is a longitudinal study of aging and Alzheimer's disease, conducted on 678 of the older School Sisters of Notre Dame in Mankato, Minnesota, starting in the late 1980s (Danner, Snowdon, & Friesen, 2001). While the study is ongoing, the first phase focused on nuns between the ages of 75 and 106. Among its many findings is a remarkable one that documents a direct relationship between positive emotions in early life and longevity. Nuns who were found to have been optimistic in their early years typically continued to be optimistic in old age. Statistical analysis also revealed that being in the top quartile of optimism increased longevity by approximately 9.3 years over being in the bottom quartile. Pessimism, therefore, is a more powerful morbidity factor than either smoking or alcoholism—a startling finding.

Another study with Mayo Clinic Minnesota Multiphasic Personality Inventory (MMPI) data similarly attributed substantial increments of longevity to those with a happy disposition (Maruta, Colligan, Malinchoc, & Offord, 2000; Seligman, 2000a). Contrary to some popular beliefs that attribute longevity to restraint and reserve, a positive disposition is a much better determinant of long life than is a negative one. While long life has never been the objective of mindfulness practice, it may turn out to be one of its benefits.

Enhanced Cooperation and Cognitive Functioning

In the comprehensive literature on negative emotions, long-standing correlations have been established between particular negative emotions and the urges associated with them. These urges have often been referred to as *specific action tendencies*. The action tendency linked with anger, for example, is the urge to attack, and that associated with fear is the urge to escape. Historically, positive emotions have also been linked with specific action tendencies, but the linkages have never been particularly heuristic or convincing. Contentment, for example, has been associated with inaction and joy with free activation, but these associations are not very specific or meaningful. Sensing that something was fundamentally askew in the study of positive emotions, Barbara Fredrickson (2003) set out to discover whether there was an entirely different calculus for them. From the point of view of traditional psychology, the findings from her controlled studies are revolutionary.

Fredrickson challenged the assumption that positive emotions were necessarily linked to specific action tendencies, as negative emotions were. An action orientation, it turns out, narrows the field of cognitive focus. Under the negative conditions of threat, this narrowing has adaptive advantages, because it leads to unambiguous and timely responsiveness. Negative emotions, therefore, perform key functions for survival. Fredrickson hypothesized, however, that positive emotions might be associated with a different set of tendencies.

She found, in fact, that positive emotions broaden the thought–action repertoire. Joy, for example, urges one to play and expand; contentment, to savor and amplify. Furthermore, play positively affects the ability to concentrate and ally with others, and it allows one to build resources that are more permanent than the playful states of mind that led to them. These findings led Fredrickson (2003; Fredrickson & Branigan, in press) to what she calls the *broaden and build theory* of positive emotions. Positive emotions, in contrast to negative ones, increase resources and social responsibility. They also trigger growth and prevent stagnation. In almost direct correspondence to these findings, the ultimate growth triggered by the middle period teachings of virtue in Buddhist psychology is the arising of compassion. For mindfulness practitioners, this particular development becomes a powerful engine for personal transformation and for increased social involvement.

There are further advantages to positive emotion. Fredrickson found that individuals who were happy performed cognitive tasks with greater alacrity, greater accuracy, and greater creativity than those who were unhappy. She also found that positive emotions helped people to assimilate a much wider range of experience than did negative ones (because they broaden and build). They also tended to expand individualistic self-definitions into more relational ones that included elements of the community.

Of particular significance, Fredrickson found that positive emotions have the unique capacity to undo the effects of destructive, negative ones. She calls this *the undoing hypothesis* and suggests that it is the reason behind increased longevity in happy individuals. Resilient people do not dwell on negative experiences. Instead, they consistently mix negative emotions with positive ones, and they recover from negative emotional states more rapidly as a result (Fredrickson, 2003; Tugade & Fredrickson, 2004). Every parent of a young child can cite abundant support for this hypothesis. While it works at the level of emotional alchemy for adults, it works at the simple level of distraction for children. With a distraught child, for example, a funny story or a pleasant game can often shift the child's mood dramatically.

Seligman's Evolutionary Hypotheses

Generalizing from the work of Barbara Fredrickson and Robert Wright (2001), Seligman (2003) muses that negative and positive emotions have had very different evolutionary purposes. He hypothesizes that negative emotions have been associated with survival of the fittest—with the zero-sum-game aspects of existence. In earlier periods of human history, competition for scarce resources was omnipresent, and life was more elemental. Even now, however, zero-sum scenarios exist in life, and one person's gains often result in another's losses. Competitive sports marvelously symbolize this common human struggle.

Seligman associates positive emotions with what he calls non-zero-sum, or positive-sum, games. Human institutions—in fact, much of human history—results from the non-zero-sum legacy. With positive-sum games, the benefits that accrue to one member of a group can be shared by all other members. One person's gain is not another's loss. If this book proves to be useful to its readers, for example, the authors will not be diminished in the process. All will benefit. Similarly, the effort expended by those on the *bodhisattva* path is directed in the positive-sum direction. One's own well-being becomes a by-product of working diligently for the benefit of others.

The Pursuit of Happiness

Seligman's (2002b) seminal work *Authentic Happiness* is about the use of positive psychology for attaining enduring fulfillment—for attaining what the Dalai Lama called "the very purpose of life." There are three pillars of positive psychology in his thinking: the study of positive emotion, the study of positive traits (most notably the strengths and virtues), and the study of positive institutions, such as democratic government and robust family life. These latter institutions, he says, support the virtues, and the virtues, in turn, support the positive emotions. Seligman also posits that there are five fundamental avenues for increasing happiness. One of these has to do with enhancing past experience, another, with enhancing future experience, and the third, with enhancing experience in the present.

Enhancing Past Experience

In his study of depression, Seligman (2003) gradually came to understand that the stories we tell ourselves about the past have a great deal to do with the way we feel about it. This understanding has become a cornerstone of cognitive-behavioral treatment. Subsequently, in his study of positive psychology, Seligman found that very happy individuals were typically grateful about many things in their history. Their gratitude served to make positive past experiences more vivid for them, and they seemed to be happier as a result. Based on this finding, many of his students wrote gratitude letters to persons that they had never explicitly thanked for various good deeds. The result was an almost universal spike in positive feeling about the past, and he concluded that the practice of gratitude, where appropriate, actually enhances one's experience of personal history (Seligman, 2003). Although the effectiveness of this intervention has not yet been documented through controlled experimentation, abundant effort is currently going into testing and validating the efficacy of this and many other positive psychology procedures.

Another technique that serves to enhance positive emotion about the past is forgiveness (Seligman, 2002b). Letting go of grudges and the desire for revenge enhances feelings about negative events. Forgiveness is a complex emotion, and its practice is a process, never a one-shot deal. It is also not a formula for forgetting; the old adage "forgive and forget" is not operative here. Forgiveness is not meant to be a universal recommendation regarding negative events, and it is not always a good idea to communicate it. Telling someone who does not think that he has harmed you that you have forgiven him is not likely to increase tranquility. Forgiveness, therefore, must sometimes be closely held. This position corresponds to the mindfulness instruction to "sit with" rather than "act on" certain emotions.

A final technique for enhancing positive emotion about the past is to increase one's awareness of it, to count one's blessings (Seligman, 2003). We have an inborn tendency to remember uncompleted tasks (about which we often feel negatively) and to forget those that we have finished (about which we often feel positively). As a result, we are unconsciously biased toward retaining negative memories. This proclivity has undoubtedly had its evolutionary advantages, particularly during hostile epochs of human history. It was first identified by a Russian psychologist, who gave the behavior its name in 1927—the Zeigarnik effect (Savitsky, Medvec, & Gilovich, 1997). Under current circumstances, nevertheless, it behooves us to count our blessings with regularity, and this can be done with a few moments of reflection each day.

The enhancement of past experience in positive psychology can augment the practice of mindfulness. Mindfulness meditation weans one's attention away from the past and focuses it on the present, and this is particularly helpful when dwelling on past experience has become habitual or obsessive. Mindfulness practice, however, does not endeavor to tamper directly with our experience of the past. Positive psychology exercises, on the other hand, attempt to reorganize our view of the past, and they can actually enhance the efficacy of mindfulness practice in focusing on the present. Since preoccupation with the past often occurs because of unfinished, negative memories (the Zeigarnik effect), exercises that redirect our attention to positive memories help to break this preoccupation. Once the preoccupation has been broken, it becomes easier for a meditator to maintain attention on the present. He or she can notice negative memories in passing, without becoming engulfed by them.

Enhancing Future Experience

The positive emotions about the future that increase the prospects of happiness are optimism, hope, and faith. The enemy of such happiness is catastrophic thinking, and the principal antidote for it is the practice of disputation (Seligman, 2002b). This is the cognitive therapy technique of identifying exaggerated, negative anticipations and marshaling evidence and reason to dispute them. We are all remarkably skillful at disputing the claims of others, particularly when they insult us. For some strange reason, however, when we insult ourselves, we often believe what we say. Successful disputation, in part, involves undoing our tendency to succumb to our own negative projections. Once we have learned to do this with some consistency, we can also usually meet the negative influences of the external world with more equanimity.

Mindfulness practice in the early stages, incidentally, is a crash course in overcoming exactly this kind of negativity. It challenges *all* thoughts, not just negative ones, with the simple instruction to notice them and to return attention to the breath. Strong negative thoughts (which tend to be recurrent) naturally receive repeated challenges, and in mindfulness practice, they are typically met at the "front gate," before we can begin ruminating on them.

Enhancing Present Experience: Pleasure

The greatest possibilities for increasing happiness are to be found in the present. We are all intimately familiar with the most common approach: the pursuit of pleasure. It may be the only thing that comes to mind for most of us when happiness is mentioned. The capacity for experiencing pleasure turns out to have a powerful genetic component. Some people are naturally bubbly, and others are not. In more scientific terms, we all have a *set point* above which we are not likely to be able to stabilize our experience (Lucas, Clark, Georgellis, & Diener, 2003). The good news, however, is that each set point has a range associated with it, and living near the top of one's range is possible for everyone. This range is not really as large as we might expect, however. Contrary to what is suggested by advertising, for a given individual, the possibilities for pleasure are not unlimited.

Another limiting factor associated with the pursuit of pleasure is known as the *hedonic treadmill*. This principle causes us to adapt to both good and bad events by taking them for granted after a short period of time (Ryan & Deci, 2001; Seligman, 2002b). Although most of us often think that good fortune will change our lives permanently for the better, in most instances, even very dramatic positive events yield an emotional high of only several weeks' duration. Similarly, dramatic negative events do not destroy us in the ways that we often imagine they will (absent serious depression). In several weeks' time, most of us have returned from the doldrums to baseline. Pleasure and displeasure are very temporary and fickle. The pursuit of pleasure, therefore, while eminently worthwhile, is not a basket into which one should put all of one's resources.

Savoring is the principal method of increasing one's experience of pleasure. A number of techniques work quite well for this purpose, regardless of where one's set point resides. They are divided into those that prolong pleasure and those that intensify it. All of them are connected in some fashion with slowing down the experience of time. Techniques for prolonging pleasure are:

- Sharing it with others.
- Building and storing memories and images.
- Self-congratulation.
- Sharpening and articulating.
- Comparing and contrasting it with what others may feel.
- Absorption.

Techniques for intensifying pleasure are:

- Blocking out interference.
- Enhancing attention through mindfulness.

While the enhancement of pleasure is abundantly desirable, its ultimate success is limited by set points and the hedonic treadmill. Mindfulness practice has always intuitively understood and accepted these limitations, and it has never really endeavored to prolong or intensify pleasure (even though it sometimes does this as a matter of course). More importantly, it has realized that the pursuit of pleasure is usually coupled for most individuals with the endeavor to avoid pain. Unfortunately, as we have seen in earlier chapters, the attempt to avoid pain produces all kinds of suffering. In enhancing pleasure, therefore, positive psychologists would do well to steer clear of this habitual pairing.

Enhancing Present Experience: Engagement

Although the experience of pleasure is limited by the factors mentioned earlier, the possibilities for engagement are virtually limitless, and they do not favor one temperament over another. Engagement is the experience of being absorbed in one's activities, and high levels of attainment can be sustained over long periods. There is no hedonic treadmill for engagement, nor is there a refractory period associated with reentering it after a previous experience of engagement has ended. The principal researcher associated with the study of engagement is Csikszentmihalyi (1991), who coined the term *flow* to describe it.

According to Czikszentmihalyi, with the experience of pleasure, one is intimately aware of oneself and one's feeling state. In the case of en-

gagement, the opposite turns out to be true. Complete engagement results in the absence of a detached sense of self-awareness, as well as the
absence of conscious feeling states. One becomes joined seamlessly with
one's activity in a flow state in which the passage of time occurs largely
outside of awareness. This timeless state has been celebrated far and
wide in literature, as well as in different spiritual traditions. One of the
more well-known popular books about it is Robert Pirsig's (1974) *Zen
and the Art of Motorcycle Maintenance.* Flow is also often mentioned as
one of the fruitions of diligent mindfulness practice. Although it is sometimes discussed in esoteric terms, there is nothing ultimately inaccessible
or remote about it. Children, for example, become immersed in flow all
the time.

Nonetheless, engagement is not a free ride. It is earned through joining one's talents with energy and one-pointedness of attention. In this
sense, it is what Seligman (2002b) refers to as a *gratification* in contrast
to a pleasure, and he believes that flow actually has the evolutionary
purpose of building emotional capital for the future. According to
Csikszentmihalyi (1991), there are a number of criteria for entering into
the flow state. One salient criterion is that flow is attained when one's
greatest strength is met with one's greatest challenge. It is important, of
course, for the strength level and the challenge level to be balanced. If
the strength level is too high, boredom may result; if the challenge level
is too high, there is the danger of feeling overwhelmed.

The issue of strength needs definition here. Seligman (2002b) is
talking about fundamental human attributes that cut across culture and
ethnicity. These are positive attributes that appear to be native to the human species, and not capacities that are developed and honed specifically through training. Additionally, he is talking about qualities that are
enduring throughout the life span. In contradistinction, traditional mental health is founded primarily on a deficit model that delineates what is
wrong with individuals. The *Diagnostic and Statistical Manual of Mental Disorders* (DSM-IV-TR; American Psychiatric Association, 2000) is a
comprehensive catalogue of such mental difficulties, the large majority
of which are characterized by symptoms that may be transient.

When beginning the study of positive psychology, Seligman (2002b)
enlisted the help of Chris Peterson in the ambitious project of cataloging
human strengths and virtues. Peterson realized that positive psychology
would need its own version of a diagnostic and statistical manual and
developed a volume, *Character Strengths and Virtues* (Peterson &
Seligman, 2004), to meet this need. It endeavors to identify those characteristics that are common to all spiritual traditions and cultures. One of
the central criteria for a strength is that it is regarded as an end in itself,
not as a means to an end. Also, a strength cannot be squandered in the

way that a talent might be. Gratitude is an example. Another criterion of strengths is that they are very easily employed in positive-sum—as opposed to zero-sum—scenarios.

Peterson catalogued 24 strengths that are subdivided into six superordinate categories of virtue. The six virtues are wisdom and knowledge, courage, humanity, justice, temperance, and transcendence. There are several specific strengths associated with each of them. For example, the strengths pertaining to wisdom and knowledge are creativity, curiosity, open-mindedness, love of learning, and perspective (wisdom itself). For each person, several of these strengths tend to be predominant, and Seligman calls these the *signature strengths*. There is even a web-based strength survey (Seligman, 2004b), which uses a forced-choice assessment tool to assist individuals in identifying their signature strengths. Seligman (2002b) hypothesizes that greatest satisfaction occurs when an individual is exercising them. This is particularly true with regard to the experience of engagement or flow. He also posits that individuals are likely to make more progress when they employ their strengths in tackling problems than when they struggle to overcome their weaknesses. Of course, the two approaches are not mutually exclusive. Further discussion of the strengths and virtues, and their similarity to those practiced on the *bodhisattva* path follow in the final section of this chapter.

Enhancing Present Experience: Meaning

As with engagement, the possibilities for increasing happiness through the experience of meaning are boundless. Meaning arises from practicing engagement for a purpose that is larger than oneself or one's narrow concerns. The energy for the development of all major institutions, both physical and conceptual, emanates from the pervasive human quest for meaning. All spiritual and philosophical traditions, furthermore, put meaning at their center. In order to facilitate this quest effectively and consciously, Seligman (2002b) says that one needs to put one's signature strengths into play for a purpose that benefits others. This is the practice of engagement, but with a vision that transcends narrow personal goals. Meaning is a calling that has been elevated to a mission. As described earlier in other terms, such a pursuit of meaning is also at the heart of the *bodhisattva* path.

Summation

Seligman (2003) offers a final cryptic footnote with regard to the cultivation of happiness. Borrowing from language that we have heard all our lives, he postulates that the *full life* is greater than the sum of it parts—

greater than the summation of pleasures, engagements, and meaning. This is nothing new. What is arresting, though, is that he also postulates that the *empty life* is less than the sum of its parts. Misfortunes and good fortunes, in other words, may both be synergistic rather than merely additive. Whether true or not, this suggestion is provocative and may kindle positive motivation. Taking the Four Noble Truths to heart has a similar effect.

THERAPY VERSUS PERSONAL TRANSFORMATION

Expanding the View

Although an overt alliance between mindfulness meditation and positive psychology has not yet been investigated widely in the literature, the possibilities for cross-fertilization are abundant. As mentioned earlier, mindfulness practice is the ultimate happiness project. It is not a frontal assault, though, and was never intended to be. Happiness, instead, is the result of living a virtuous and unselfish life, as laid out in *bodhisattva* discipline. The causality, in other words, is indirect. Seligman (2003) states it another way, asserting that happiness is largely a welcome side effect that results from the exercise of one's highest capacities. Engagement and meaning, after all, are rewards in themselves.

The Color of Money

Therapy is defined as the remedial treatment of a bodily or mental disorder. This definition, while limited, describes a great deal of what normally transpires in the therapy office. At the same time, many psychotherapists are closet positive psychologists, and they would not agree that their work is limited to the treatment of mental illness. Until now, however, mainstream psychology has not had much to offer them in this regard. They have consequently sought assistance elsewhere, drawing on the mindfulness tradition or other spiritual and personal experiences. Furthermore, when billing insurance companies for services, many therapists face a dilemma. Insurance companies pay for medically necessary treatment, not for transformative, positive personal growth. Considering that insurance, by definition, is a bulwark against unexpected misfortune, this is arguably the way that it should be.

Seligman (2003) has begun to argue that the exercise of positive psychology falls more into a coaching model than into a therapy model. Many coaches say the same. There is much to be said for this distinction, but a problem arises at the boundary between mental difficulty and mental well-being. In a normal therapy hour with a high functioning patient, a therapist might reasonably cross this boundary back and forth a number of times. Should insurance pay for a third of the work, half, none, or the full freight? It is a thorny problem, and payment for services unfortunately cannot be separated entirely from the delivery of them. In the mindfulness tradition, fortunately, this dilemma has never existed, because (1) the tradition itself is all-inclusive and has not been partitioned into arenas of mental difficulty and mental well-being, and (2) services have been largely free, with payment for them seldom entering the equation.

Prospects for a New Synergy

The problematic issue of reimbursement remains unsettled at the boundary between mental illness and mental health, and we will not resolve it here. The boundary between therapy and personal transformation, however, is becoming far more fluid, and it may no longer be necessary to pretend that there is an important watershed between them. Mindfulness discipline has always crossed the line between illness and health without a passport, and there is good reason to think that medical model psychology and positive psychology can learn to do the same thing. Medical model psychology resonates a great deal with early period Buddhist psychology, and positive psychology resonates equally well with middle and late period teachings. While the compatibilities between Western psychology and the three periods are being illuminated, though, it is important to remember that the three periods themselves are overlapping and interrelated. They cannot ultimately be separated from one another. Perhaps medical model psychologists and positive psychologists will learn over time to honor their own unseverable connections. Additionally, mindfulness practice and positive psychology may begin to develop an invigorating partnership.

Parallels in Ethical Thinking between Positive and Buddhist Psychologies

Recall the differences in ethical perspectives between Western and Buddhist psychologies that were discussed briefly in Chapter 2. Seligman's (2003) thorough grounding in empirical psychology provides a possible bridge here. He feels that the role for a scientific discipline is to *describe*, not to *prescribe*. Psychology, therefore, can describe what the rest of the culture attempts to prescribe. It can point out the documented advantages of virtue, as well as the documented disadvantages of its absence. This is precisely the attitude that Buddhist psychology has taken toward its ethical rules: They are not commandments, but rather are practical guidelines designed to reduce suffering. Instead of prescribing ethical conduct, a positive psychologist will be able to invite a patient to see the consequences of different actions for him- or herself.

Parallels between Positive Psychology and the Early Period

Several chapters of this book have documented fruitful uses of mindfulness meditation in the practice of traditional psychotherapy. For the most part, these currents have flowed from the early period teachings about suffering, the cause of suffering, and the possibilities for overcoming suffering. The literature is exploding, and in all likelihood, we are only at the beginning of this joint venture.

No discussion of the benefits of mindfulness meditation in psychotherapy can overlook the importance of being in the present moment. Mindfulness practice, after all, is quintessentially a discipline for paying attention to what is actually going on, not what went on yesterday or what will go on tomorrow, just what is going on right now. "Be Here Now" is a familiar pop psychology mantra, but it could not have become as popular as it is without having bestowed some actual value. Learning to reign in one's attention and gently focus it on the present is a skill that delivers untold benefits.

There is, nevertheless, a potential pitfall associated with focusing naively on the present, and many mindfulness practitioners have been trapped by it. Both traditional and positive psychologies can be of assistance here. The past does exist in our memories, and it is powerful. Diligent psychotherapy patients and mindfulness practitioners alike benefit greatly from opening the border between past and present experience, and creating good, constructive commerce between them. Being present in the sense of sweeping the past under the rug is not a recipe for well-being; finding a proper balance is key. This call for balance is expressed in the Buddhist concept of the "middle way," which cautions against extremes in all endeavors.

Similar thinking can be applied to the relationship between the present moment and the future. Again, the future exists in our projections. Mindfulness meditation practice teaches us how to avoid being kidnapped by these projections, but complete avoidance of future mindedness is also not a recipe for well-being. Goldberg (2001), a student of the neuropsychologist Alexander Luria, posits that the history of human culture and institutions is paralleled by the development of the frontal lobes of the brain. These are the brain structures associated with executive functioning, with the capacities to plan a sequence of activities for a particular purpose and to carry them out. The frontal lobes, in other words, mediate the boundary between present and future. Individuals with executive functioning deficits such as attention-deficit/hyperactivity disorder and frontal dementia suffer enormously. They are captives of the present moment and cannot reliably or consistently project the future. In focusing on the present, therefore, mindfulness meditation practitioners should not endeavor to ignore the future, as some naive adherents unfortunately do. As mentioned earlier, the real issue is one of avoiding being held hostage by thoughts of the future. Straddling the boundary between the two times with balance is the goal, and it is assisted by the positive psychology technique of disputation.

Parallels between Positive Psychology and the Middle Period

Glimpses of emptiness are familiar to all students of meditation, even beginners. Additionally, most therapists value and practice compassion even if they have never heard of mindfulness. The profound experience of no-self and the spontaneous arising of compassion in its wake, however, are subjects addressed most eloquently in the middle period teachings. They are also experiences denied to the beginner. Traditional psychology finds some familiar ground here, nevertheless, particularly among therapists. The *bodhisattva* path has been explicitly embraced by many psychotherapists, particularly those who are also mindfulness meditation practitioners. The path may be less attractive to traditional therapy patients, however, because the *bodhisattva* is one who consciously begins to put others before him- or herself; individuals struggling with serious mental difficulties are not necessarily prepared to take this step. Positive psychology clients, on the other hand, may be open to this expansion of loyalties, and there is very good reason for pursuing it. Research shows that helping professionals with heartfelt commitments typically benefit even more from their helping efforts than those whom they attempt to serve (Seligman, 2003).

The cultivation of positive emotion is a huge part of *bodhisattva* discipline. Not only is it valued in itself, but it is also recognized, as the Dalai Lama (Dalai Lama & Cutler, 1998) notes, as a powerful antidote for negative emotion. As discussed earlier, Fredrickson arrives at the same conclusion with her undoing hypothesis (Tugade & Fredrickson, 2004). Another of Fredrickson's findings parallels middle period mindfulness practices. Her "broaden and build" theory of positive emotion is a positive-sum scenario for human interaction (Fredrickson & Branigan, in press). The *bodhisattva* path itself can be thought of as the unparalleled positive-sum adventure. Part of the *bodhisattva* discipline is that of explicitly replacing negative, zero-sum thoughts with positive, non-zero-sum intentions. A conscientious student overtly attempts to make this substitution whenever negative emotions arise. For example, if anger arises, one attempts to practice patience and replace feelings of anger with those of understanding and clarity. It is an enormous undertaking, but when seen from the perspective of zero-sum and non-zero-sum paradigms, the wisdom of it becomes clear.

The actual cultivation of positive emotion in the middle period teachings comes through the practice of the six virtues of generosity, discipline, patience, exertion, meditative action, and wisdom. Just as in positive psychology, the principal vehicles for both engagement and meaning are the signature strengths and virtues. In positive psychology, they are regarded as innate, but the middle period teachings suggest that they can actually be cultivated. The possibility of such cultivation could be of great interest to positive psychologists.

Peterson (2004) suggests, furthermore, that enduring personality characteristics may have more do with one's innate profile of strengths and virtues than with one's transient deficits. He posits that the real psychopathologies may be due to lacunae in one's strength and virtue repertoire rather than due to a collection of transitory, DSM-type symptoms. If this turns out to be true, then the possibility of cultivating strength and virtue could prove to be of unparalleled benefit. The cultivation of virtue, in other words, could become powerful medicine for the treatment of mental illness as well as for the pursuit of happiness.

Parallels between Positive Psychology and the Late Period

The concept of *buddhanature* has always been more attractive to Western audiences than the diligent exercise of discipline or the experience of emptiness, but it is critical to remember that buddhanature is a late period teaching and cannot be properly comprehended without a thorough grounding in the teachings of the early and middle periods. Buddhist teachers have recognized this issue and caution against the tremendous egotism that arises when one attempts to short-circuit one's mindfulness training (Trungpa, 1973). If there is one overarching principle that supports all mindfulness practice, it is that there are no shortcuts.

Keeping this general caveat in mind, a few synergies between positive psychology and late period mindfulness disciplines can be illuminated. It is worth noting, initially, that Seligman (2003) takes the professional stance that human beings are fundamentally good. This position is entirely consonant with the concept of buddhanature, but it flies in the face of much Western thinking (see Chapter 2). The doctrine of original sin is deeply embedded in our culture, and the legacy of Freud's aggressive instinct is also powerful. There have been many attempts to buck this tide over the past half-century, Heinz Kohut's (1978) being one of the most articulate. He argued that human beings are fundamentally good, and he believed that the darker side of their natures is secondary.

It is easy to hold the view that human beings are fundamentally good if one has had a relatively easy life, and if one has had little experience with the grimmer aspects of human existence. For individuals as accomplished and knowledgeable about human misery as Seligman and Kohut, however, coming to such a view is far from a given. It is, in all likelihood, a measured accomplishment that has arisen out of thorough reflection and hard work. Such individuals, in other words, have probably undergone their own versions of early and middle period experience, arriving in good health at the late period. From the point of view of Buddhist late period teaching, this is actually the way it should be. The most powerful and liberating ideas cannot necessarily be handed out on the street corner with any mature hope that they will have tangible and enduring effect. In this sense, they are what is known as *self-secret* in the Buddhist tradition. At face value, they may or may not appear to be profound, but as one grows in understanding, their profundity deepens. The vast wisdom contained in them, in fact, becomes limited only by one's own capacities to tap them.

Another late period parallel with psychology seems to come with age and slowing down. Many of life's journeys are circular, ultimately bringing one back to his or her point of origin. Such journeys are necessary in spite of their circularity. Without them, we would often fail to appreciate what we have had all along. In psychotherapy, as in mindfulness practice, there is no real need to go anywhere. Everything is right here, right now. Everything is complete, even in its incompleteness. This is what it means to say that reality can only be held in an open hand. Letting go is the only way, like following the breath out into space in mindfulness meditation.

An Overarching Parallel: The Importance of Training

For those who practice psychotherapy professionally, the importance of academic training, continuing education, and supervision are universally acknowledged. These help to support ongoing development, as well as to confront and minimize self-deception. For those who aspire to practice mindfulness meditation with diligence, there are similar requirements, although they are less formally codified. Traditionally, all of the many Buddhist schools held that a living teacher and a community of fellow practitioners were indispensable for those who wished to travel the path of mindfulness practice extensively. While one may have only very episodic contact with such a teacher and community, at every stage of mindfulness practice, guides are considered crucial for avoiding the endless possibilities for self-deception. It is important to recognize that it is extremely difficult to undergo the development described in this chapter without such guidance.

Coda

As we conclude this rich exchange between Western psychology and Buddhist mindfulness practice, it will be useful to carry a few key concepts with us. At the level of early period understanding, it will be useful to remember that suffering cannot be avoided. In fact, suffering must be embraced in order to overcome it, and psychotherapy can often benefit immeasurably from an alliance with mindfulness in this enterprise.

At the level of middle period understanding, it will be useful to remember that unselfishness is the most felicitous path to well-being. Compassionately attuning to the pain of others can become spontaneous, and when it does, it turns into powerful medicine. This altruistic stance, moreover, is abundantly salutary for the person taking it. It is the definitive positive-sum proposition, but it must be entered into without equivocation. Pretending to be unselfish will not work.

At the level of late period understanding, it will be useful to remember that maturity, training, and hard work are assumed. Uninformed, inherited positive beliefs about human nature and potential may serve as valuable guides and inspiration, but if they are harvested as fruit straight from the tree, rather than learned through direct experience, they are likely to do more harm than good.

Simultaneously, there is an opportunity for awakening in every moment, and such awakening emanates from meeting each life event completely as it is. Often this is quite painful (e.g., witnessing one's failure as a friend) and does not feel like "awakening" at all. Each moment, nevertheless, contains power and wisdom if it is met and appreciated fully on its own terms. Although paradoxical, herein lies the magic of uncovering one's own fundamental goodness, as well as the goodness inherent in all phenomena. Conventional labels for experience that were once so critically important in one's life start to fade away, and all experience, instead, begins to seem somewhat astonishing—like the wonder of being alive itself. Maintaining an unobstructed view of this wonder is a very tall order, however, and it requires the stamina and spirit of a warrior. Furthermore, this gentle warrior needs to avoid extremes and travel the middle way with a patient, steady gait. This is a path that courts the sunshine of basic goodness and leads to pervasive transformation.

APPENDICES

Resources for the Clinician

The following are selected resources to help the interested clinician learn more about the application of mindfulness and Buddhist psychology to psychotherapy.

MINDFULNESS-ORIENTED PSYCHOTHERAPY

Books

Epstein, M. (1995). *Thoughts without a thinker: Psychotherapy from a Buddhist perspective*. New York: Basic Books.

Hayes, S. C., Follette, V. M., & Linehan, M. M., (Eds.). (2004). *Mindfulness and acceptance: Expanding the cognitive-behavioral tradition*. New York: Guilford Press.

Hayes, S. C., Strosahl, K. D., & Wilson, K. G. (1999). *Acceptance and commitment therapy: An experiential approach to behavior change*. New York: Guilford Press.

Kabat-Zinn, J. (1990). *Full catastrophe living*. New York: Delacorte Press.

Linehan, M. (1993). *Cognitive-behavioral treatment of borderline personality disorder*. New York: Guilford Press.

Magid, B. (2002). *Ordinary mind: Exploring the common ground of Zen and psychotherapy*. Boston: Wisdom Publications.

Molino, A. E. (1998). *The couch and the tree*. New York: North Point Press.

Segal, Z. V., Williams, J. M. G., & Teasdale, J. D. (2002). *Mindfulness-based cognitive therapy for depression: A new approach to preventing relapse*. New York: Guilford Press.

Websites

Mindfulness-based stress reduction: *www.umassmed.edu/cfm*

Dialectical behavior therapy: *www.behavioraltech.com*

Acceptance and commitment therapy: *www.acceptanceandcommitmenttherapy. com*

Institute for Meditation and Psychotherapy: *meditationandpsychotherapy.org*

Mindfulness and Acceptance Special Interest Group of the Association for Advancement of Behavior Therapy: *listserv.kent.edu/archives/mindfulness/ html*

MINDFULNESS PRACTICE

Books

Aronson, H. (2004). *Buddhist practice on Western ground: Reconciling Eastern ideals and Western psychology.* Boston: Shambhala.

Beck, C, (1989). *Everyday Zen: Love and work.* San Francisco: HarperSanFrancisco.

Brach, T. (2003). *Radical acceptance: Embracing your life with the heart of a Buddha.* New York: Bantam/Dell.

Dalai Lama, & Cutler, H. (1998). *The art of happiness: A handbook for living.* New York: Riverhead.

Goldstein, J. (1993). *Insight meditation: The practice of freedom.* Boston: Shambhala.

Goldstein, J., & Kornfield, J. (1987). *Seeking the heart of wisdom.* Boston: Shambhala.

Goleman, D. (2003). *Destructive emotions: How can we overcome them?* New York: Bantam/Dell.

Gunaratana, B. (2002). *Mindfulness in plain English.* Somerville, MA: Wisdom Publications.

Hanh, T. N. (1987). *The miracle of mindfulness.* Boston: Beacon Press. (Original published in 1975)

Kabat-Zinn, J. (1994). *Wherever you go there you are: Mindfulness meditation in everyday life.* New York: Hyperion.

Kabat-Zinn, J. (2005). *Coming to our senses: Healing ourselves and the world through mindfulness.* New York: Hyperion.

Kornfield, J. (1993). *A path with heart: A guide through the perils and promises of spiritual life.* New York: Bantam.

Lama Surya Das. (1997). *Awakening the Buddha within: Tibetan wisdom for the Western world.* New York: Broadway.

Rosenberg, L. (1998). *Breath by breath: The liberating practice of insight meditation.* Boston: Shambhala.

Salzberg, S. (1995). *Lovingkindness: The revolutionary art of happiness.* Boston: Shambhala.

Smith, J. (Ed.). (1998). *Breath sweeps mind: A first guide to meditation practice.* New York: Riverhead Books.

Meditation Training Centers

Non-Buddhist

Center for Mindfulness in Medicine, Healthcare, and Society, University of Massachusetts Medical School, 55 Lake Avenue North, Worcester, MA 01655; *www.umassmed.edu/cfm/mbsr*

Vipassana

Barre Center for Buddhist Studies, 149 Lockwood Road, Barre, MA 01005; *www.dharma.org*
Insight Meditation Society, 1230 Pleasant Steet, Barre, MA 01005; *www.dharma. org*
New York Insight, P.O. Box 1790, Murray Hill Station, New York, NY 10156; *www.nyimc.org*
Spirit Rock Meditation Center, P.O. Box 909, Woodacre, CA 94973; *www. spiritrock.org*

Tibetan

Naropa University, 2130 Arapahoe Avenue, Boulder, CO 80302; *www.naropa. edu*
Shambhala Mountain Center, 4921 County Road 68-C, Red Feather Lakes, CO 80545; *www.shambhalamountain.org*

Zen

San Francisco Zen Center, 300 Page Street, San Francisco, CA 94102; *www.sfzc. com*
Zen Center of Los Angeles, 923 South Normandie Avenue, Los Angeles, CA 90006; *www.zcla.org*
Zen Mountain Monastery, P. O. Box 197, Mt. Tremper, NY 12457; *www.mro.org/ zmm/zmmhome/*

BUDDHIST PSYCHOLOGY

Books

Batchelor, S. (1997). *Buddhism without beliefs.* New York: Riverhead Books.
Bodhi, B. (Ed.). (1999). *A comprehensive manual of Abhidhamma.* Seattle: Buddhist Publication Society.

Fleischman, P. (1999). *Karma and chaos: New and collected essays on vipassana meditation*. Seattle: Vipassana.
Johansson, R. (1979). *The dynamic psychology of early Buddhism*. New York: Humanities Press.
Kalupahana, D. (1987). *The principles of Buddhist psychology*. Albany: State University of New York Press.
Nyanaponika, T. (1996). *The heart of Buddhist meditation*. Boston: Weiser Books. (Original work published 1965)
Rahula, W. (1986) *What the Buddha taught*. New York: Grove Press.

Websites

Audiovisual materials of all kinds: *www.soundstrue.com*

Mindfulness teacher talks: *www.dharmaseed.org*

Buddhist journal (USA): *www.tricycle.com*

Journal for mindfulness practitioners: *www.inquiringmind.com*

Buddhism and science: *www.mindandlife.org*

Thich Nhat Hanh and Buddhist links: *www.iamhome.org*

Glossary of Terms
in Buddhist Psychology

ANDREW OLENDZKI

TWO KINDS OF MEDITATION

Many different forms of meditation are practiced in the Buddhist and non-Buddhist traditions of Asia. The two practices most prevalent in the earliest teachings of the Buddha are as follows:

    1. *Concentration* (calming, *samatha* in Pali). Focusing the mind on a single object to the exclusion of other objects fosters concentration, or a "one-pointed" mode of mental function. As distracting thoughts or sensations arise, one abandons giving attention to those objects and gently returns awareness to the primary object of experience (the breath, a word or phrase, etc.). As the mind steadies on one particular aspect of the phenomenal field, it gains tranquility, stability and power.

    2. *Mindfulness* (insight, *vipassana*). In mindfulness meditation, one allows awareness to move from one object to another as stimuli present themselves in experience. When this is done in a sustained manner, it leads to insight into the subjective construction of experience, and into the three characteristics of existence.

THE THREE CHARACTERISTICS OF EXISTENCE

Construed as three fundamental attributes of the human condition, the three characteristics are normally obscured from view by distortions of perception, thought, and view, and are revealed through careful and disciplined investigation of experience. Insight into these characteristics contributes to wisdom.

1. *Impermanence* (*anicca*). The stream of consciousness that makes up the subjective flow of human awareness and, hence, the world constructed by the mind is actually composed of very brief episodes of cognitive activity that arise and pass away with great rapidity. More generally, it refers to the observation that all conditioned phenomena are unenduring.

2. *Suffering* (*dukkha*). This word is used in a very broad and existential manner in the Buddhist tradition. It refers not only to the inevitability of physical pain, injury, illness, aging, and death, but also to the more subtle psychological distress resulting from the fundamental insatiability of desire. Not getting what one wants, having to cope with what one does not want, and confusion about conflicting desires are all encompassed by the word *suffering*.

3. *Non-self* (*anatta*). Ever a source of perplexity, the Buddhist insight of non-self is not denying that there are unique and more or less stable patterns of personality that develop throughout a person's lifetime. Rather it points out that these patterns are *just* patterns of conditioning and learned behaviors, and lack any essence or numinous core. The reflex toward "ownership" of thoughts, feelings, sensations, and so on (these are *mine*, this is *me*) is unwarranted, maladaptive, and the source of a host of psychological difficulties.

THE THREE ROOT CAUSES

These are the three unwholesome underlying tendencies of human behavior, from which all the other afflictive emotions are derived.

1. *Greed*. Also known as craving, wanting, or attachment, greed is the impulse to reach for or hold on to something that is desirable. It is a reflexive response to the feeling tone of pleasure. The corresponding wholesome underlying tendency is non-greed, which manifests as generosity or renunciation.

2. *Hatred*. Also referred to as aversion or ill will, hatred involves pushing away, denying, or attacking something that is experienced as undesirable. It is usually generated as a response to pain or displeasure. Greed and hatred are the bipolar expressions of desire. The corresponding wholesome underlying tendency is non-hatred or "lovingkindness" (see later).

3. *Delusion*. Also referred to as ignorance or confusion, delusion is used in a technical way in Buddhist thought to denote blindness to certain facets of real-

ity, such as the three characteristics and the construction of experience. The wholesome underlying tendency that corresponds to and balances delusion is wisdom.

THE THREE KINDS OF FEELING

The word *feeling* in Buddhist thought refers to a hedonic tone rather than to the more complex emotions the word denotes in English. One of the three feeling tones is always present in every moment, accompanying both physical and mental experience.

1. *Pleasant feeling.* Arising from contact between a sense object and a sense organ, a feeling of pleasure may arise. It is always a very brief and very specific event, conditioned by the particular sense modality and one's underlying attitude toward the particular object.

2. *Unpleasant feeling.* Also arising from contact between a particular sense object and organ, a feeling of displeasure or pain may arise. Both pleasure and pain give rise to a response of wanting or not wanting the sensation to continue. This feeling is distinguishable from the ensuing response.

3. *Neither-pleasant-nor-unpleasant feeling.* Sometimes careful attention will reveal a sensation as pleasant or unpleasant, while at other times, one can be aware of feeling tone that is neutral, neither pleasant nor unpleasant.

THE FOUR NOBLE TRUTHS

A basic organizing principle of Buddhist doctrine, the four truths taught by the Buddha are considered noble because they help raise one's understanding above the level of automatic response into the realm of transformation through wisdom. Based upon an ancient medical lore, the truths may be taken as analogous to a physician's diagnosis, etiology, prognosis, and treatment plan for a patient afflicted with a disease.

1. *Suffering.* The term *suffering* is used in a broad sense to point out a fundamental unsatisfactoriness to the human condition (see earlier). Much of our effort works to obscure this truth, but, as with all healing, an important first step is to face the nature of the affliction with honesty and courage.

2. *The origination of suffering.* All human suffering has a simple and consistent cause: desire. Whenever there is a disequilibrium between what is arising in experience and what one *wants* to have happen, suffering is inevitable.

3. *The cessation of suffering.* Understanding the causal interdependence of these first two truths, suffering can be brought to cessation simply by the

elimination of desire. Unpleasant thoughts and sensations may still exist and are in fact invariably part of all experience, but by changing one's attitude of resistance to what is unpleasant, suffering can be reduced and even eliminated.

4. *The path leading to the cessation of suffering.* Many different strategies and programs for bringing suffering to an end have been developed over Buddhism's 2,500 years. Traditionally, the healing program is articulated as the "Noble Eight-fold Path."

THE EIGHTFOLD PATH

These eight guidelines for living one's life and holding oneself in the moment constitute a broad ethical context for development in the Buddhist tradition. The word "right" is used before each one, not to impose a rigid normative mold, but more in the sense of "appropriate" or "well-tuned." These eight dimensions are to be practiced in parallel, and each supports and reinforces the others.

1. *Right view.* This is the first element in the series but also culminates the list. At the near end of the progression, one needs a certain amount of confidence in the teachings to put them into practice, and one needs to be pointing in the right direction for any journey to be effective. At the far end of the path, right view refers to awakening fully to "seeing things as they really are."

2. *Right intention.* In Buddhist psychology, intention is the principle tool of transformation. When intention is skillfully crafted in each moment, it guides the mind wisely to its state in the next moment and, thus, like the rudder of a ship, can be used to navigate through the changes of arising and passing experience. It is also sometimes known as "right aim."

3. *Right speech.* Since speech molds and reflects the quality of thoughts, it becomes quite important that one's habits of speech are truthful, helpful, kind, and free of selfish and manipulative motives. Right speech is used for healing and education, and never for harmful or divisive purposes.

4. *Right action.* Traditionally, right action is expressed in terms of living by five ethical precepts: not killing, not stealing, not lying, not misbehaving sexually, and not indulging in intoxicants. Each of these precepts is open to more or less strict interpretation, depending on one's level of commitment (e.g., for a monastic versus a layperson).

5. *Right livelihood.* This is also construed traditionally as a series of ethical constraints upon a layperson's mode of livelihood, and culminates in the monastic code of living for monks and nuns. Laypeople should avoid professions that involve killing, for example, and mendicants should keep their intentions pure as they wander for alms.

6. *Right effort.* Right effort primarily involves the mindful cultivation of wholesome states both before and after they arise in experience, and the deliberate abandoning of unwholesome states, also both before and after they occur. It describes a level of mental hygiene that is quite scrupulous and requires considerable ongoing attentiveness to the quality of the inner life.

7. *Right mindfulness.* When mindfulness is well developed, following the guidelines of the foundations of mindfulness (see below), it is said to be right mindfulness, which means applying attention carefully and evenly to phenomena as they appear.

8. *Right concentration.* This calls for the steady application of one-pointed awareness from time to time, outside of everyday activities, and is particularly encouraged as a tool for development in Buddhist psychology. Regular meditation is a foundational aspect of the eightfold path.

THE FOUR FOUNDATIONS OF MINDFULNESS

Basic instructions for the cultivation of mindfulness are given in this classical form. Each category is considered a "foundation" in the sense of providing a basis for practicing those techniques of mind training that have to do with being fully aware, in the present moment, of one sensory or thought object at a time, and of understanding thereby the changeable and ultimately selfless nature of phenomenological experience.

1. *Mindfulness of body.* Beginning with sitting in a quiet place with legs crossed and back straight, mindfulness practice commences with deliberate awareness of breathing, of the tranquilization of body and mind, and with attention to the bodily sensations arising in conjunction with bodily postures, movements, and activities.

2. *Mindfulness of feelings.* The practice progresses by focusing present moment, nonconceptual awareness upon the feeling tone running through all arising and passing experience. Whether each moment is accompanied by a pleasant, an unpleasant, or a neutral feeling, the practitioner seeks to know with great precision the feeling tone of the experience.

3. *Mindfulness of mind.* Shifting attention from bodily sensations and feelings to the purely mental sphere, the meditator is directed to bring awareness to the quality of mind as it arises and passes away moment by moment. This is done by noticing whether any of the three unwholesome roots (greed, hatred, and delusion) are present, or whether they are absent.

4. *Mindfulness of mental objects.* An even more detailed and nuanced investigation of mental events involves noticing the presence, absence, and changing dynamic of a number of other factors outlined in Buddhist psychology: hindrances, aggregates, sense spheres, factors of awakening, and noble truths. It

is not a discursive analysis of these factors, but rather an experiential and intuitive exploration of the texture of the phenomenal landscape.

THE FOUR LIMITLESS QUALITIES
OF HEART (*BRAHMA VIHARAS*)

There are four qualities of heart that are particularly healing and can be developed using a form of concentration meditation that focuses on each of the four unique mental states. These meditations are also called *divine abidings* in a figurative sense, insofar as they involve elevating the mind to very subtle and sublime states. They are classically presented by analogy to a mother's feelings toward her child:

1. *Lovingkindness* (*metta*). As a mother would feel boundless lovingkindness to her newborn babe, wishing deeply for its health and well-being, a person deliberately cultivates and develops the same quality of universal and selfless love toward all beings, by focusing the mind unswervingly on intentions such as "May they be happy," "May they be well."

2. *Compassion* (*karuna*). As a mother would respond to a child who is sick or injured, so also a meditator can intentionally develop an attitude of compassion that meets the experience of suffering with the wish for all beings to be safe, secure, and healed of their afflictions. Compassion is a particular state of mind that can be singled out and cultivated by concentration and absorption.

3. *Sympathetic joy* (*mudita*). The quality of mind that responds to the good fortune of others with happiness and goodwill rather than with jealousy or envy is called sympathetic joy. This state, too, can be deliberately strengthened by practice, and is similar to a mother's response to her grown son leaving home to marry or pursue his profession. An unselfish perspective is a key ingredient of this absorption.

4. *Equanimity* (*upekkha*). As a mother might listen to her grown son recount his various business decisions, neither being attracted to nor repelled by any particular outcome as long as he is healthy and happy, so the tradition describes the state of mind called equanimity. It is not a detachment due to distancing from phenomena, nor a desensitized neutrality of feeling, but is rather an advanced state of being able to embrace both pleasant and unpleasant experience, without the responses usually conditioned by desire.

THE SEVEN FACTORS OF AWAKENING

These seven states of mind or attitudes are particularly helpful in gaining the sort of insight into experience that Buddhist psychology encourages; each factor therefore contributes greatly to the development of wisdom. In some formulations of the teaching, each one of these factors provides the basis for the natural unfolding of the next in an organic process of development.

1. *Mindfulness.* This is the practice of being fully aware in the present moment, without self-judgment or other forms of linguistic and conceptual overlay, of the arising and passing away of phenomena in the field of direct experience.

2. *Investigation.* This is willingness and ability to bring interest, enthusiasm, and an attitude of detailed exploration to experience. The states investigated are the arising and passing of the awareness of sensory objects, mental objects, and whatever else may be unfolding in the moment.

3. *Energy.* When mental effort is brought to a situation, there is the application of energy. It is not the counterproductive striving or straining to attain a goal, but involves the diligent and consistent application of awareness to the present moment.

4. *Joy.* Often the mind and body can become exuberant and appear to bubble over with happiness, contentment, or thrill. Though many people are more familiar with this experience when it is induced in unwholesome ways, the positive and transformative value of wholesome joy is an important quality of mind in Buddhist psychology and is to be cultivated.

5. *Tranquility.* Of equal value is the deep serenity that can emerge in the mind and body when there is an absence of conflict, distress, or suffering. This tranquility is not the opposite of joy, for the two can easily coexist. Rather than a tranquility that reduces energy, it is described more as a quality of mental luminescence that emerges as the mind becomes unified, stable, and focused.

6. *Concentration.* As described earlier, concentration involves a one-pointed attentiveness over time to a particular sensation or object to the exclusion of others.

7. *Equanimity.* Also described earlier, equanimity is the quality of mental equipoise in which the mind is neither attracted to a pleasant object nor averse to an unpleasant object.

References

Adler, A. (2002). The neurotic character. In H. Stein (Ed.) & C. Koen (Trans.), *The collected clinical works of Alfred Adler* (Vol. 1). San Francisco: Alfred Adler Institutes of San Francisco and Northwestern Washington. (Original work published 1927)

Agency for Health Care Policy and Research. (1994). *Acute low back problems in adults: Clinical Practice Guideline No. 14* (AHCPR Publication No. 95–0642). Rockville, MD: Public Health Service, U.S. Department of Health and Human Services.

Alexander C., Langer E., Newman R., Chandler H., & Davies J. (1989). Transcendental meditation, mindfulness, and longevity: An experimental study with the elderly. *Journal of Personality and Social Psycholology, 57*(6), 950–964.

Alexander, F. (1931). Buddhist training as an artificial catatonia. *Psychoanalytic Review, 18,* 129–145.

American Psychiatric Association. (1952). *Diagnostic and statistical manual of mental disorders* (1st ed.). Washington, DC: Author

American Psychiatric Association. (1994). *Diagnostic and statistical manual of mental disorders* (4th ed.). Washington, DC: Author.

American Psychiatric Association. (2000). *Diagnostic and statistical manual of mental disorders* (4th ed., text rev.). Washington, DC: Author.

Antony, M. (2002). Enhancing current treatments for anxiety disorders. *Clinical Psychology: Science and Practice, 9*(1), 91–94.

Antony, M., & Swinson, R. (2000). *Phobic disorders and panic in adults: A guide to assessment and treatment.* Washington, DC: American Psychological Association.

Aranow, P. (1998, July). Some parallels between meditation and psychotherapy. In *Psychotherapy and meditation: Cultivating insight and compassion.* Symposium conducted by the New England Educational Institute, Eastham, MA.

Arnow, B., & Constantino, M. (2003). Effectiveness of psychotherapy and combination treatment for chronic depression. *Journal of Clinical Psychology* *59*(8), 893–905.

Aron, E. (1996). *The highly sensitive person*. New York: Broadway Books.

Astin, J. (1997). Stress reduction through mindfulness meditation. Effects on psychological symptomatology, sense of control, and spiritual experiences. *Psychotherapy and Psychosomatics, 66*(2), 97–106.

Atwood, G., & Stolorow, R. (1984). *Structures of subjectivity: Explorations in psychoanalytic phenomenology*. Hillsdale, NJ: Analytic Press.

Auerbach, H., & Johnson, M. (1977). Research on the therapist's level of experience. In A. S. Gurman & A. M. Razin (Eds.), *Effective psychotherapy: A handbook of research*. New York: Pergamon Press.

Austin, J. (1998). *Zen and the brain*. Cambridge, MA: MIT Press.

Bach, P., & Hayes, S. (2002). The use of acceptance and commitment therapy to prevent the rehospitalization of psychotic patients: A randomized controlled trial. *Journal of Consulting and Clinical Psychology, 70*(5), 1129–1139.

Baer, R. (2003). Mindfulness training as a clinical intervention: A conceptual and empirical review. *Clinical Psychology: Science and Practice, 10*(2), 125–142.

Bandura, A. (1977). Self-efficacy: Toward a unifying theory of behavioral change. *Psychological Review, 84*, 191–215.

Bandura, A. (1982). Self-efficacy mechanisms in human agency. *American Psychologist, 37*, 122–147.

Barkley, R. A., & Benton, C. M. (1998). *Your defiant child: Eight steps to better behavior*. New York: Guilford Press.

Barlow, D. H. (2002). *Anxiety and its disorders: The nature and treatment of anxiety and panic* (2nd ed.). New York: Guilford Press.

Barlow, D., & Wilson, R. (2003, May). *Treatment of panic disorder*. Paper presented at a conference of the Milton Erickson Foundation on Brief Treatment of Anxiety Disorders, Boston, MA.

Barnouw, V. (1973). *Culture and personality* (rev. ed.). Homewood, IL: Dorsey Press.

Bastis, M. (2000). *Peaceful dwelling: Meditations for healing and living*. Boston: Tuttle.

Batchelor, S. (1997). *Buddhism without beliefs*. New York: Riverhead Books.

Beck, A. (1976). *Cognitive therapy and the emotional disorders*. New York: International Universities Press.

Beck, A., Emery, G., & Greenberg, R. (1985). *Anxiety disorders and phobias: A cognitive perspective*. New York: Basic Books.

Beck, A. T., Rush, A. J., Shaw, B. F., & Emery, G. (1987). *Cognitive therapy of depression*. New York: Guilford Press.

Becker, D., & Shapiro, D. (1981). Physiological responses to clicks during Zen, Yoga, and TM meditation. *Psychophysiology, 18*(6), 694–699.

Becker, E. (1973). *The denial of death*. New York: Free Press.

Beckham, J., Crawford, A., Feldman, M., Kirby, A., Hertzberg, M., Davidson, J., et al. (1997). Chronic posttraumatic stress disorder and chronic pain in Vietnam combat veterans. *Journal of Psychosomatic Research, 43*(3), 379–389.

Beebe, B., & Lachmann, F. (1998). Co-constructing inner and relational processes:

Self and mutual regulation in infant research and adult treatment. *Psychoanalytic Psychology, 15*(4), 480–516.

Beecher, H. K. (1946). Pain in men wounded in battle. *Annals of Surgery, 123*(1), 95–105.

Bennett-Goleman, T. (2001). *Emotional alchemy.* New York: Harmony Books.

Benson, H. (1975). *The relaxation response.* New York: Morrow.

Benson, H., & Klipper, M. (2000). *The relaxation response.* New York: Avon.

Benson, H., Beary, J., & Carol, M. (1974). The relaxation response. *Psychiatry, 37,* 37–46.

Bergman, S. (1990). *Men's psychological development: A relational perspective.* (Work in Progress, No. 48)., Wellesley, MA: Stone Center Working Paper Series.

Bhikku Bodhi. (Ed.). (2000). *A comprehensive manual of Abhidhamma.* Seattle: BPS Pariyatti Editions.

Bhikku, T. (Trans.). (2004a). *Raja Sutta* [The King]. In *Khuddaka Nikaya, Udana* 47. Retrieved July 27, 2004, from *www.accesstoinsight.org/canon/sutta/khuddaka/udana/ud5–01.html*

Bhikku, T. (Trans.). (2004b). *Salllatha Sutta* [The Arrow]. In *Samyutta Nikaya XXXVI6.* Retrieved July 18, 2004, from *www.accesstoinsight.org/canon/sutta/samyutta/sn36–006.html#shot*

Bickman, L. (1999). Practice makes perfect and other myths about mental health services. *American Psychologist, 54*(11), 965–979.

Bien, T., & Bien, B. (2002). *Mindful recovery: A spiritual path to healing from addiction.* New York: Wiley.

Bigos, S., Battie, M., Spengler., Fisher, L., Fordyce, W., Hansson, T., et al. (1991). A prospective study of work perceptions and psychosocial factors affecting the report of back injury. *Spine, 16*(1), 1–6.

Bion, W. (1967). Notes on memory and desire. *Psychoanalytic Forum, 2,* 271–80.

Bishop, S. (2002). What do we really know about mindfulness-based stress reduction? *Psychosomatic Medicine, 64,* 71–84.

Bishop, S., Lau, M., Shapiro, S., Carlson, L., Anderson, N., Carmody, J., et al. (2004). Mindfulness: A proposed operational definition. *Clinical Psychology: Science and Practice, 11*(3), 230–241.

Blanchard, E. (1993). Irritable bowel syndrome. In R. J. Gatchel & E. B. Blanchard (Eds.), *Psychophysiological disorders.* Washington, DC: American Psychological Association.

Blatt, S. (2004). *Experiences of depression: Theoretical, clinical and research perspectives.* Washington, DC: American Psychological Association.

Block, J., & Wulfert, E. (2000). Acceptance and change: Treating socially anxious college students with ACT or CBGT. *Behavior Analysis Today, 1,* 3–11.

Boccio, F. (2004). *Mindfulness yoga.* Somerville, MA: Wisdom Publications.

Bogart, G. (1991). The use of meditation in psychotherapy: A review of the literature. *American Journal of Psychotherapy, 45,* 383–413.

Bohart, A., Elliott, R., Greenberg, L., & Watson, J. (2002). Empathy. In J. C. Norcross (Ed.), *Psychotherapy relationships that work.* New York: Oxford University Press.

Bohus, M., Haaf, B., Stiglmayr, C., Pohl, U., Bohme, R., & Linehan, M. (2000).

Evaluation of inpatient dialectical-behavioral therapy for borderline personality disorder—a prospective study. *Behaviour Research and Therapy, 38*(9), 875–887.

Bohus, M., Haaf, B., Simms, T., Limberger, M., Schmahl, C., Unckel, C., et al. (2004). Effectiveness of inpatient dialectical behavioral therapy for borderline personality disorder: A controlled trial. *Behaviour Research and Therapy, 42*(5), 487–499.

Bonadonna, R. (2003). Meditation's impact on chronic illness. *Holistic Nurse Practitioner, 17*(6), 309–319.

Bond, F., & Bunce, D. (2000). Mediators of change in emotion-focused and problem-focused worksite stress management interventions. *Journal of Occupational Health Psychology, 5,* 156–163.

Boorstein, S. (1994). Insight: Some considerations regarding its potential and limitations. *Journal of Transpersonal Psychology, 26*(2), 95–105.

Borkevec, T. (1987). Relaxation-induced panic (RIP): When resting isn't peaceful. *Integrative Psychiatry, 5*(2), 104–106.

Borkovec, T. (2002). Life in the future versus life in the present. *Clinical Psychology: Science and Practice, 9*(1), 76–80.

Brach, T. (2003). *Radical acceptance: Embracing your life with the heart of a Buddha.* New York: Bantam/Dell.

Brantley, J. (2003). *Calming your anxious mind.* Oakland, CA: New Harbinger.

Brazier, D. (1995). *Zen therapy.* New York: Wiley.

Bremner, J., & Charney, D. (2002). Neural circuits in fear and anxiety. In D. Stein & E. Hollander (Eds.), *Textbook of anxiety disorders.* Washington, DC: American Psychiatric Publishing.

Bremner, J., Randall, P., Scott, T., Bronen, R., Seibyl, J., Southwick, S., et al. (1995). MRI-based measurement of hippocampal volume in patients with combat-related posttraumatic stress disorder. *American Journal of Psychiatry, 152*(7), 973–981.

Breslin, F., Zack, M., & McMain, S. (2002). An information-procession analysis of mindfulness: Implications for relapse prevention in the treatment of substance abuse. *Clinical Psychology: Science and Practice, 9*(3), 275–299.

Brown, K., & Ryan, R. (2003). The benefits of being present: Mindfulness and its role in psychological well-being. *Journal of Personality and Social Psychology, 84*(4), 822–848.

Brown, K., & Ryan, R. (2004). Perils and promise in defining and measuring mindfulness: Observations from experience. *Clinical Psychology: Science and Practice, 11*(3), 242–248.

Bruner, J. (1973). *Beyond the information given: Studies in the psychology of knowing.* New York: Norton.

Buber, M. (1970). *I and thou.* New York: Scribner's.

Bunge, M. (1963). *Causality: The place of the causal principle in modern science.* New York: World Publishing Company.

Burnard, P. (1987). Meditation: uses and methods in psychiatric nurse education. *Nurse Education Today, 7,* 187–191.

Butler, S. (2004). [Quotation]. *Samuel Butler.* Retrieved July 26, 2004, from *www.thinkexist.com/english/author/x/author_4057_1.htm*

Campos, P. (2002). Special series: Integrating Buddhist philosophy with cognitive and behavioral practice. *Cognitive and Behavioral Practice, 9*, 38–40.

Carey, B. (2004, July 13). With toughness and caring, a novel therapy helps tortured souls. *New York Times*, pp. D2, D6.

Carlson, L., Speca, M., Patel, K., & Goodey, E. (2003). Mindfulness-based stress reduction in relation to quality of life, mood, symptoms of stress, and immune parameters in breast and prostate cancer outpatients. *Psychosomatic Medicine, 65*(4), 571–581.

Carlson, L., Speca, M., Patel, K., & Goodey, E. (2004). Mindfulness-based stress reduction in relation to quality of life, mood, symptoms of stress and levels of cortisol, dehydroepiandrosterone sulfate (DHEAS) and melatonin in breast and prostate cancer outpatients. *Psychoneuroendocrinology, 29*(4), 448–474.

Chah, A., Kornfield, J., & Breiter, P. (1985). *A still forest pool: The insight meditation of Achaan Chah*. Wheaton, IL: Theosophical Publishing House.

Chambless, D., Baker, M., Baucom, D., Beutler, L., Calhoun, K., Crits-Christoph, P., et al. (1998). Update on empirically validated therapies, II. *The Clinical Psychologist, 51*(1), 3–16.

Chesson, A., Anderson, W., Littner, M., Davila, D., Hartse, K., Johnson, S., et al. (1999). Practice parameters for the nonpharmacologic treatment of chronic insomnia. *Sleep, 22*(8), 1128–1133.

Christensen, A., & Jacobson, N. S. (2000). *Reconcilable differences*. New York: Guilford Press.

Chung, C.Y. (1990). Psychotherapist and expansion of awareness. *Psychotherapy and Psychsomatics, 53*(1–4), 28–32.

Cohen, N., Lojkasek, M., Muir, E., Muir, R., & Parker, C. (2002). Six-month follow-up of two mother–infant psychotherapies: Convergence of therapeutic outcomes. *Infant Mental Health Journal, 23*(4), 361–380.

Cohen, N., Muir, E., Lojkasek, M., Muir, R., Parker, C., Barwick, M., et al. (1999). Watch, wait, and wonder: Testing the effectiveness of a new approach to mother–infant psychotherapy. *Infant Mental Health Journal, 20*(4), 429–451.

Conn, S. (1998). Living in the earth: Ecopsychology, health and psychotherapy. *Humanistic Psychologist, 26*(1–3), 179–198.

Cottraux, J., Note, I., Albuisson, E., Yao, S., Note, B., Mollard, E., et al. (2000). Cognitive behavior therapy versus supportive therapy in social phobia: A randomized controlled trial. *Psychotherapy and Psychosomatics, 69*(3), 137–146.

Craske, M., & Hazlett-Stevens, H. (2002). Facilitating symptom reduction and behavior change in GAD: The issue of control. *Clinical Psychology: Science and Practice, 9*(1), 69–75.

Craven, J. (1989). Meditation and psychotherapy. *Canadian Journal of Psychiatry, 34*, 648–653.

Crits-Christoph, P. (2002). Psychodynamic–interpersonal treatment of generalized anxiety disorder. *Clinical Psychology: Science and Practice, 9*(1), 81–84.

Crits-Christoph, P., Baranacke, K., Kurcias, J., Beck, A., Carrol, K., Perry, K., et al. (1991). Meta-analysis of therapist effects in psychotherapy outcome studies. *Psychotherapy Research, 2*, 81–91.

Crombez, G., Vlaeyen, J., Heuts, P., & Lysens, R. (1999). Pain-related fear is more disabling than pain itself: Evidence on the role of pain-related fear in chronic back pain disability. *Pain, 80*(1–2), 329–339.

Csikszentmihalyi, M. (1991). *Flow: The psychology of optimal experience.* New York: HarperCollins.

Dalai Lama. (1997). *Healing anger: The power of patience from a Buddhist perspective.* Ithaca, NY: Snow Lion.

Dalai Lama, & Cutler, H. (1998). *The art of happiness.* New York: Riverhead Books.

Danner, D., Snowdon, D., & Friesen, W. (2001). Positive emotions in early life and longevity. *Journal of Personality and Social Psychology, 80*(5), 804–813.

Dass, R. (1971). *Be here now.* New York: Crown.

Davidson, R. (2003). Affective neuroscience and psychophysiology: Toward a synthesis. *Psychophysiology, 40*(5), 655–665.

Davidson, R., & Kabat-Zinn, J. (2004). Response to letter by J. Smith. *Psychosomatic Medicine, 66,* 149–152.

Davidson, R. J., Kabat-Zinn, J., Schumacher, J., Rosenkranz, M., Muller, D., Santorelli, S., et al. (2003). Alterations in brain and immune function produced by mindfulness meditation. *Psychosomatic Medicine, 65*(4), 564–570.

Davis, M. (1992). The role of the amygdala in fear and anxiety. *Annual Review of Neuroscience, 15,* 353–375.

Deatherage, G. (1975). The clinical use of "mindfulness" meditation techniques in short-term psychotherapy. *Journal of Transpersonal Psychology, 7*(2), 133–143.

Deepak, K., Manchanda, S., & Maheshwari, M. (1994). Meditation improves clinicoelectroencephalographic measures in drug-resistant epileptics. *Biofeedback and Self-Regulation, 19*(1), 25–40.

Deikman, A. (2001). Spirituality expands a therapist's horizons. Retrieved July 6, 2004, from *www.buddhanet.net/psyspir3.htm*

Delmonte, M. (1984). Physiological responses during meditation and rest. *Biofeedback and Self-Regulation, 9*(2), 181–200.

Delmonte, M. (1986). Meditation as a clinical intervention strategy: A brief review. *International Journal of Psychosomatics, 33*(3), 9–12.

Delmonte, M. (1987). Constructivist view of meditation. *American Journal of Psychotherapy, 41*(2), 286–298.

Delmonte, M. (1988). Personality correlates of meditation practice: Frequency and dropout in an outpatient population. *Journal of Behavioral Medicine, 11*(6), 593–597.

Devine, D., & Fernald, P. (1973). Outcome effects of receiving a preferred, randomly assigned, or nonpreferred therapy. *Journal of Consulting and Clinical Psychology, 41*(1), 104–107.

Deyo, R., Rainville, J., & Kent, D. (1992). What can the history and physical examination tell us about low back pain? *Journal of the American Medical Association, 268*(6), 760–765.

Dickinson, E. (2004). Dickinson/Higginson correspondence: Late 1872. "Dickinson Search," *Dickinson Electronic Archives.* Online. Institute for Advanced Technology in the Humanities (IATH), University of Virginia. Retrieved July

21, 2004, from *jefferson.village.virginia.edy/cgi-bin/at-dickinsonsearch.cgi* (Original work published 1872)

Doi, T. (1962). Morita therapy and psychoanalysis. In A. Molino (Ed.), *The couch and the tree: Dialogues in psychoanalysis and Buddhism.* New York: North Point Press.

Duncan, B., Hubble, M., & Miller, S. (1997). *Psychotherapy with "impossible" cases: The efficient treatment of therapy veterans.* New York: Norton.

Duncan, B., & Miller, S. (2000). *The heroic client: Doing client-centered, outcome-informed therapy.* San Francisco: Jossey-Bass.

Efran, J., Germer, C., & Lukens, M. (1986). Contextualism and psychotherapy. In R. Rosnow & M. Georgoudi (Eds.), *Contextualism and understanding in behavioral science.* New York: Praeger.

Ehlers, A., Clark, D., Hackmann, A., McManus, F., Fennell, M., Herbert, C., et al. (2003). A randomized controlled trial of cognitive therapy, a self-help booklet, and repeated assessments as early interventions for posttraumatic stress disorder. *Archives of General Psychiatry, 60*(10), 1024–1032.

Eliot, T. S. (1930/1963). Ash Wednesday. In *Collected Poems 1909–1962 by T. S. Eliot.* New York: Harcourt.

Ellis, A. (1962). *Reason and emotion in psychotherapy.* New York: Lyle Stuart.

Engler, J. (1986). Therapeutic aims in psychotherapy and meditation. In K. Wilber, J. Engler, & D. Brown (Eds.), *Transformations of consciousness.* Boston: Shambhala.

Epstein, M. (1995). *Thoughts without a thinker.* New York: Basic Books.

Epstein, M. (1998). *Going to pieces without falling apart.* New York: Broadway Press.

Epstein, M., & Lieff, J. (1981). Psychiatric complications of meditation practice. *Journal of Transpersonal Psychology, 13*(2), 137–147.

Faber, A., & Mazlish, E. (1999). *How to talk so kids will listen and listen so kids will talk.* New York: Avon.

Fields, R. (1992). *How the swans came to the lake: The narrative history of Buddhism in America.* Boston: Shambala.

Fishman, B. (2002). *Emotional healing through mindfulness meditation.* Rochester, VT: Inner Traditions.

Flavell, J., & Ross, L. (1981). *Social cognitive development: Frontiers and possible futures.* New York: Cambridge University Press.

Flor, H., Turk, D., & Birbaumer, N. (1985). Assessment of stress-related psychophysiological reactions in chronic back pain patients. *Journal of Consulting and Clinical Psychology, 53*(3), 354–364.

Foa, E., Franklin, M., & Kozak, M. (1998). Psychosocial treatments for obsessive–compulsive disorder: Literature review. In R. Swinson, M. Anthony, S. Rachman, & M. Richter (Eds.), *Obsessive–compulsive disorder: Theory, research, and treatment.* New York: Guilford Press.

Fonagy, P. (2000). Attachment and borderline personality disorder. *Journal of the American Psychoanalytic Association, 48*(4), 1129–1146.

Frank, J. (1961). *Persuasion and healing: A comparative study of psychotherapy.* London: Oxford University Press.

Fraser, R., Sandhu, A., & Gogan, W. (1995). Magnetic resonance imaging findings 10 years after treatment for lumbar disc herniation. *Spine, 20*(6), 710–714.

Fredrickson, B. (2003). The value of positive emotions. *American Scientist, 91,* 330–335.

Fredrickson, B., & Branigan, C. (in press). Positive emotions broaden the scope of attention and thought–action repertoires. *Cognition and Emotion.*

Freud, S. (1961a). Recommendations to physicians practicing psychoanalysis. In J. Strachey (Ed. and Trans.), *The standard edition of the complete psychological works of Sigmund Freud* (Vol. 21). London: Hogarth Press. (Original work published 1912)

Freud, S. (1961b). Civilization and its discontents. In J. Strachey (Ed. and Trans.), *The standard edition of the complete psychological works of Sigmund Freud* (Vol. 21). London: Hogarth Press. (Original work published 1930)

Freud, S. (1961c). Beyond the pleasure principle. In J. Strachey (Ed. and Trans.), *The standard edition of the complete psychological works of Sigmund Freud* (Vol. 18). London: Hogarth Press. (Original work published 1920)

Freud, S., & Breuer, J. (1961). Studies on hysteria. In J. Strachey (Ed. and Trans.), *The standard edition of the complete psychological works of Sigmund Freud* (Vol. 2). London: Hogarth Press. (Original work published 1895)

Friedman, M., & Whisman, M. (2004). Implicit cognition and the maintenance and treatment of major depression. *Cognitive and Behavioral Practice, 11,* 168–177.

Friedman, S., Hatch, M., & Paradis, C. (1993). Dermatological disorders. In R. J. Gatchel & E. B. Blanchard (Eds.), *Psychophysiological disorders.* Washington, DC: American Psychological Association.

Fritz, G., & Miezwa, J. (1983). Meditation: A review of literature relevant to therapist behavior and personality. *Psychotherapy in Private Practice, 1*(3), 77–87.

Fromm, E., Suzuki, D. T., & DeMartino, R. (1960). *Zen Buddhism and psychoanalysis.* New York: Harper & Row.

Furmark, T., Tillfors, M., Marteinsdottir, I., Fischer, H., Pissiota, A., Langstroem, B., et al. (2002). Common changes in cerebral blood flow in patients with social phobia treated with citalopram or cognitive-behavioral therapy. *Archives of General Psychiatry, 59*(5), 425–433.

Gallese, V. (2001). The "shared manifold" hypothesis: From mirror neurons to empathy. *Journal of Consciousness Studies, 8*(5–7), 33–50.

Garfield, S. (1981). Critical issues in the effectiveness of psychotherapy. In C. E. Walker (Ed.), *Clinical practice of psychology.* Elmsford, NY: Pergamon.

Gendlin, E. T. (1996). *Focusing-oriented psychotherapy: A manual of the experiential method.* New York: Guilford Press.

Gifford, E., Hayes, S., & Strosahl, K. (2004). *Examples of ACT components.* Retrieved July 23, 2004, from *www.acceptanceandcommitmenttherapy.com/resources/components.html*

Gilbert, P. (2001). *Overcoming depression: A step-by-step approach to gaining control over depression.* New York: Oxford University Press.

Gilligan, C. (1982). *In a different voice.* Cambridge, MA: Harvard University Press.

Goffman, E. (1971). *Relations in public*. New York: Harper Colophon.

Goisman, R., Rogers, M., Steketee, G., Warshaw, M., Cuneo, P., & Keller, M. (1993). Utilization of behavioral methods in a multicenter anxiety disorders study. *Journal of Clinical Psychiatry, 54*(6), 213–218.

Goldberg, E. (2001). *The executive brain: Frontal lobes and the civilized mind*. Oxford, UK: Oxford University Press.

Goldenberg, D., Kaplan, K., Nadeau, M., Brodeur, C., Smith, S., & Schmid, C. (1994). A controlled study of a stress-reduction, cognitive-behavioral treatment program in fibromyalgia. *Journal of Musculoskeletal Pain, 2*, 53–66.

Goldstein, J. (1993). *Insight meditation: The practice of freedom*. Boston: Shambhala.

Goldstein, J. (2002). *One dharma: The emerging western Buddhism*. New York: HarperCollins.

Goldstein, J. (2004, Spring). Fear, pain . . . and trust. *Insight Journal*, pp. 9–12.

Goleman, D. (1977). *The varieties of meditative experience*. New York: Dutton.

Goleman, D. (1988). *The meditative mind: The varieties of meditative experience*. New York: Tarcher/Putnam Books.

Goleman, D. (2003). *Destructive emotions: How can we overcome them?* New York: Bantam/Dell.

Goleman, D., & Schwartz, G. (1976). Meditation as an intervention in stress reactivity. *Journal of Consulting and Clinical Psychololology, 44*(3), 456–66.

Goodale, I., Domar, A., & Benson, H. (1990). Alleviation of premenstrual syndrome symptoms with the relaxation response. *Obstetrics and Gynecology, 75*(4), 649–655.

Gratacos, M., Nadal, M., Martin-Santos, R., Pujana, M. A., Gago, J., Peral, B., et al. (2001). A polymorphic genomic duplication on human chromosome 15 is a susceptibility factor for panic and phobic disorders. *Cell, 106*(3), 367–379.

Green, R. (2001). *The explosive child: A new approach for understanding and parenting easily frustrated, chronically inflexible children*. New York: HarperCollins.

Greist, J., & Baer, L. (2002). Psychotherapy for obsessive–compulsive disorder. In D. Stein & E. Hollander (Eds.), *Textbook of anxiety disorders*. Washington, DC: American Psychiatric Publishing.

Groopman, J. (2004, January 26). The grief industry. *The New Yorker*, pp. 30–32, 34–36, 38.

Grossman, P., Niemann, L., Schmidt, S., & Walach, H. (2004). Mindfulness-based stress reduction and health benefits: A meta-analysis. *Journal of Psychosomatic Research, 57*(1), 35–43.

Gunaratana, B. (2002). *Mindfulness in plain English*. Somerville, MA: Wisdom Publications.

Guzman, J., Esmail, R., Karjalainen, K., Malmivaara, A., Irvin, E., & Bombardier, C. (2001). Multidisciplinary rehabilitation for chronic low back pain: Systematic review. *British Medical Journal, 323*(7322), 1186–1187.

Hall, H., McIntosh, G., Wilson, L., & Melles, T. (1998). Spontaneous onset of back pain. *Clinical Journal of Pain, 14*(2), 129–133.

Hanh, T. N. (1976). *The miracle of mindfulness*. Boston: Beacon Press.

Hanh, T. N. (1992). *Peace is every step*. New York: Bantam.

Hanh, T.N. (1997). *Teachings on love*. Berkeley, CA: Parallax Press.

Hartranft, C. (2003). *The Yoga-Sutra of Pantajali.* Boston: Shambala.

Hayes, S. (2002a). Acceptance, mindfulness, and science. *Clinical Psychology: Science and Practice, 9*(1), 101–106.

Hayes, S. (2002b). Buddhism and acceptance and commitment therapy. *Cognitive and Behavioral Practice, 9,* 58–66.

Hayes, S. C., Bissett, R., Korn, Z., Zettle, R., Rosenfarb, I., Cooper, L., et al. (1999). The impact of acceptance versus control rationales on pain tolerance. *Psychological Record, 49,* 33–47.

Hayes, S. C., Follette, V. M., & Linehan, M. M. (Eds.). (2004). *Mindfulness and acceptance: Expanding the cognitive-behavioral tradition.* New York: Guilford Press.

Hayes, S. C., Strosahl, K. D., & Wilson, K. G. (1999). *Acceptance and commitment therapy: An experiential approach to behavior change.* New York: Guilford Press.

Hayes, S., & Feldman, G. (2004). Clarifying the construct of mindfulness in the context of emotion regulation and the process of change in therapy. *Clinical Psychology: Science and Practice, 11*(3), 255–262.

Hayes, S., Masuda, A., Bissett, R., Luoma, J., & Guerrero, L. (2004). DBT, FAP, and ACT: How empirically oriented are the new behavior therapy technologies? *Behavior Therapy, 35,* 35–54.

Hayes, S., Strosahl, K., & Houts, A. (Eds.). (2005). *A practical guide to acceptance and commitment therapy.* New York: Springer.

Hebert, R., & Lehmann, D. (1977). Theta bursts: An EEG pattern in normal subjects practicing the transcendental meditation technique. *Electroencephalography and Clinical Neurophysiology, 42,* 397–405.

Heiman, J., & Meston, C. (1997). Empirically validated treatment for sexual dysfunction. *Annual Review of Sex Research, 8,* 148–194.

Henley, A. (1994). When the iron bird flies: A commentary on Sydney Walter's "Does a systemic therapist have Buddha nature?" *Journal of Systemic Therapies, 13*(3), 50–51.

Ho, K., Moody, G., Peng, C.-K., Mietus, J., Larson, M., Levy, D., et al. (1997). Predicting survival in heart failure case and control subjects by use of fully automated methods for deriving nonlinear and conventional indices of heart rate dynamics. *Circulation, 96,* 842–848.

Horney, K. (1945). *Our inner conflicts: A constructive theory of neurosis.* New York: Norton.

Horney, K. (1998). Free associations and the use of the couch. In A. Molino (Ed.), *The couch and the tree: Dialogues in psychoanalysis and Buddhism.* New York: North Point Press. (Original work published 1952)

Hull, A. (2002). Neuroimaging findings in post-traumatic stress disorder: Systematic review. *British Journal of Psychiatry, 181,* 102–110.

Ivanov, P., Rosenblum, M., Peng, C.-K., Mietus, J., Havlin, S., Stanley, B., et al. (1996). Scaling behaviour of heartbeat intervals obtained by wavelet-based time-series analysis. *Nature, 383,* 323–327.

Jacobson, E. (1938). *Progressive relaxation.* Chicago: University of Chicago Press.

Jacobson, N., Christensen, A., Prince, S., Cordove, & Eldridge, K. (2000). Integrative behavioral couple therapy: An acceptance-based, promising new treatment for couple discord. *Journal of Consulting and Clinical Psychology, 68,* 351–355.

Jensen, M. , Brant-Zawadzki, M., Obucowski, N., Modic, M., Malkasian, D., & Ross, J. (1994). Magnetic resonance imaging of the lumbar spine in people without back pain. *New England Journal of Medicine, 331*(2), 69–73.

Johnson, J., Germer, C., Efran, J., & Overton, W. (1988). Personality as a basis for theoretical predilections. *Journal of Personality and Social Psychology, 55*(5), 824–835.

Jordan, J. V. (2003). *Qualities of presence in the therapy relationship.* Paper presented at the Jean Baker Miller Training Institute, Wellesley College, Wellesley, MA.

Jordan, J. V. (1991). Empathy and self boundaries. In J. V. Jordan, A.G. Kaplan, J. B. Miller, I. P. Stiver, & J. L. Surrey, *Women's growth in connection: Writings from the Stone Center.* New York: Guilford Press.

Jordan, J. V. (Ed.). (1997). *Women's growth in diversity: More writings from the Stone Center.* New York: Guilford Press.

Jordan, J. V., Kaplan, A. G., Miller, J. B., Stiver, I. P., & Surrey, J. L. (1991). *Women's growth in connection: Writings from the Stone Center.* New York: Guilford Press.

Jung, C. G. (1992). Psychological commentary on the *Tibetan Book of Great Liberation.* In D. Meckel & R. Moore (Eds.), *Self and liberation: The Jung–Buddhism dialogue.* New York: Paulist Press. (Original work published 1939)

Kabat-Zinn, J. (1982). An outpatient program in behavioral medicine for chronic pain patients based on the practice of mindfulness meditation: Theoretical considerations and preliminary results. *General Hospital Psychiatry, 4*(1), 33–47.

Kabat-Zinn, J. (1990). *Full catastrophe living: Using the wisdom of your body and mind to face stress, pain, and illness.* New York: Dell.

Kabat-Zinn, J. (1994). *Wherever you go there you are: Mindfulness meditation in everyday life.* New York: Hyperion.

Kabat-Zinn, J. (2000). Indra's net at work: The mainstreaming of Dharma practice in society. In G. Watson, S. Batchelor, et al. (Eds.), *The psychology of awakening: Buddhism, science, and our day-to-day lives.* York, ME: S. Weiser.

Kabat-Zinn, J. (Speaker). (2002a). *Guided mindfulness meditation: Body scan meditation.* (Compact disc recording). Stress Reduction CDs and Tapes, P.O. Box 547, Lexington, MA 02420.

Kabat-Zinn, J. (Speaker). (2002b). *Guided mindfulness meditation: Sitting meditation* (Compact disc recording). Stress Reduction CDs and Tapes, P.O. Box 547, Lexington, MA 02420.

Kabat-Zinn, J. (Speaker). (2002c). *Guided mindfulness meditation: Mountain meditation/lake meditation.* (Compact disc recording). Stress Reduction CDs and Tapes, P.O. Box 547, Lexington, MA 02420.

Kabat-Zinn, J., Lipworth, L., & Burney, R. (1985). The clinical use of mindfulness meditation for the self-regulation of chronic pain. *Journal of Behavioral Medicine, 8*(2), 163–190.

Kabat-Zinn, J., Lipworth, L., Burney, R., & Sellers, W. (1987). Four-year follow-up of a meditation-based program for the self-regulation of chronic pain: Treatment outcomes and compliance. *Clinical Journal of Pain, 2*, 159–173.

Kabat-Zinn, J., Massion, A. O., Kristeller, J., Peterson, L., Fletcher, K. E., Pbert, L., et al. (1992). Effectiveness of a meditation-based stress reduction program in the treatment of anxiety disorders. *American Journal of Psychiatry, 149*(7), 936–943.

Kabat-Zinn, J., Wheeler, E., Light, T., Skillings, A., Scharf, M., Cropley, T. G., et al. (1998). Influence of a mindfulness meditation-based stress reduction intervention on rates of skin clearing in patients with moderate to severe psoriasis undergoing phototherapy (UVB) and photochemotherapy (PUVA). *Psychosomatic Medicine, 60*(5), 625–632.

Kabat-Zinn, M., & Kabat-Zinn, J. (1998). *Everyday blessings: The inner work of mindful parenting.* New York: Hyperion.

Kabat-Zinn, J. (2003). Mindfulness-based interventions in context: Past, present, and future. *Clinical Psychology: Science and Practice, 10*(2), 144–156.

Kabat-Zinn, J. (2005). *Coming to our senses: Healing ourselves and the world through mindfulness.* New York: Hyperion.

Kaplan, K., Goldenberg, D., & Galvin-Nadeau, M. (1993). The impact of a meditation-based stress reduction program on fibromyalgia. *General Hospital Psychiatry, 15*, 284–289.

Kasamatsu, A., & Hirai, T. (1973). An electroencephalographic study on the Zen meditation (Zazen). *Journal of the American Institute of Hypnosis, 14*(3), 107–114.

Kawai, H. (1996). *Buddhism and the art of psychotherapy.* College Station: Texas A&M University Press.

Keller, M., Yonkers, K., Warshaw, M., Pratt, L., Gollan, J., Massion, A., et al. (1994). Remission and relapse in subjects with panic disorder and panic with agoraphobia: A prospective short interval naturalistic follow-up. *Journal of Nervous and Mental Disease, 182*(5), 290–296.

Kelly, G. (1955). *The psychology of personal constructs.* New York: Norton.

Kendall, P. (Ed.). (2003). *Clinical Psychology: Science and Practice* [full issue], *10*(2).

Keown, D. (2000). *Contemporary Buddhist ethics.* Surrey, UK: Curzon Press.

Kessler, R., Sonnega, A., Bromet, E., Hughes, M., & Nelson, C. (1995). Posttraumatic stress disorder in the National Comorbidity Survey. *Archives of General Psychiatry, 52*(12), 1048–1060.

Kinnell, G. (1980). Saint Francis and the sow. In *Mortal acts mortal words.* Boston: Houghton Mifflin.

Kirsch, I. (1990). *Changing expectations; A key to effective psychotherapy.* Pacific Grove, CA: Brooks/Cole.

Kjaer, T., Bertelsen, C., Piccini, P., Brooks, D., Alving, J., & Lou, H. (2002). Increased dopamine tone during meditation-induced change of consciousness. *Brain Research and Cognitive Brain Research, 13*(2), 255–259.

Kleinman, A., Kunstadter, P., Alexander, E., Russell, G., & James, L. (Eds.). (1978). *Culture and healing in Asian societies: Anthropological, psychiatric and public health studies.* Cambridge, MA: Schenkman.

Koerner, K., & Linehan, M. (2000). Research on dialectical behavior therapy for patients with borderline personality disorder. *Psychiatric Clinics of North America, 23*(1), 151–67.

Kohut, H. (1977). *The restoration of the self.* New York: International Universities Press.

Kohut, H. (1978). *The search for the self: Selected writings of Heinz Kohut: 1950–1978.* New York: International Universities Press.

Kori, S., Miller, R., & Todd, D. (1990). Kinesiophobia: A new view of chronic pain behavior. *Pain Management, 3,* 35–43.

Kramer, J. (2003). *Buddha Mom: The journey through mindful mothering.* New York: Tarcher.

Kristeller, J., & Hallett, C. (1999). An exploratory study of a meditation-based intervention for binge eating disorder. *Journal of Health Psychology, 4*(3), 357–363.

Kübler-Ross, E. (1977). *On death and dying: What the dying have to teach doctors, nurses, clergy, and their own families.* New York: Simon & Schuster.

Kuhn, T. (1970). *The structure of scientific revolutions.* Chicago: University of Chicago Press.

Kutz, I., Borysenko, J., & Benson, H. (1985). Meditation and psychotherapy: A rationale for the integration of dynamic psychotherapy, the relaxation response, and mindfulness meditation. *American Journal of Psychiatry, 142*(1), 1–8.

Kutz, I., Leserman, J., Dorrington, C., Morrison, C., Borysenko, J., & Benson, H. (1985). Meditation as an adjunct to psychotherapy. *Psychotherapy and Psychosomatics, 43,* 209–218.

Ladner, L. (2004). *The lost art of compassion: Discovering the practice of happiness in the meeting of Buddhism and psychology.* New York: HarperCollins.

Lambert, M., & Barley, D. (2002). Research summary on the therapeutic relationship and psychotherapy outcome. In J. C. Norcross (Ed.), *Psychotherapy relationships that work.* New York: Oxford University Press.

Lambert, M., & Bergin, A. (1994). The effectiveness of psychotherapy. In A. E. Bergin & S. L. Garfield (Eds.), *Handbook of psychotherapy and behavior change* (4th ed.). New York: Wiley.

Lambert, M. J. (1992). Psychotherapy outcome research; Implications for integrative and eclectic theories. In J. C. Norcross & M. R. Goldfried (Eds.), *Handbook of psychotherapy integration.* New York: Basic Books.

Landreth, G. (2002). *Play therapy: The art of the relationship.* New York: Brunner-Routledge.

Langer, E. (1989). *Mindfulness.* Cambridge, MA: Da Capo Press.

Lazar, S., Bush, G., Gollub, R., Fricchione, G., Khalsa, G., & Benson, H. (2000). Functional brain mapping of the relaxation response and meditation. *NeuroReport, 11*(7), 1581–1585.

Lazar, S. (2004). [*Breathing rate correlated with years of mindfulness meditation*]. Unpublished raw data.

Lazarus, A. (1993). Tailoring the therapeutic relationship, or being an authentic chameleon. *Psychotherapy, 30,* 404–407.

LeDoux, J. (1995). Emotion: Clues from the brain. *Annual Review of Psychology, 46,* 209–235.

LeDoux, J. (2000). Emotion circuits in the brain. *Annual Review of Neuroscience,* 23, 155–184.

Lee, D. (1959). *Freedom and culture.* Englewood Cliffs, NJ: Prentice Hall.

Lee, R., & Martin, J. (1991). *Psychotherapy after Kohut: A textbook of self-psychology.* Hillsdale, NJ: Analytic Press.

Lehmann, D., Faber, P. Achermann, P., Jeanmonod, D., Gianotti, L., & Pizzagalli, D. (2001). Brain sources of EEG gamma frequency during volitionally meditation-induced, altered states of consciousness, and experience of the self. *Psychiatry Research,* 108(2), 111–121.

Lehrer, P., Sasaki, Y., & Saito, Y. (1999). Zazen and cardiac variability. *Psychosomatic Medicine,* 61(6), 812–821.

Leiblich, A., McAdams, D., & Josselson, R. (2004). *Healing plots: The narrative basis of psychotherapy.* Washington, DC: American Psychological Association Books.

Lesh, T. (1970). Zen meditation and the development of empathy in counselors. *Journal of Humanistic Psychology* 10(1), 39–74.

Libet, B. (1999). Do we have free will? In B. Libet, A. Freeman, & K. Sutherland (Eds.), *The volitional brain: Towards a neuroscience of free will.* Thorverton, UK: Imprint Academic.

Linehan, M., Armstrong, H., Suarez, A., Allmon, D., & Heard, H. (1991). A cognitive-behavioral treatment of chronically parasuicidal borderline patients. *Archives of General Psychiatry,* 48, 1060–1064.

Linehan, M. (1993a). *Cognitive-behavioral treatment of borderline personality disorder.* New York: Guilford Press.

Linehan, M. (1993b). *Skills training manual for treating borderline personality disorder.* New York: Guilford Press.

Linehan, M., Schmidt, H., Dimeff, L., Craft, J., Katner, J., & Comtois, K. (1999). Dialectical behavior therapy for patients with borderline personality disorder and drug-dependence. *American Journal on Addiction,* 8, 279–292.

Linehan, M., Dimeff, L., Reynolds, S., Comtois, K., Welch, S., Heagerty, P., & Kivlahan, D. R. (2002). Dialectical behavior therapy versus comprehensive validation therapy plus 12–step for the treatment of opioid dependent women meeting criteria for borderline personality disorder. *Drug and Alcohol Dependence,* 67(1), 13–26.

Linton, S. (1997). A population-based study of the relationship between sexual abuse and back pain: Establishing a link. *Pain,* 73(1), 47–53.

Logsdon-Conradsen, S. (2002). Using mindfulness meditation to promote holistic health in individuals with HIV/AIDS. *Cognitive and Behavioral Practice,* 9, 67–72.

Lopez, F. (2000). Acceptance and commitment therapy (ACT) in panic disorder with agoraphobia: A case study. *Psychology in Spain,* 4(1), 120–128.

Lou, H., Kjaer, T., Friberg, L., Wildschiodtz, G., Holm, S., & Nowak, M. (1999). A 15O-H2O PET study of meditation and the resting state of normal consciousness. *Human Brain Mapping,* 7(2), 98–105.

Luborsky, L., Crits-Christoph, P., McLellan, T., Woody, G., Piper, W., Imber, S., et al. (1986). Do therapists vary much in their success?: Findings from four outcome studies. *American Journal of Orthopsychiatry,* 51, 501–512.

Luborsky, L., Rosenthal, R., Diguer, L., Andrusyna, T., Berman, J., Levitt, J., et al. (2002). The dodo bird is alive and well—mostly. *Clinical Psychology: Science and Practice, 9*(1), 2–12.

Luborsky, L., Singer, B., & Luborsky, L. (1975). Comparative studies of psychotherapies: Is it true that "everyone has won and all must have prizes"? *Archives of General Psychiatry, 32,* 992–1008.

Lucas, R. E., Clark, A. E., Georgellis, Y., & Diener, E. (2003). Reexamining adaptation and the set point model of happiness: Reactions to changes in marital status. *Journal of Personality and Social Psychology, 84*(3), 527–539.

Lynch, T., Morse, J., Mendelson, T., & Robins, C. (2003). Dialectical behavior therapy for depressed adults: A randomized pilot study. *American Journal of Geriatric Psychiatry, 11*(1), 33–45.

Ma, S., & Teasdale, J. (2004). Mindfulness-based cognitive therapy for depression: Replication and exploration of differential relapse prevention effects. *Journal of Consulting and Clinical Psychology, 72*(1), 31–40.

Macy, J., & Brown, M. (1998). *Coming back to life: Practices to reconnect our lives, our world.* Gabriola Island, BC, Canada: New Society.

Magid, B. (2002). *Ordinary mind: Exploring the common ground of Zen and psychotherapy.* Somerville, MA: Wisdom Publications.

Maharaj, N. (1997). *I am that: Talks with Sri Nisargadatta* (M. Frydman, Trans.). New York: Aperture.

Malik, M., & Camm, A. J. (Eds.). (1995). *Heart rate variability.* Armonk, NY: Futura.

Mallinckrodt, B. (1996). Change in working alliance, social support, and psychological symptoms in brief therapy. *Journal of Counseling Psychology, 43*(4), 448–455.

Mancini, C., van Ameringen, M., Szatmari, P., Fugere, C., & Boyle, M. (1996). A high-risk pilot study of the children of adults with social phobia. *Journal of the American Academy of Child and Adolescent Psychiatry, 35,* 1511–1517.

Markowitz, J. (2002). *Interpersonal psychotherapy for dysthymic disorder.* Washington, DC: American Psychiatric Press.

Marlatt, A. (2002). Buddhist philosophy and the treatment of addictive behavior. *Cognitive and Behavioral Practice, 9,* 44–50.

Marlatt, G., & Kristeller, J. (1999). Mindfulness and meditation. In W. R. Miller (Ed.), *Integrating spirituality into treatment.* Washington, DC: American Psychological Association.

Marotta, S. (2003). Unflinching empathy: Counselors and tortured refugees. *Journal of Counseling and Development, 81,* 111–114.

Martin, J. (1997). Mindfulness: A proposed common factor. *Journal of Psychotherapy Integration, 7*(4), 291–312.

Martin, J. (1999). *The Zen path through depression.* New York: HarperCollins.

Maruta, T., Colligan, R., Malinchoc, M., & Offord, K. (2000). Optimists vs. pessimists: Survival rate among medical patients over a 30-year period. *Mayo Clinic Proceedings, 75,* 140–143.

Maslach, C., & Leiter, M. (1997). *The truth about burnout: How organizations cause personal stress and what to do about it.* San Francisco: Jossey-Bass.

Maslow, A. H. (1966). *The psychology of science:* A *reconnaissance.* New York: Harper & Row.

Masters, W. (1970). *Human sexual inadequacy.* New York: Little, Brown.

Masters, W., & Johnson, V. (1966). *Human sexual response.* Philadelphia: Lippincott, Williams & Wilkins.

Mattson, M. (1995). Patient–treatment matching. *Alcohol Health and Research World, 18,* 287–295.

May, R. (1967). *The art of counseling.* New York: Abingdon Press.

Mayer, T., Gatchel, R., Mayer, H., Kishino, N. D., Keeley, J., & Mooney, V. (1987). A prospective two-year study of functional restoration in industrial low back injury: An objective assessment procedure. *Journal of the American Medical Association, 258*(13), 1763–1767.

McCullough, J. (2000). *Treatment for chronic depression: Cognitive behavioral analysis system of psychotherapy.* New York: Guilford Press.

McIntyre, R., & O'Donovan, C. (2004). The human cost of not achieving full remission in depression. *Canadian Journal of Psychiatry, 49,* 10S-16S.

McQuaid, J., & Carmona, P. (2004). *Peaceful mind: using mindfulness and cognitive behavioral psychology to overcome depression.* Oakland, CA: New Harbinger.

Melzack, R., & Wall, P. (1965). Pain mechanisms: a new theory. *Science, 150*(699), 971–979.

Mennin, D., Heimberg, R., Turk, C., & Fresco, D. (2002). Applying an emotion regulation framework to integrative approaches to generalized anxiety disorder. *Clinical Psychology: Science and Practice, 9*(1), 85–90.

Metzler, C., Biglan, A., Noell, J., Ary, D., & Ochs, L. (2000). A randomized controlled trial of a behavioral intervention to reduce high-risk sexual behavior among adolescents in STD clinics. *Behavior Therapy, 31,* 27–54.

Meyer, B., Pilkonis, P., Krupnick, J., Egan, M., Simmens, S., & Sotsky, S. (2002). Treatment expectancies, patient alliance, and outcome: Further analyses from the National Institute of Mental Health Treatment of Depression Collaborative Research Program. *Journal of Consulting and Clinical Psychology, 70*(4), 1051–1055.

Miller, J. B. (1976). *Toward a new psychology of women.* Boston: Beacon Press.

Miller, J. B., & Stiver, I. (1997). *The healing connection.* Boston: Beacon Press.

Miller, J. J. (1993). The unveiling of traumatic memories and emotions through mindfulness and concentration meditation: Clinical implications and three case reports. *Journal of Transpersonal Psychology, 25*(2), 169–176.

Miller, J. J., Fletcher, K., & Kabat-Zinn, J. (1995). Three-year follow-up and clinical implications of a mindfulness meditation-based stress reduction intervention in the treatment of anxiety disorders. *General Hospital Psychiatry, 17,* 192–200.

Miller, S., Duncan, B., & Hubble, M. (1997). *Escape from Babel: Toward a unifying language for psychotherapy practice.* New York: Norton.

Molino, A. (Ed.). (1998). *The couch and the tree.* New York: North Point Press.

Murphy, M., Donovan, S., & Taylor, E. (1997). *The physical and psychological effects of meditation: A review of contemporary research with a comprehensive bibliography, 1931–1996* (2nd ed.). Sausalito, CA: The Institute of Noetic Sciences.

Murphy, S. (2002). *One bird one stone.* New York: Renaissance Books.

Myers, D. (2000). The funds, friends, and faith of happy people. *American Psychologist, 55*(1), 56–67.

Nanamoli, B. (Trans.), & Bodhi, B. (Ed.). (1995a). Bhayabherava Sutta: Fear and dread. In *The middle length discourses of the Buddha.* Boston: Wisdom Publications.

Nanamoli, B. (Trans.), & Bodhi, B. (Ed.). (1995b). *The middle length discourses of the Buddha.* Boston: Wisdom.

Napthali, S. (2003). *Buddhism for mothers: A calm approach to caring for yourself and your children.* Crows Nest, Australia: Allen & Unwin Pty.

National Institute of Mental Health. (2001). *The invisible disease: Depression* (NIH Publication No. 01-4591). Retrieved April 9, 2004, from *www.nimh.nih.gov/publicat/invisible.cfm*

Narrow, W. (1998). *One-year prevalence of depressive disorders among adults 18 and over in the U.S.: NIMH ECA prospective data.* Unpublished, cited in *NIMH Fact Sheet on Depression*, 2001.

Neff, K. (2003). The development and validation of a scale to measure self-compassion. *Self and Identity, 2*(3), 223–250.

Newberg, A., Alavi, A., Baime, M., Pourdehnad, M., Santanna, J., & d'Aquili, E. (2001). The measurement of regional cerebral blood flow during the complex cognitive task of meditation: A preliminary SPECT study. *Psychiatry Research, 106*(2), 113–122.

Newman, J. (1994). Affective empathy training with senior citizens using Zazen (zen) meditation. *Dissertation Abstracts International, 55*(5–A), no. 1193.

Norcross, J. (Ed.). (2001). Empirically supported therapy relationships: Summary report of the Division 29 Task Force. *Psychotherapy, 38*(4), 345–356.

Norcross, J. (Ed.). (2002). *Psychotherapy relationships that work: Therapist contributions and responsiveness to patient needs.* New York: Oxford University Press.

Norcross, J. C., & Beutler, L. E. (1997). Determining the therapeutic relationship of choice in brief therapy. In J.N. Butcher (Ed.), *Personality assessment in managed health care: A practitioner's guide.* New York: Oxford University Press.

Nyanaponika T. (1998). *Abhidhamma studies.* Boston: Wisdom Publications. (Original work published 1949)

Nyanaponika T. (1965). *The heart of Buddhist meditation.* York Beach, ME: Red Wheel/Weiser.

Nyanaponika T. (1972). *The power of mindfulness.* San Fransisco: Unity Press.

Olendzki, A. (2002, Spring). Skinny Gotami and the mustard seed. *Insight Journal*, p. 40.

Palfai, T., & Wagner, E. (2004). Special series: Current perspectives on implicit processing in clinical disorders: Implications for assessment and intervention. *Cognitive and Behavioral Practice, 11*, 135–138.

Patterson, G. (1977). *Living with children: New methods for parents and teachers.* Champaign, IL: Research Press.

Pearl, J., & Carlozzi, A. (1994). Effect of meditation on empathy and anxiety. *Perceptual and Motor Skills, 78*, 297–298.

Pecukonis, E. V. (1996). Childhood sex abuse in women with chronic intractable back pain. *Social Work in Health Care, 23*(3), 1–16.

Peng, C., Mietus, J., Liu, Y., Khalsa, G., Douglas, P., Benson, H., et al. (1999). Exaggerated heart rate oscillations during two meditation techniques. *International Journal of Cardiology, 70*, 101–107.

Pennebaker, J. (1997). *Opening up: The healing power of expressing emotions.* New York: Guilford Press.

Pennebaker, P., Keicolt-Glaser, J., & Glaser R. (1988). Disclosure of traumas and immune function: Health implications for psychotherapy. *Journal of Consulting and Clinical Psychology, 56*(2), 239–245.

Pepper, S. (1942). *World hypotheses.* Berkeley: University of California Press.

Peterson, C., & Seligman, M. (2004). *Character strengths and virtues.* London: Oxford University Press.

Pieper, S., & Hammill, S. (1995). Heart rate variability: Technique and investigational applications in cardiovascular medicine. *Mayo Clinic Procedings, 70*, 955–964.

Pirsig, R. (1974). *Zen and the art of motorcycle maintenance: An inquiry into values.* New York: Morrow.

Rainville, J., Sobel, J., Hartigan, C., Monlux, G., & Bean, J. (1997). Decreasing disability in chronic back pain through aggressive spine rehabilitation. *Journal of Rehabilitation Research and Development, 34*(4), 383–393.

Rabten, G., & Batchelor, S. (1983). *Echoes of voidness.* Somerville, MA: Wisdom Publications.

Rauch, S., Cora-Locatelli, G., & Geenberg, B. (2002). Pathogenesis of obsessive–compulsive disorder. In D. Stein & E. Hollander (Eds.), *Textbook of anxiety disorders.* Washington, DC: American Psychiatric Publishing.

Raue, P., Golfried, M., & Barkham, M. (1997). The therapeutic alliance in psychodynamic–interpersonal and cognitive-behavioral therapy. *Journal of Consulting and Clinical Psychology, 65*(4), 582–587.

Reibel, D., Greeson, J., Brainard, G., & Rosenzweig, S. (2001). Mindfulness-based stress reduction and health-related quality of life in a heterogeneous patient population. *General Hospital Psychiatry, 23*(4), 183–192.

Reik, T. (1949). *Listening with the third ear.* New York: Farrar, Straus.

Reiman, J. (1985). The impact of meditative attentional training on measures of select attentional parameters and on measures of client perceived counselor empathy. *Dissertation Abstracts International, 46*(6–A), 1569.

Reynolds, D. (2003). Mindful parenting: A group approach to enhancing reflective capacity in parents and infants. *Journal of Child Psychotherapy, 29*(3), 357–374.

Riedesel, B. (1983). Meditation and empathic behavior: A study of clinically standardized meditation and affective sensitivity. *Dissertation Abstracts International, 43*(10–A), 3274.

Rizzolatti, G., Fadiga, L., Fogassi, L., & Gallese, V. (1996). Premotor cortex and the recognition of motor actions. *Cognitive Brain Research, 3*, 131–141.

Robins, C. (2002). Zen principles and mindfulness practice in dialectical behavior therapy. *Cognitive and Behavioral Practice, 9*(9), 50–57.

Robins, C., & Chapman, A. (2004). Dialectical behavior therapy: Current status, recent developments, and future directions. *Journal of Personality Disorders, 18*(1), 73–89.

Robins, L., Helzer, J., Weissman, M., Orvaschel, H., Gruengerge, E., Burke, J., et al. (1984). Lifetime prevalence of specific psychiatric disorders in three sites. *Archives of General Psychiatry, 41*, 949–958.

Robinson, M., & Riley, J. (1999). The role of emotion in pain. In R. J. Gatchel & D. C. Turk (Eds.), *Psychosocial factors in pain: Critical perspectives.* New York: Guilford Press.

Roemer, L., & Orsillo, S. (2002). Expanding our conceptualization of and treatment for generalized anxiety disorder: Integrating mindfulness/acceptance-based approaches with existing cognitive-behavioral models. *Clinical Psychology: Science and Practice, 9*(1), 54–68.

Roemer, L., & Orsillo, S. (2003). Mindfulness: A promising intervention strategy in need of further study. *Clinical Psychology: Science and Practice, 10*(2), 172–178.

Rogers, C. (1961). *On becoming a person,* New York: Houghton Mifflin.

Rosenbaum, R. (1999). *Zen and the heart of psychotherapy.* New York: Plenum Press.

Rosenzweig, S., Reibel, D., Greeson, J., Brainard, G., & Hojat, M. (2003). Mindfulness-based stress reduction lowers psychological distress in medical students. *Teaching and Learning in Medicine, 15*(2), 88–92.

Ross, J. (2002). Consumer considerations. In D. Stein & E. Hollander (Eds.), *Textbook of anxiety disorders.* Washington, DC: American Psychiatric Publishing.

Roth, B., & Stanley, T. (2002). Mindfulness-based stress reduction and healthcare utilization in the inner city: Preliminary findings. *Alternative Therapy and Health Medicine, 8*(1), 60–62, 64–66.

Rubin, J. (1996). *Psychotherapy and Buddhism.* New York: Plenum Press.

Russell, P. (1996). [*Process with involvement: The interpretation of affect*]. Unpublished draft manuscript, Smith College, Northampton, MA.

Ryan, R., & Deci, E. (2001). On happiness and human potentials: A review of research on hedonic and eudaimonic well-being. *Annual Review Psychology, 52*; 141–166.

Safer, D., Telch, C., & Agras, W. (2001). Dialectical behavior therapy for bulimia nervosa. *American Journal of Psychiatry, 158*, 632–634.

Safran, J. E. (2003). *Psychoanalysis and Buddhism.* Boston: Wisdom Publications.

Salzberg, S. (1995). *Lovingkindness: The revolutionary art of happiness.* Boston: Shambhala.

Sapolsky R. (1998). *Why zebras don't get ulcers: An updated guide to stress, stress related diseases, and coping.* New York: Freeman.

Savitsky, K., Medvec, V., & Gilovich, T. (1997). Remembering and regretting: The Zeigarnik effect and the cognitive availability of regrettable actions and inactions. *Personality and Social Psychology Bulletin, 23*, 248–257.

Saxe, G., Hebert, J., Carmody, J., Kabat-Zinn, J., Rosenzweig, P., Jarzobski, D., et al. (2001). Can diet in conjunction with stress reduction affect the rate of increase in prostate specific anigen after biochemical recurrence of prostate cancer? *Journal of Neurology, 166*(6), 2202–2207.

Sayadaw, M. (1971). *Practical insight meditation: Basic and progressive stages.* Kandy, Sri Lanka: Forest Hermitage.

Schacht, T. (1991). Can psychotherapy education advance psychotherapy integration?: A view from the cognitive psychology of expertise. *Journal of Psychotherapy Integration, 1,* 305–320.

Scheel, M., Hanson, W., & Razzhavaikina, T. (2004). The process of recommending homework in psychotherapy: A review of therapist delivery methods, client acceptability, and factors that affect compliance. *Psychotherapy: Theory, Research, Practice, Training, 41*(1), 38–55.

Schmidt, A., & Miller, J. (2004, Fall). Healing trauma with meditation. *Tricycle,* pp. 40–43.

Schneider, K., & Leitner, L. (2002). Humanistic psychotherapy. In M. Hersen & W. Sledge (Eds.), *Encyclopedia of psychotherapy* (Vol. 1). New York: Elsevier Science/Academic Press.

Schneider, K. (2003). Existential-humanistic psychotherapies. In A. S. Gurman & S. B. Messer (Eds.), *Essential psychotherapies: Theory and practice.* New York: Guilford Press.

Schneider, R., Staggers, F., Alexander, C., Sheppard, W., Rainforth, M., Kondwani, K., et al. (1995). A randomised controlled trial of stress reduction for hypertension in older African Americans. *Hypertension, 5,* 820–827.

Schnurr, P., Friedman, M., Foy, D., Shea, M., Hsieh, F., Lavori, P., et al. (2003). Randomized trial of trauma-focused group therapy for posttraumatic stress disorder: Results from a Department of Veterans Affairs cooperative study. *Archives of General Psychiatry, 60*(5), 481–489.

Schonstein, E., Kenny, D., Keating, J., & Koes, B. (2003). Work conditioning, work hardening and functional restoration for workers with back and neck pain. *Cochrane Database Systematic Review, 1,* CD001822.

Schultz, J., & Luthe, W. (1959). *Autogenic training: A psychophysiologic approach in psychotherapy.* New York: Grune & Stratton.

Schwartz G. (1990). Psychobiology of repression and health: A systems approach. In J. L. Singer (Ed.), *Repression and dissociation: Defense mechanisms and personality styles: Current theory and research.* Chicago: University of Chicago Press.

Schwartz, J. (1996). *Brain lock.* New York: Regan Books.

Schwartz, J., & Begley, S. (2002). *The mind and the brain: Neuroplasticity and the power of mental force.* New York: HarperCollins.

Schwartz, J., Stoessel, P., Baxter, L., Martin, K., & Phelps, M. (1996). Systematic changes in cerebral glucose metabolic rate after successful behavior modification treatment of obsessive–compulsive disorder. *Archives of General Psychiatry, 53*(2), 109–113.

Segal, Z., Vincent, P., & Levitt, A. (2002). Efficacy of combined, sequential and crossover psychotherapy and pharmacotherapy in improving outcomes in depression. *Journal of Psychiatry and Neuroscience, 27*(4), 281–290.

Segal, Z. V., Williams, J. M. G., & Teasdale, J. D. (2002). *Mindfulness-based cog-*

nitive therapy for depression: A new approach to preventing relapse. New York: Guilford Press.

Segall, S. (2003). *Encountering Buddhism: Western psychology and Buddhist teachings.* Albany: State University of New York Press.

Seligman, M. (1995). The effectiveness of psychotherapy: The *Consumer Reports* study. *American Psychologist, 50*(12), 965–974.

Seligman, M. (2002a). Optimism, pessimism, and mortality. *Mayo Clinic Proceedings, 75*(2), 133–134.

Seligman, M. (2002b). *Authentic happiness: Using the new positive psychology to realize your potential for lasting fulfillment.* New York: Free Press.

Seligman, M. (2003). *Vanguard authentic happiness teleclass—24 weeks.* Retreived October 26, 2004, from *www.authentichappiness.com*

Seligman, M. (2004a). *Dr. Martin E. P. Seligman's bio.* Retrieved October 26, 2004, from *www.psych.upenn.edu/seligman/bio.htm*

Seligman, M. E. P. (2004b). *VIA Signature Strengths Survey.* Retreived on October 26, 2004, from *www.authentichappiness.com*

Seligman, M., & Csikszentmihalyi, M. (2000). Positive psychology. An introduction. *American Psychologist, 55*(1), 5–14.

Selye, H. (1956). *The stress of life.* New York: McGraw-Hill.

Shahrokh, N., & Hales, R. (Eds.). (2003). *American Psychiatric glossary* (8th ed.). Washington, DC: American Psychiatric Publishing.

Shapiro, D. (1992). Adverse effects of meditation: A preliminary investigation of long-term meditators. *International Journal of Psychosomatics, 39*, 62–66.

Shapiro, D., & Shapiro, D. (1982). Meta-analysis of comparative therapy outcome studies: A replication and refinement. *Psychological Bulletin, 92*, 581–604.

Shapiro, S., Bootzin, R., Figueredo, A., Lopez, A., & Schwartz, G. (2003). The efficacy of mindfulness-based stress reduction in the treatment of sleep disturbance in women with breast cancer: An exploratory study. *Journal of Psychosomatic Research, 54*(1), 85–91.

Shapiro, S., Schwartz, G., & Bonner, G. (1998). Effects of mindfulness-based stress reduction on medical and premedical students. *Journal of Behavioral Medicine, 21*(6), 581–599.

Shoham-Salomon, V., & Rosenthal, R. (1987). Paradoxical interventions: A meta-analysis. *Journal of Consulting and Clinical Psychology, 55*, 22–28.

Siegel, D. J. (1999). *The developing mind: Toward a neurobiology of interpersonal experience.* New York: Guilford Press.

Siegel, R. D., Urdang, M., & Johnson, D. (2001). *Back sense: A revolutionary approach to halting the cycle of back pain.* New York: Broadway Books.

Singer-Kaplan, H. (1974). *New sex therapy: Active treatment of sexual dysfunctions.* New York: Crown.

Singh, N., Wahler, R., Adkins, A., & Myers, R. (2003). Soles of the feet: A mindfulness-based self-control intervention for aggression by an individual with mild mental retardation and mental illness. *Research in Developmental Disabilities, 24*(3), 158–169.

Skinner, B. F. (1974). *About behaviorism.* New York: Knopf.

Smith, J. (2004). Alterations in brain and immune function produced by mindfulness meditation: Three caveats. *Psychosomatic Medicine, 66*, 148–152.

Smith, J. (Ed.). (1998). *Breath sweeps mind: A first guide to meditation practice.* New York: Riverhead Books.

Smith, J. C. (1975). Meditation as psychotherapy: A review of the literature. *Psychological Bulletin, 82*(4), 558–564.

Smith, M., & Neubauer, D. (2003). Cognitive behavior therapy for chronic insomnia. *Clinical Cornerstone, 5*(3), 28–40.

Solomon, A. (2001). *The noonday demon: An atlas of depression.* New York: Scribner.

Speca, M., Carlson, L., Goodey, E., & Angen, M. (2000). A randomized, wait-list controlled clinical trial: The effect of a mindfulness meditation-based stress reduction program on mood and symptoms of stress in cancer outpatients. *Psychosomatic Medicine, 62*(5), 613–622.

Stein, G. (1993). Sacred Emily. In *Geography and Plays.* Madison: University of Wisconsin Press. (Original work published in 1922)

Stern, D. (2003). The present moment. *Psychology Networker, 27*(6), 52–57.

Stern, D. (2004). *The present moment in psychotherapy and everyday life.* New York: Norton.

Sternberg, R. (2000). Images of mindfulness. *Journal of Social Issues, 56*(1), 11–26.

Stevenson, W., & Erdman, D. (Eds.). (1971). *Blake: The complete poems.* London: Longman.

Stile, J., Lerner, J., Rhatigan, L., Plumb, C., & Orsillo, S. (2003, November). *Mindfulness as an underlying mechanism of empathic concern.* Poster session presented at the annual meeting of the Association for Advancement of Behavior Therapy, Boston, MA.

Stiver, I., Rosen, W., Surrey, J., & Miller, J. (2001). Creative moments in relational–cultural therapy. In *Work in progress, No. 92.* Wellesley, MA: Stone Center Working Paper Series.

Styron, W. (1990). *Darkness visible: A memoir of madness.* New York: Vintage Books.

Suler, J. (1993). *Contemporary psychoanalysis and Eastern thought.* Albany: State University of New York Press.

Sussman, M. (1992). *A Curious calling: Unconscious motivations for practicing psychotherapy.* Northvale, NJ: Aronson.

Suzuki, S. (1973). *Zen mind, beginner's mind.* New York: John Weatherhill.

Sweet, M., & Johnson, C. (1990). Enhancing empathy: The interpersonal implications of a Buddhist meditation technique. *Psychotherapy: Theory, Research, Practice, Training, 27*(1), 19–29.

Tacon, A., McComb, J., Caldera, Y., & Randolph, P. (2003). Mindfulness meditation, anxiety reduction, and heart disease: A pilot study. *Family and Community Health, 26*(1), 25–33.

Teasdale, J., Moore, R., Hayhurst, H., Pope, M., Williams, S., & Segal, Z. (2002). Metacognitive awareness and prevention of relapse in depression: Empirical evidence. *Journal of Consulting and Clinical Psychology, 70*(2), 275–287.

Teasdale, J., Segal, Z., & Williams, J. (1995). How does cognitive therapy prevent depressive relapse and why should attentional control (mindfulness) training help? *Behaviour Research and Therapy, 33*, 25–39.

Teasdale, J., Segal, Z., Williams, J., Ridgeway, V., Soulsby, J., & Lau, M. A. (2000). Prevention of relapse/recurrence in major depression by mindfulness-based cognitive therapy. *Journal of Consulting and Clinical Psychology, 68*(4), 615–623.

Telch, C., Agras, W., & Linehan, M. (2001). Dialectical behavior therapy for binge eating disorder. *Journal of Consulting and Clinical Psycholology, 69*(6), 1061–1065.

Thakar, V. (1993). *Contact with Vimala Thakar, No. 33.* Mt. Abu, India: Author.

Thomas, L. (1995). *The lives of a cell: Notes of a biology watcher.* New York: Penguin.

Thompson, E. (2001). Empathy and consciousness. In E. Thompson (Ed.), *Between ourselves: Second-person issues in the study of consciousness.* Thorverton, UK: Imprint Academic.

Thomson, R. (2000). Zazen and psychotherapeutic presence. *American Journal of Psychotherapy, 54*(4), 531–548.

Toneatto, T. (2002). A metacognitive therapy for anxiety disorders: Buddhist psychology applied. *Cognitive and Behavioral Practice, 9*(1), 72–78.

Tremlow, S. (2001). Training psychotherapists in attributes of mind from Zen and psychoanalytic perspectives: Part II. Attention, here and now, nonattachment, and compassion. *American Journal of Psychotherapy, 55*(1), 22–39.

Tronick, E. (1989). Emotions and emotional communication in infants. *American Psychologist, 44*(2), 112–119.

Trungpa, C. (1973). *Cutting through spiritual materialism.* Boston: Shambhala Publications.

Trungpa, C. (1984). *Shambhala: The sacred path of the warrior.* Boston: Shambhala.

Trungpa, C. (1992). *Transcending madness: The experience of the six bardos.* Boston: Shambhala.

Tugade, M. M., & Fredrickson, B. L. (2004). Resilient individuals use positive emotions to bounce back from negative emotional experiences. *Journal of Personality and Social Psychology, 86*, 320ˆ333.

Tullberg T., Grane, P., & Isacson J. (1994). Gadolinium enhanced magnetic resonance imaging of 36 patients one year after lumbar disc resection. *Spine, 19*(2), 176–182.

Urbanowski, F., & Miller, J. (1996). Trauma, psychotherapy, and meditation. *Journal of Transpersonal Psychology, 28*(1), 31–47.

Valentine, E., & Sweet, P. (1999). Meditation and attention: A comparison of the effects of concentrative and mindfulness meditation on sustained attention. *Mental Health, Religion and Culture. 2*(1), 59–70.

VanderKooi, L. (1997). Buddhist teachers' experience with extreme mental states in Western meditators. *Journal of Transpersonal Psychology, 29*(1), 31–46.

Volinn, E. (1997). The epidemiology of low back pain in the rest of the world: A review of surveys in low middle income countries. *Spine, 22*(15), 1747–1754.

Vythilingum, B., & Stein, D. (2004). Specific phobia. In D. Stein (Ed.), *Clinical manual of anxiety disorders.* Washington, DC: American Psychiatric Publishing.

Waddell, G., Newton, M., Henderson, I., & Somerville, D. (1993). A fear-avoidance beliefs questionnaire (FABQ) and the role of fear-avoidance beliefs in chronic low back pain and disability. *Pain, 52*(2), 157–168.

Wallace, R., Benson, H., & Wilson, A. (1971). A wakeful hypometabolic physiological state. *American Journal of Physiology, 221*(3), 795–799.

Wampold, B. (2001). *The great psychotherapy debate: Models, methods, and findings.* Mahwah, NJ: Erlbaum.

Wampold, B., Mondin, G., Moody, M., Stitch, F., Benson, K., & Ahn, H. (1997). A meta-analysis of outcome studies comparing bona fide psychotherapies: Empirically, "All must have prizes." *Psychological Bulletin, 122*(3), 203–215.

Warkentin, J. (1972). The paradox of being alive and intimate. In A. Burton, *Twelve therapists.* San Francisco: Jossey-Bass.

Watts, A. (1963). *Psychotherapy: East and West.* New York: New American Library.

Wells, A. (1997). *Cognitive therapy of anxiety disorders.* Chichester, UK: Wiley.

Wells, A. (2002). GAD, metacognition, and mindfulness: An information processing analysis. *Clinical Psychology: Science and Practice, 9*(9), 95–100.

Welwood, J. (2000). *Toward a psychology of awakening.* Boston: Shambhala.

Westen, D. (1999). *Psychology: Mind, brain and culture* (2nd ed.). New York: Wiley.

Westen, D. (2000a). Commentary: Implicit and emotional processes in cognitive-behavioral therapy. *Clinical Psychology: Science and Practice, 7*(4), 386–390.

Westen, D. (2000b). The efficacy of dialectical behavior therapy for borderline personality disorder. *Clinical Psychology: Science and Practice, 7*(1), 92–94.

White, M., & Epston, D. (1990). *Narrative means to therapeutic ends.* New York: Norton.

Williams, J., Teasdale, J., Segal, Z., & Soulsby, J. (2000). Mindfulness-based cognitive therapy reduces overgeneral autobiographical memory in formerly depressed patients. *Journal of Abnormal Psychology, 109*(1), 150–155.

Williams, K., Kolar, M., Reger, B., & Pearson, J. (2001). Evaluation of a wellness-based mindfulness stress reduction intervention: A controlled trial. *American Journal of Health Promotion, 15*(6), 422–432.

Winnicott, D. W. (1971). *Playing and reality.* New York: Basic Books.

Witkiewitz, K., & Marlatt, G. A. (2004). Relapse prevention for alcohol and drug problems: That was Zen, this is Tao. *American Psychologist, 59*(4), 224–235.

Witooonchart, C., & Bartlet, L. (2002). The use of a meditation programme for institutionalized juvenile delinquents. *Journal of the Medical Association of Thailand, 85*(2), 790–793.

World Health Organization. (2003). *International classification of diseases for hospitals,* (Vols. 1–3, 6th ed., 9th rev.). Geneva, Switzerland: Author.

Wright, R. (2001). *Nonzero: The logic of human destiny.* New York: Vintage.

Wylie, M. (2004, January/February). The limits of talk. *Psychotherapy Networker,* pp. 30–41, 67.

Yaari, A., Eisenberg, E., Adler, R., & Birkhan, J. (1999). Chronic pain in Holocaust survivors. *Journal of Pain and Symptom Management, 17*(3), 181–187.

Yehuda, R., & Wong, C. (2002). Pathogenesis of posttraumatic stress disorder and acute stress disorder. In D. Stein & E. Hollander (Eds.), *Textbook of anxiety disorders.* Washington, DC: American Psychiatric Publishing.

Young, J. E., Klosko, J. S., & Weishaar, M. E. (2003). *Schema therapy: A practitioner's guide.* New York: Guilford Press.

Young-Eisendrath, P., & Muramoto, S. (2002). *Awakening and insight: Zen Buddhism and psychotherapy.* New York: Taylor & Francis.

Zettle, R., & Hayes, S. (1986). Dysfunctional control by client verbal behavior: The context of reason-giving. *Analysis of Verbal Behavior, 4,* 30–38.

Zettle, R., & Raines, J. (1989). Group cognitive and contextual therapies in treatment of depression. *Journal of Clinical Psychology, 45,* 438–445.

Zettle, R. (2003). Acceptance and commitment therapy (ACT) vs. systematic desensitization in treatment of mathematics anxiety. *The Psychological Record, 53,* 197–215.

Zetzel, E. (1970). *The capacity for emotional growth.* New York: International Universities Press.

Index